INTEGRATION STRATEGIES FOR STUDENTS WITH HANDICAPS

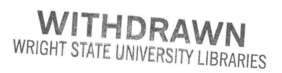

INTEGRATION STRATEGIES FOR STUDENTS WITH HANDICAPS

edited by

Robert Gaylord-Ross, Ph.D.
Department of Special Education
San Francisco State University

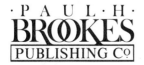
·P A U L·H·
BROOKES
PUBLISHING Co

Baltimore • London • Toronto • Sydney

Paul H. Brookes Publishing Co.
Post Office Box 10624
Baltimore, Maryland 21285-0624

Typeset by Brushwood Graphics, Inc., Baltimore, Maryland.
Manufactured in the United States of America by
The Maple Press Company, York, Pennsylvania.

Library of Congress Cataloging-in-Publication Data

Integration strategies for students with handicaps.

   Bibliography: p.
   Includes index.
   1. Handicapped children—Education—United States.   2. Mainstreaming
in education—United States.   I. Gaylord-Ross, Robert.
LC4031.I58   1989   371.9   88-35365
ISBN 1-55766-010-7

CONTENTS

CONTRIBUTORS

The Editor

Robert Gaylord-Ross, Ph.D., Department of Special Education, San Francisco State University, San Francisco, CA 94132

Professor **Robert Gaylord-Ross** is Coordinator of the Vocational Special Education Program at San Francisco State University. He is a Fullbright Senior Research Fellow. He has directed a number of research, demonstrations grants dealing with disabled youth in the areas of vocational education, social skills, and behavior management. He has published numerous chapters and articles and has been a Consulting Editor for the journals: *Career Development for Exceptional Individuals, Education and Training of the Mentally Retarded, Exceptional Children,* and the *Journal of The Association for Persons with Severe Handicaps.* His other books have included: (with J. Holvoet) *Strategies for Educating Students with Severe Handicaps* (Little, Brown, 1988); *Vocational Education for Persons with Handicaps* (Mayfield, 1988); *Issues and Research in Special Education, Volume 1* (Teachers College Press, 1989); and (with S. Sacks & L. Kekelis) *The Social Development of Visually Impaired Students* (American Foundation for the Blind, 1990).

The Chapter Authors

Michael P. Brady, Ph.D., Department of Educational Psychology, College of Education, University of Houston, Houston, TX 77204-5874

Michael Bullis, Ph.D., Teaching Research Division, Oregon State System of Higher Education, 345 North Monmouth Avenue, Monmouth, OR 97361

Philippa H. Campbell, Ph.D., Family Child Learning Center, Children's Hospital of Akron, 90 West Overdale Drive, Tallmadge, OH 44278

Vicki R. Casella, Department of Special Education, San Francisco State University, 1600 Holloway Avenue, San Francisco, CA 94132

Joy Casey-Black, M.S., Division of Special Education and Rehabilitation, Syracuse University, 805 South Crouse Avenue, Syracuse, NY 13210

Philip C. Chinn, Professor of Special Education, Division of Special Education, California State University, Los Angeles, Los Angeles, CA 90032

Addie Comegys, B.A., P.O. Box 491, Wenham, MA 01984

Linda Davern, M.S., Division of Special Education and Rehabilitation, Syracuse University, 805 South Crouse Avenue, Syracuse, NY 13244-2280

Donald H. Doorlag, Department of Special Education, San Diego State University, San Diego, CA

Alison Ford, Ph.D., Division of Special Education and Rehabilitation, Syracuse University, 805 South Crouse Avenue, Syracuse, NY 13244-2280

Mary Frances Hanline, Ph.D., Assistant Professor, Florida State University, Department of Special Education, Education Building 209, Tallahassee, FL 32306

Marci J. Hanson, Ph.D., Professor, Department of Special Education, San Francisco State University, 1600 Holloway Avenue, San Francisco, CA 94132

Laurie Hayden, M.A., Educational Service District 101, West 1025 Indiana Street, Spokane, WA 99205

David W. Johnson, Cooperative Learning Center, University of Minnesota, 202 Pattee Hall, 150 Pillsbury Drive, S.E., Minneapolis, MN 55455

Roger T. Johnson, Cooperative Learning Center, University of Minnesota, 202 Pattee Hall, 150 Pillsbury Drive, S.E., Minneapolis, MN 55455

Peter Knoblock, Ph.D., Division of Special Education and Rehabilitation, Syracuse University, 805 South Crouse Avenue, Syracuse, NY 13210

James A. Knoll, Ph.D., Human Services Research Institute, 2336 Massachusetts Avenue, Cambridge, MA 02140

Mary A. McEvoy, Ph.D., Department of Special Education, P.O. Box 328, George Peabody College, Vanderbilt University, Nashville, TN 37203

Lynn Mineur, M.A., Clearwater Economic Development Association, 1626-B 6th Avenue North, Lewiston, ID 83501

Charles A. Peck, Ph.D., Department of Counseling, Psychology, Washington State University–Vancouver, 1800 McLoughlin, Vancouver, WA 98663

Karen Peterson, Ph.D., Department of Child and Family Studies, Washington State University, Pullman, WA 99164

Maximino Plata, Department of Psychology and Special Education, East Texas State University, Commerce, TX 75428

Maureen P. Reardon, M.A., J.D., San Mateo County Office of Education, Visually Impaired Program, 3601 Curtiss Street, San Mateo, CA 94403

John W. Reiman, Ph.D., Teaching Research Division, Oregon State System of Higher Education, 345 North Monmouth Avenue, Monmouth, OR 97361

Sherrill A. Richarz, Ed.D., Department of Child and Family Studies, Washington State University, Pullman, WA 99164

Sharon Zell Sacks, Ph.D., Department of Special Education, San Francisco State University, 1600 Holloway Avenue, San Francisco, CA 94132

Steven J. Taylor, Ph.D., Center on Human Policy, Syracuse University, 724 Comstock Avenue, Syracuse, NY 13244

Mary Wandschneider, M.A., Department of Child and Family Studies, Washington State University, Pullman, WA 99164

Peggy B. Wilson, Department of Special Education, San Francisco State University, 1600 Holloway Avenue, San Francisco, CA 94132

William C. Wilson, Ph.D., Department Chair, Department of Special Education, San Francisco State University, 1600 Holloway Avenue, San Francisco, CA 94132

FOREWORD

The history of special education can be summarized quite well in two words: *progressive inclusion*. Over the last century and a half in the United States, the education of disabled children has come forward gradually from total exclusion into, first, residential schools, and then progressively into special day schools, special day classes in regular schools, part-time resource rooms, and the mainstream classes of regular schools. Virtually all disabled students now are in an educational program of some kind, but integration of disabled and nondisabled students within the schools is still incomplete. *Integration Strategies for Students with Handicaps* represents both a prediction and a commitment that for the future, *progressive inclusion* will continue to be the trend. The book has been produced at a critical time, one of great tension and momentum in efforts to achieve the fuller integration of disabled students in the schools.

Some changes toward integration come quickly and easily, at least in the sense that they involve no great technical difficulties. For example, implementing the decision that persons of all races could sit wherever they wished on public busses presented no technical problems. The attitudinal and moral aspects of the change were difficult, but the technical aspects were not. Such is not the case in moving toward integration of disabled and nondisabled students in the schools. There is much to be learned by educators, and still more yet to be discovered, about how to create effective integrated school programs. This book represents, more thoroughly than any other compilation known to me, the state of the art in integration of disabled students in the schools. It should be enormously helpful in preparation programs for teachers, school administrators, school psychologists, and others employed in the schools; and it should be helpful to parents and the public in general in setting expectations for school programs.

Some years ago, in a speech at a convention of the American Association of Colleges for Teacher Education, Professor Brody of the University of Illinois introduced the concept of *consensus doctorum*; it was the foundation principle for all of the professions, he said. Briefly, consensus doctorum means that in setting standards for services in any field that involves high competence, complexity, and judgment, one convenes the chief custodians of knowledge in the field and asks them to assert a standard based on the well-confirmed knowledge of the day. For instance, if one wants to know about qualities and standards of air-worthiness of aircraft, one would assemble experts in that field and ask them what it takes to offer reasonable safety in flight. Sometimes the standards are made explicit only in court, after some disaster; but one must hope that the standards will be laid out carefully in developmental contexts (in schools, for example) rather than to wait upon the courts. One aspect of this developmental effort is the creating of a solid literature for the field.

In assembling this book, Gaylord-Ross has convened people who are among the chief custodians of knowledge regarding integration of disabled students in the schools. They (the authors) were not asked to write all they know, nor to speculate extensively about what might be tried in the future, but to summarize in practical terms what can be done in the schools today. This is a state-of-the-art statement derived in accordance with the consensus doctorum principle. It is clear to me that if one judged practices of most schools of today against the state of the art as specified in this book, there would be a considerable negative discrepancy. There is room for much catch-up or improvement in the integration of disabled students in the schools. The challenge is to bring educators to mastery and implementation of the state of the art.

There is the important matter of negotiating with mainstream educators for a more integrated arrangement for education of disabled pupils, but there is also a need to avoid segregating subgroups of disabled pupils from each other. Sometimes narrowly framed categorical programs force separations among disabled students that are unjustified. There are new opportunities to avoid these kinds of separations as *early education* programs expand; then we must hope and try for continuing programs in the elementary schools and higher levels of schooling where separations of all kinds are held to a minimum.

Just as wars are too important to be left to the generals, so the matter of integrated schooling is too important to be left just to educators. Professional educators have very important and special contributions to make, but they must join with parents and enter the rhetoric of the community to make the case for integrated education. Finally, the community as a whole must make a judgment of the validity of the case and then join in the adaptations that are necessary in integrated models of schools and community life. In fact, not all educators are agreed on integration polices and strategies. Everywhere work is required to move progressively toward more inclusive arrangements in the schools, in other institutions and in the community-in-general. This need is recognized and treated fully in this text.

The changes required are not all straight-on rational matters. Deeply felt value differences are involved, resources will need to be redirected, patterns of communication will need to be changed, many people will need to change their attitudes and learn new skills, the validity of new ideas will be challenged, people will need to work with new partners in new arrangements, opportunities for creativity in the new arrangements will need to be provided, and strong leadership will be required. To achieve such deep changes, it may be necessary to creat new forums for discussion and planning and new informal judiciaries for dealing with problems and complaints. Let there be no mistake; the work before us in creating more integrated environments is challenging indeed.

There is much discussion in these days of late 20th century about the general restructuring of schools. But "regular" educators talk of new structures for elementary and secondary education, with almost no mention of disabled students. It's strange that this should happen when one teacher out of eight in the United States is employed in special education. If we add the school psychologists, school social workers, occupational therapists, and other professional personnel who work mainly with handicapped students, we come to a total of about 400,000 professional employees in U.S. schools—about one-sixth of the total number of professional school employees. It would seem hard to disregard an enterprise of that size. Yet that is the problem. Not only are disabled children left to the side; so are their teachers. Even the literature regarding special and regular education has become separated. Thus, special efforts will be required to enter the case for integrated education into the broader discussions about restructuring the schools.

The forms of integration described and advocated in this book cannot be achieved by special educators alone. It will be necessary for "regular" educators to join in the process of creating new and more inclusive programs that encompass literally all students. This book deserves broad attention as we seek to connect the integration movement and the more general efforts for restructuring the schools.

I have read this book with much personal interest and profit. As one reads the many accounts of integrated schooling provided in this book, one has a sense of great moral and intellectual victory. What is being diminished is exclusion and segregation; what is being advanced is inclusion and integration. This book contributes to a highly worthy and very human enterprise.

Maynard C. Reynolds
Professor, Special Education
University of Minnesota

To Alexa

INTEGRATION STRATEGIES FOR STUDENTS WITH HANDICAPS

INTRODUCTION

Robert Gaylord-Ross

Integration Strategies for Students with Handicaps is a textbook that provides practical information about persons with disabilities. It should serve as an introductory text for regular education and special education teachers in training. It can also be used in an advanced methods course that addresses particular types of disabilities and teaching approaches.

This volume is quite different from a typical introductory book. Most "intro" books offer broad surveys of the characteristics of different types of disabilities. Some may have a research focus in presenting the latest empirical findings. The present text has taken the tactic of emphasizing a description of *actual teaching techniques*. The authors believe that beginning students need a text that will provide them with effective procedures that they can use in real classroom settings. The core of each chapter, therefore, describes a number of such techniques that have been tried and validated in the field. The chapters also provide related information about the characteristics of individuals with different types of disabilities, but the major emphasis is on instructional techniques.

OVERVIEW OF INTEGRATION

Almost all professionals in the field agree that enabling students to attain independence is the most important goal for special education programs. Full independence or partial independence ultimately means performing successfully in normal environments. In the past, persons with disabili-

ties have often been placed in large state hospitals, segregated all-handicapped schools, and sheltered work settings. During the past 20 years, though, an "integration" movement has developed that has progressively moved persons with disabilities into regular public schools, community apartments and normal domiciles, and nonsheltered employment. Although most professionals agree upon these placements as ultimate goals, there is a difference of opinion in the field with regard to how fast one should move an individual from more segregated to more integrated placements. The Education for All Handicapped Children Act (Public Law 94-142) asserts that a student should be placed in the least restrictive environment. Often there is professional and/or parental disagreement in determining just what is the least restrictive, or most appropriate integrated setting. Fortunately, as each year passes one sees more indisputable demonstrations of disabled people succeeding in the most integrated settings (e.g., a deaf-blind youth working for pay in a pizza parlor).

It is the purpose of this book to present a number of real-life illustrations of integration. The reader should get a feel for integrated placements and activities as she or he reads about the pupils, settings, materials, teaching procedures, and evaluation design in each chapter.

A more recent development and controversy in the field has been called the regular education initiative (REI). REI is a further extension of the integration principle. It states that most handicapped pupils should spend almost all of their time in the regular education classroom. Under

1

REI, there would be few, if any, self-contained classes for handicapped students. Administratively, REI would have special education totally subsumed within regular education. That is, there would be no separate special education infrastructure of directors and other administrators. Although REI is currently quite controversial, probably some form of this "radical" integration plan will emerge in future years. The current text provides numerous examples of how REI can be implemented in actual school districts and classrooms.

ORGANIZATION OF CHAPTERS

Most chapters in the text are organized into four parts. An introduction provides an overview to the type of disability or the instructional process to be addressed. Often disability characteristics or research findings are presented here. The second section describes the author's educational model for service delivery. The model carefully addresses how integration will be accomplished. It also sets a context for the subsequent instructional activities. The model section, in particular, tries to show how specific activities would fit within a comprehensive integration system. The core of the chapter consists of a description of five or six instructional activities. The reader should be able to relate these activities to actual pupils they have known or will know in the future. At minimum, the reader will get a sense of the educational process of disabled persons. The final section reviews the material in the chapter and suggests future directions for research and practice. In addition, study questions are included. Instructors and students may use these questions for homework assignments or class review.

OVERVIEW OF
SECTIONS AND CHAPTERS

The book is divided into three sections. The first section of the book addresses the education of students with different types of disabilities. The authors describe characteristics of the disabilities, and illustrate effective integration models and activities. For example, until the passage of PL 94-142, students with severe disabilities were, by and large, not served by the public school system. Children either stayed at home or attended privately run schools. The new federal law guaranteed all students, no matter how severe their handicaps, a free and appropriate education. Even though all students subsequently received an education, most were placed in segregated schools (i.e., schools serving only handicapped pupils). A major movement in this field, led by Lou Brown and The Association for Persons with Severe Handicaps, was to advocate for integrated school programs. Alison Ford was originally a teacher in Madison, Wisconsin, one of the pioneer sites for such integrated education. In Chapter 1, Ford and Davern describe a wide array of integration activities. They give particular attention to friendship development among severely disabled and nondisabled peers.

The largest group (approximately 80%) of special education students have mild or learning handicaps. In some ways this group has provided the most challenges to the field. Because the curriculum and ability level of the learning handicapped student overlaps considerably with nondisabled students, there are differences in opinion with regard to how much time the learning handicapped student should spend in a regular or in a special class. As stated earlier, proponents of the regular education initiative feel that almost 100% of the student's time should be in the regular class. In Chapter 2, Doorlag presents a number of activities that successfully mainstream the learning handicapped pupil into regular settings. The activities should be pertinent for special and regular educators alike.

When the public thinks of the term *disability,* they usually associate it with persons having physical or sensory impairments. Physically disabled persons often have a wide range of medical and mobility problems. Originally, this necessitated their placement in highly supervised, segregated programs. Over time, it has been shown that students with severe impairments can be served in integrated settings. For example, an earlier barrier to integration was the contention that special therapy services could only be efficiently provided in segregated, therapeutic settings. Campbell's transdisciplinary model, in Chapter 3, has professionals learn to implement some of the specialized skills of other professionals. Such transdisciplinary implementation permits a treatment to be delivered for greater time periods and in different situations with a number of persons, and thus allows for the successful integration of students with physical disabilities. Campbell also emphasizes the importance of involving nondisabled peers in facilitating interactions with and enabling the integration of students with physical disabilities. Several activities illustrate ways in which teachers, other professionals, and parents can help to initiate and sustain the process of integration.

Visually impaired students have often been limited in their social interaction skills. They may have difficulty reading social cues or maintaining a proper physical distance during conversations. Such impairment-related social difficulties do not preclude school and community integration. In Chapter 4, Sacks and Reardon describe a set of activities that socially engage the visually impaired student in the public school. For instance, social skills training is often the enabling activity that teaches students how to participate in prolonged interactions.

Each disability group offers its own particular challenges in integration. While hearing impaired individuals are certainly capable of being integrated, many have chosen to form educational and social groupings almost exclusively with other persons with hearing impairments. That is, a hearing impaired or Deaf culture has been defined by its participants. Members of the culture are quite sensitive to the oppression of their culture by the majority hearing culture. Reiman and Bullis, in Chapter 5, delineate a model for integration that respects and balances integration in both cultures.

Such biculturalism is an appealing approach for those with disability, ethnic, and racial differences.

Students with behavior disorders are probably considered the most intrusive on their surrounding environment. In general, persons with disabilities often evoke the empathy of others—yet the person who steals, assaults, or deceives usually elicits the enmity of those around him or her. Although there has been a general trend toward integrating students with disabilities, in many cases students with behavior disorders are being increasingly segregated in residential and school facilities. In Chapter 6, Casey-Black and Knoblock present a number of integration activities based on sound behavioral and curricular approaches. Fortunately, there is a technology to teach and support such pupils. Yet, behaviorally disordered students often have few advocates. This, coupled with the appearance of highly intrusive behaviors, often leads to incarceration or other further segregation.

Undoubtedly the largest influx of students with special needs is coming from the migration of ethnic groups from Asia and Latin America. Bilingual and bicultural special education is a rapidly emerging field, probably fraught with more questions than answers. As with persons with hearing impairments, issues arise as to how one can balance the culture of origin with the mainstream culture's values and behaviors. In Chapter 7, Plata and Chinn describe a wide range of activities that adapt curricula for bicultural students. Undoubtedly successful integration strategies for bicultural students will further develop. It is likely that the more critical issues of bicultural education will evolve at a political level. That is, citizens and politicians of a conservative political persuasion have rejected and tried to eliminate bilingual education. Since previous immigrants were immediately forced to assimilate within the Anglo-dominant culture, conservative thinkers feel that there should be similar expectations for current emigrés. Proponents of bilingualism and biculturalism feel that their approach offers a balance between two diverse cultures, while enabling individuals to maintain their historical identity.

They also feel that such approaches offer a more effective way to teach academic and other school-related curricula, as the student gradually acquires the new language and culture.

The second section of the book offers innovative techniques in integration. It concerns generic integration services, those that cut across a particular type of disability. The services often entail heterogeneous groupings of persons with different types of disabilities (or no disabilities), functioning level, and age. An increasing data base is emerging that such heterogeneous groupings allow students to learn and perform successfully, as well as serve as a vehicle for social integration.

Historically, the first integration attempts were carried out with preschoolers (Bricker, 1982). In fact, most of the empirical research demonstrating social integration has been conducted in university-based, early childhood classrooms (e.g., Shores, 1987). Although early childhood research has been in the vanguard, required preschool services lagged behind mandated services for school-age, handicapped pupils. Just recently, PL 99-457 has encouraged the development of preschool services in each of the participating states. It is not yet clear how widespread these services will ultimately be. In Chapter 8, Hanson and Hanline review some of the history and recent developments in early childhood special education. They describe a number of activities that involve not only students, but parents as well. In fact, early childhood programs have a very strong parent involvement component. Parent involvement, like transdisciplinary planning, guarantees that instruction will be carried out across many settings and persons. This increases the chances that the learned tasks will generalize and be maintained.

Early childhood special education has operated on the premise that the earlier a child receives intervention, the greater the likelihood that the child's growth and development will accelerate. The past 30 or more years of research have largely supported the efficacy of early childhood intervention. That is, the earlier and more intensive a child's program, the more likely the child's level of functioning will increase. In some cases the person might grow up to not be disabled at all. More likely, the person might improve cognitively or socially so that he or she might, for example, read at a significantly higher level.

The field of vocational special education is typically associated with services at the higher end of the age spectrum. Career and vocational education usually means training for a job during adolescence. Yet, effective career education programs encompass the life span; they begin at an early age and continue through adulthood.

The vocational special education field has been recently fueled by the federal initiative to successfully "transition" disabled youth from school to adulthood. In 1984 Public Law 98-199 established a transition initiative to increase the rate of employment for school leavers and disabled adults (Will, 1984). Some exciting developments have appeared with the "supported employment" of persons with severe disabilities. Until recently, this population was thought incapable of non-sheltered work. It has been shown, though, with the presence of a teacher or job coach at the work site, that individuals with severe disabilities can be productive workers. In Chapter 9, Gaylord-Ross describes a wide range of vocational activities that should prepare the student for successful employment. Interestingly, persons with mild handicaps may sometimes have a poorer prognosis for job retention than individuals with severe disabilities. Thus, successful programs such as Job Club have taught clients to seek, interview for, and procure competitive employment.

Social skills training has been the best empirically documented technique to foster social integration. Influenced by the previous work of Shores and Strain, Chapter 10 authors Brady and McEvoy describe the different ways to promote social interactions between disabled and nondisabled students. Peer-mediated instruction was the earliest technique used to teach social skills. Peer-mediated instruction teaches a nondisabled student to participate in play and other social interactions. After being trained, the nondisabled peer

Nolen, Karen
10-13-99

 engages a
actions. As
abled peer
 respond-
 so forth.
Ross and
ng on the
e taught
th non-
led stu-
aviors
should
egrat-
hould
room
iors
ings

…ation is the wide
…ed and nondisabled students that a teacher may have to instruct in a particular classroom. Gerber and Semmel (1986) assert that a teacher makes a cognitive decision either to advance the average level of the class's performance or to reduce the difference (or variance) between the highest and lowest performants. Increasing the mean achievement of the class usually leads to spending less time with lower achieving students. Reducing pupil variance involves spending more time with these lower performing students (at the expense of the average or above-average pupils). In either case there is a perplexing puzzle to be solved by the classroom teacher. In fact, one solution in the past was to refer the disabled student out of the regular class into a special class. This referral led to a reduction in pupil variance (cognitive and behavioral) and made the class more manageable for the teacher in terms of curriculum focus and behavioral discipline.

The regular education initiative, as well as the least restrictive environment principle, calls for disabled students to spend maximal proportions of their school day in the regular classroom. Given the problem of pupil variance just mentioned, cooperative learning offers an appealing solution to classroom integration. Cooperative learning entails the formation of mixed-level groups of students to accomplish particular tasks. A group of four to eight students may contain individuals who are gifted, average achievers, low achievers, mildly handicapped, and moderately handicapped. The group must accomplish a particular task, such as publishing a school newsletter. A division of labor is organized so that different students engage in different talks according to their abilities. The group is rewarded as a whole for task completion. Thus, everyone is dependent on each other to attain a superordinate goal. In Chapter 11, Johnson and Johnson show that such cooperative groups can accomplish academic and other tasks. Most important, cooperative groups should promote intense and amicable interactions among its members. Students with disabilities, for example, are respected for their necessary contribution to the group endeavor. Such numerous cooperative interactions with one's peers contrasts with a lecture-format class where most of the interactions are from the teacher to the student (or with a seat-work format where the student works quietly and alone on some worksheets). Conceivably, much or part of a class's time could be spent in such cooperative groupings. Social integration would certainly be fostered under these circumstances.

Perhaps the most promising breakthrough in special education will lie in the innovations and applications of new technologies. Microcomputers have certainly been the new technology receiving the most attention. Microcomputers have been adapted so they are accessible to persons with sensory and physical impairments. Software has been developed that is particularly effective for persons with cognitive impairments. The "interactive" characteristics of the computer have been enhanced so that the student receives corrective feedback and emits creative solutions to challenging problems.

Yet, microcomputers have sometimes been criticized for isolating the student from peers and teachers. Such man-machine interactions will not necessarily produce a socially skillful individual.

Some research by Semmel has shown computers are mostly used for isolated drill-and-practice routines with special education students.

In Chapter 12, Wilson, Casella, and Wilson describe an array of activities that capitalizes on the dynamic properties of microcomputers. These activities demonstrate how curricula are adapted by the microcomputer to enhance instructional power. They also show how the interactive problem-solving capabilities of the computer can be assessed. Most important, Wilson et al. make clear that the computer does not necessarily entail isolated, individual work with a machine. There are a number of ways that small group encounters and active social exchanges may revolve around the computer. Thus, the computer may not only be a powerful learning tool, but also an effective agent to promote social integration.

The third section deals with the ecology of delivering services to persons with disabilities. More and more, investigators are looking beyond the purview of the individual to the macrosystem in which the person functions. Such ecobehavioral transactions play a role in determining issues dealing with labeling, placement, treatment effectiveness, and so forth. Thus, the book concludes by examining the total system as it transacts upon and affects the individual.

Peck, Richarz, Peterson, Hayden, Mineur, and Wandschneider, in Chapter 13, begin this macrosystem analysis by describing how systems change efforts may evolve in early childhood education. There are many concerns, of parents and professionals alike, as an integrated system evolves. Peck et al. describe this evolution through qualitative or anthropological research methodology. This approach permits the researcher to view the world through the eyes of its participants. Findings thereby uncovered will enable professionals to develop more powerful systems change interventions.

When converting to an integrated system, a question always arises as to at what level the change should begin. Historically, parents have often provided the initial impetus to rock the foun-

dations of the status quo. In other cases, individual teachers may move their students toward more integrated and community-based training experiences. Probably, though, it is ultimately imperative for top-level administrators to support and lead systems change efforts if there is to be any lasting and substantial effect. In many ways the tone as well as the policy is set by one or more administrators. Administrators have too often been reactive rather than active leaders of change. In Chapter 14, Wilson advances a model for administrative systems change. He states how to involve all of the different factors (e.g., parents) in integration efforts. The chapter carefully articulates administrative roles in facilitating the regular education initiative.

When examining the macrosystem of service delivery, it becomes important to consider the community. Independent living for disabled adults primarily means both surviving and enjoying life in the community. In terms of instruction, research is showing that a substantial amount of training needs to occur in the criterion community environment. Disabled students typically do not generalize from an artificial or school setting to real community contexts such as shopping malls, banks, and restaurants. At minimum, teachers need to coordinate their efforts with key community members such as parents and recreational providers. What is learned at school should be practical at home (and vice-versa). Chapter 15, by Taylor and Knoll, advances a model for a continuum of community services. New program models such as self-advocacy are described; self-advocacy permits disabled consumers to make choices in determining goals and life-styles for themselves. The encouragement of choice making in the community should maximize the independence of persons with disabilities.

PL 94-142 guarantees the legal right of parents to participate in the planning of the educational program of their child. This process is formalized in the individualized education program (IEP). Although parent participation has grown since the passage of this law in 1975, there is still too little involvement of parents in the educational process. Educators and administrators often give only lip service to parent involvement. In Chapter 16, Comegys presents a personalized view of her daughter and of her own role as a parent in the educational process. While differing considerably in style from the other chapters, it offers an inspirational account of parent-child involvement.

SUMMARY

Integration Strategies for Students with Handicaps offers a tested set of integration activities for the reader. The introductory student should get a sense of effective teaching practices to use with disabled students. General background information should also introduce the reader to the latest developments in curricula and methods in the special education field. Because of its activity focus, the book should also serve as a reference for practitioners in the field. The study questions should be useful for both introductory and advanced students. Overall, it is hoped that the book will serve as a force in its own right—to promote and maximize integration for students with handicaps.

REFERENCES

Bricker, D. (1982). *The rate and quality of social behavior of severely handicapped students in integrated and nonintegrated settings.* Paper presented at the Integration Evaluation Project Conference, Educational Testing Service, Princeton, NJ.

Gaylord-Ross, R., & Haring, T. (1987). Social integration research for adolescents with severe handicaps. *Behavioral Disorders, 12,* 269–275.

Gerber, M., & Semmel, M. (April, 1986). *Mainstreaming and social interaction.* Paper presented at the annual meeting of the California Association of Professors of Special Education, Lake Tahoe, California.

McConnell, S.R. (1987). Entrapment effects and the generalization and maintenance of social skills training for elementary school students with behavioral disorders. *Behavioral Disorders, 12,* 252–263.

Semmel, M. (April, 1986). *Mainstreaming and social interaction.* Paper presented at the annual meeting of the California Association of Professors of Special Education, Lake Tahoe, California.

Shores, R.E. (1987). Overview of research on social interaction: A historical and personal perspective. *Behavioral Disorders, 12,* 233–241.

Will, M. (1984). *Supported employment: An OSERS position paper.* Washington DC: U.S. Department of Education.

STRATEGIES FOR SPECIFIC DISABILITIES

CHAPTER 1

Moving Forward with School Integration
Strategies for Involving Students with Severe Handicaps in the Life of the School

Alison Ford and Linda Davern

"Are your students integrated?" is a question that teachers of students with severe handicaps are frequently asked. Years ago, the meaning of this question was readily understood. More than likely the inquirer simply wanted to know whether the students were attending a regular public school with peers who were not handicapped. If they were, they were considered integrated. If they were not, that is, if they attended a "special" school in which only students with handicaps were enrolled, they were considered segregated.

Through just a one-word response to the integration question, much was communicated about the quality of the students' education. Responding "yes" to the integration question meant that students with severe handicaps could potentially have access to many critical *opportunities* such as attending a school closer to home, being surrounded by nonhandicapped peers and thereby being exposed to effective language and social models,

having a chance to make friends in the neighborhood, being challenged by ever-increasing expectations, and being in a place where the sights and sounds have a rich and spontaneous quality. Responding "no" to the integration question meant that students were confined to a sheltered existence in simulations of real schools—places where they would have no regular contact with nonhandicapped peers.

Although the integration question continues to be posed today, the inquirer can no longer assume that a common understanding of the term *integration* exists. A simple "yes" or "no" does not tell the full story as it did when integration meant mere enrollment in a regular school. Now when the question "Are your students integrated?" is posed, one is likely to hear a variety of answers such as:

"Do you mean integrated in a regular school or *class*?"

Preparation of this chapter was supported in part by Grant No. G008530151 awarded to Syracuse University from the Office of Special Education and Rehabilitative Services, U.S. Department of Education. The opinions expressed herein do not necessarily reflect the position or policy of the U.S. Department of Education, and no official endorsement should be inferred. The authors' appreciation is expressed to the students, parents, teachers, assistants, and administrators at Edward Smith, Salem Hyde, and Hughes Elementary Schools; Levy, Grant, Lincoln, and Huntington Middle Schools; and Fowler, Henninger, and Nottingham High Schools for shaping their ideas about the activities presented in this chapter.

"It depends on what you call integration. My students are in a special class but they go to gym
  and art with nonhandicapped students."
"Only partially; most of the time they are grouped
  with students with handicaps."
"Yes, but they could be integrated more."
"35% of the time."

These responses suggest an interpretation of what
integration means that goes far beyond the establishment of special classes in regular school settings. The integration question is now weighted
with the years of experience accumulated by
teachers who have educated students with severe
handicaps in regular schools, as well as the changing expectations of parents and advocates. (See,
for example, Biklen [1985], Biklen, Ferguson,
and Ford [in press], Forest [1987b], Stainback and
Stainback [1984], Strully and Strully [1985], and
Thousand et al. [1986].) Increasingly, this question is being rephrased in the following ways:

"Have the students become a part of the school?"
"Are the students fully accepted as members of
  the student body?"
"Are they active participants?"
"Do the students feel a sense of belonging to the
  school?"

Here, the term *integration* is interchangeable with
the phrases "a part of," "fully accepted," "active
participant," and "a sense of belonging."

Another important message can be discerned
from the teachers' remarks. They communicate a
sense of dissatisfaction with the separateness that
continues to characterize their students' educational programs. Although the students are being
educated in the same school as their nonhandicapped peers, they have made a point of qualifying the involvement by mentioning the "special
class" status and "partial" inclusion of their students within the school. Their dissatisfaction
prompts one to wonder what it will take for them
to become satisfied with their students' integration—What is "true" integration? Will these
teachers know it when they see it?

The authors suspect that integration is like
many complex social phenomena in that it seems
easier to describe what it is not than what it is. For
example, one knows that integration is not separate buses, different school hours, and separate
classes. One knows that full integration has not
been achieved when students' pictures are routinely overlooked when the school yearbook is
compiled or when their names never appear on
computerized class lists. And, one knows that integration has not been reached when not one student with severe handicaps participates in an extracurricular activity, a school play, a graduation
ceremony, or a homecoming dance.

An increased sensitivity to the meaning of
school integration has brought about new and interesting challenges for teachers. No longer feeling satisfied with the marginal status that students
with severe handicaps have had within schools,
teachers are creating strategies and designing activities to remedy the problem. Regular education
colleagues, school administrators, and committed
parents and community members are also becoming actively involved in moving forward with
school integration.

INTEGRATION ACTIVITIES

Five descriptions of activities or program innovations follow. Collectively, they represent but a
small sampling of the many steps that committed
individuals can take to move forward with school
integration. The authors' purpose in presenting
these activities is more to stimulate thinking about
furthering integration than to recommend the exact steps or activities to undertake in one's school.
In developing these descriptions, they have drawn
upon their own involvement with schools, along
with discussions with parents, teachers, and prac-
ticum students about the changing meaning of integration. Some of these activities or program innovations may still be at the idea stage, others may
have advanced to the planning and implementation stage. The actual stage of development does

not matter greatly. The greater concern is whether these activities and program innovations offer a vision of a more complete school—a school in which all students belong, including students with the most severe handicaps (Biklen, 1985).

Activity-Based Lessons

James Schubert is a student teacher in a fourth-grade class at Weyland Elementary School. The class to which he has been assigned is unique in at least one important respect: There are two students with severe handicaps enrolled full time in the class. For almost 10 years now, the school has been recognized for its model programs that fully integrate students with severe handicaps in kindergarten through sixth-grade classes. It was because of the school's reputation that James requested a student-teaching assignment at Weyland. He was committed to creating a classroom climate in which students with very diverse learning needs could be educated together; he saw this unique teaching assignment as a chance to follow through on this commitment.

The Challenge

Although the school and classroom philosophy is one of learning together, James noticed that during math and reading periods the two students with severe handicaps were always pulled aside for separate skill instruction. Since reading and math activities occupied a large percentage of the school day, the amount of time the students were actually separated from their nonhandicapped peers was substantial. The justification for a separate group stemmed from the considerable discrepancy between the proficiencies of the two students with severe handicaps and those expected of typical fourth graders. For example, Shawn, one of the two students with severe handicaps, was learning how to match coins to money cards (each card had a graphic representation of a coin). The purpose of this activity was to help Shawn determine how much money he needed for frequently purchased items in school or at the grocery store.

Jerry, the other student, was learning basic money-counting skills and how to use a calculator for purchasing items. Most of the other fourth graders were learning how to multiply and divide three to four digit numbers. How could a teacher include Jerry and Shawn with the other students and still appropriately challenge each member of the group?

The Solution

Jerry and Shawn, like many students with severe handicaps, learn best when they are expected to apply skills in direct, hands-on experiences. James knew that while other fourth graders could learn in more indirect ways (e.g., by listening to lectures, completing worksheets, discussing a real-life math problem), their motivation increased when he involved them in a related activity. In light of this observation, James decided to devise a math activity that could be used to teach Jerry and Shawn the skills they needed to learn as well as address the skill areas covered in the fourth grade math curriculum. His idea was to operate a hot chocolate business.

The Hot Chocolate Business

Each day during math time, Shawn and Jerry were assigned to The Hot Chocolate Business. Other groups of students—four at a time—were assigned on a rotating basis following a schedule devised by James and the classroom teacher. On Mondays, Tuesdays, and Thursdays, James held the math sessions in the classroom. On Wednesdays, the students walked 2 blocks to a grocery store where they purchased the supplies needed for the business, and on Fridays they opened The Hot Chocolate Business for sales during recess.

A typical classroom lesson was outlined in a manner that would allow James to accomplish several objectives: 1) to teach the *application* of the math concept that the nonhandicapped students were currently working on from the fourth-grade curriculum, 2) to teach Jerry how to count money and use his calculator to determine the affordability of items, and 3) to teach Shawn how to match real coins to graphic representations of coins on money cards. In addition to the money skills that Shawn and Jerry would learn from such a lesson, it is important to acknowledge that this activity also presents opportunities for the students to develop social and communication skills, and, in Shawn's case, fine motor skills. See Table 1 for a description of the lesson.

Thus it can be seen that activity-based lessons not only allow teachers to work on a variety of objectives at varying levels of proficiency, but also can make learning much more interesting for all students. The key is to not let the activity dominate the lesson, but to use it as a *backdrop* for achieving specific targeted objectives for each student. Once a student has mastered the objectives, new ones should be built into the lesson. In the above example, an activity was created that would provide the necessary challenges to both Shawn and Jerry as well as to their nonhandicapped classmates.

The Hot Chocolate Business is only one of many activity-based lessons that can be created in regular classes to enable joint participation among students with diverse learning characteristics. Some other examples follow.

Language Arts

Two hours each morning were devoted to language arts in the second-grade classroom. A portion of this time was devoted to independent reading or "reading for pleasure." Students chose their own books, read them independently, and talked about them with their peers. Tina, a student with severe handicaps, was just beginning to show signs of interest in pictures. Together, Tina and a peer chose a book. The peer then read the book to Tina and drew her attention to the pictures.

Journal Writing

After lunch each day the sixth-grade students returned to the classroom and wrote a page in their journals. Sherri, a student with severe handicaps, was paired with a different peer each day of the week. On Mondays, Carol joined Sherri in the journal-writing activity. Although Sherri could not actually write, she was able to "dictate" her message to Carol who then wrote down the appropriate word or drew the appropriate symbol in the journal. When the teacher called upon different students to read their journals, Sherri took her turn just like the others.

Computer Programming

Each week the students in this 10th-grade computer class switched partners. One week, Jesse and Nicole worked together. Nicole is a student with severe handicaps who uses a symbol board for communication purposes. One of the things that Jesse and Nicole worked on together was the design of symbols to represent some of the new messages she needed to add to her communication board. For example, one of the vocabulary items Nicole needed to add to her board was the word "sandwich." Jesse designed the image and Nicole touched the keyboard to activate the computer commands necessary to produce the desired images.

Conclusion

Typically, joint activities between students with severe handicaps and those without are confined to the "nonacademic" areas. The activities described here demonstrate how, with a measure of creativity and careful planning, activities can be designed that challenge a wide range of learners —even in the academic areas.

Community-Based Instruction

Paula, age 10, and John, 11, are students at Ross Elementary School. Both have severe handicaps, and receive community-based instruction. Community-based instruction refers to systematically teaching "life" skills in the *actual* environments in which the students will need to apply them. For young students this may include teaching the use of community services such as grocery stores and

Table 1. A description of an activity-based math lesson: The Hot Chocolate Business

The Hot Chocolate Business
Classroom session
Regular math unit:
  Division with Remainders (p. 146)
Students: Group #3: Hillery, Terry, Joseph, Bobby

Monday, 10:15–10:55
Date: 10/21
Money handling focus:
  Shawn: Matches coins to money card to purchase familiar items; prepares list for shopping
  Jerry: Adds value of coins into calculator to determine total spending money, subtracts price of item to determine "enough/not enough"

Teaching procedures	Targeted skills		
	Hillery, Terry, Joseph, Bobby	Jerry	Shawn
INTRODUCTION (10:15–10:20)			
Develops readiness for today's lesson by drawing group's attention to graph of profits from sales of hot chocolate.	Identifies components of graph (x axis, y axis).	Indicates whether sales are going up or down.	Holds graph.
Explains what students will work on during today's lesson, and why it is important: "Today we need to figure out how much money to reinvest in hot chocolate supplies, and how much profit we made last week toward our goal." (class trip to Lakeland Amusement Park)			
DIRECT INSTRUCTION (10:20–10:30)			
Demonstrates the tasks that each student will need to perform: "We know how much money we made last week. How do we figure out how many cups we sold?"	Suggests how to solve problem: Divide total receipts by price of one cup.		
"Jerry and Shawn, you are going to need to buy some more marshmallows and cups."		Observes teacher model the calculator process (adds coins to determine "money to spend"; subtracts price to determine "enough/not enough").	Observes teacher match coins to money card to cover cost of marshmallows.

(continued)

Table 1. *(continued)*

The Hot Chocolate Business
Classroom session
Regular math unit:
Division with Remainders (p. 146)
Students: Group #3: Hillery, Terry, Joseph, Bobby

Monday, 10:15–10:55
Date: 10/21
Money handling focus:
Shawn: Matches coins to money card to purchase familiar items; prepares list for shopping
Jerry: Adds value of coins into calculator to determine total spending money, subtracts price of item to determine "enough/not enough"

Teaching procedures *(continued)*	Targeted skills *(continued)*		
	Hillery, Terry, Joseph, Bobby	Jerry	Shawn
GUIDED PRACTICE (10:30–10:45)			
Communicate expectation that each student will complete problems/tasks on her or his own, and then check with other group members to see if they agree.	Divides total receipts by price of one cup of hot chocolate. Completes several "practice problems" when given hypothetical total receipt amounts.	When given some coins and an item (marshmallows or a package of cups), adds coins into calculator, then subtracts to see if enough (at least one practice trial is designed so he does *not* have enough).	With teacher assistance: Identifies money/picture card marshmallows when shown bag of marshmallows. Matches coins to card and places money in wallet for use at the store Wednesday. Identifies card of plastic cups when shown bag of cups. Matches coins to money card and pools with money for marshmallows. Places picture cards next to money in wallet. Independently: Puts extra coins back into the metal cashier's box. Looks up at graph.
Requests an estimate of how much money will need to be reinvested in supplies for next week, and a process for determining this week's profits.	Gives estimates, and subtracts estimate from last week's total receipts to determine profit.		

SUMMARY (10:45–10:55)

Requests estimate of how long it will take to reach their goal	References graph; group gives estimate.	Marks area on graph that is pointed to by other group member to record profits. Indicates whether sales went up or down.
Elicits ideas to increase sales.	Offers ideas.	Offers ideas.
Confirms plans to shop on Wednesday.		Identifies shopping day on calendar for group.
		Places coins from profit into bank wrappers with partner.
		Puts items away (in cabinet) with partner. Places wallet (for individual purchase on Wednesday) in desk.

This lesson, as well as the general idea of creating The Hot Chocolate Business, was adapted from an instructional program developed by David Smukler while he was completing an internship at Ed Smith Elementary School in Syracuse, NY.

restaurants, and related mobility skills such as street crossing. Older students may receive additional community-based instruction in areas such as home living, preparation for jobs in the community, the use of recreational facilities, and the use of public transportation.

The extent to which a particular student engages in community-based instruction depends on a variety of factors including her or his age, learning style, interests, and so forth. Since Paula and John are quite young, the bulk of their education takes place in school where they can engage in meaningful learning opportunities with other students. However, their families and teachers feel that learning community skills such as street crossing, buying a snack at the grocery store, and handling money are important skills for them to be learning now. Based on their past performance and an assessment of their skills in community environments, it appears very unlikely that these important skills would be learned without this type of instruction. Thus, for Paula and John, and students with similar learning characteristics, community-based instruction becomes an essential component of the overall educational program.

The Challenge

Although instruction in the community is a vital component of an educational program for students with severe disabilities, in practice it often results in small groups of students being separated from their nonhandicapped peers to engage in a "special" program. While it is not highly unusual for older students to leave school on a regular basis for special programs (e.g., career "apprenticeships," volunteer work, precollege programs), it is somewhat unusual for younger students to leave school on a regular basis for instructional purposes. This was the observation made by a teacher at Ross Elementary School whose responsibility it was to provide community-based instruction to Paula and John. Each Wednesday morning these students could be seen leaving the school with this teacher or an instructional assistant to receive in-

struction in travel skills and buying groceries at a nearby store. There were community-based sessions held on other days as well to teach these students the use of places such as the public library and restaurants. When asked why these students were separated from their nonhandicapped peers for these community-based activities, the teacher replied, "Because they need to learn and apply skills in real-life settings." But upon reflection, she began to question whether Paula and John actually needed to be separated from others in order to receive this type of instruction. Could not other students benefit from learning in the community? How could she make her community-based instruction less "special" in the sense that only students with handicaps participated, and more "special" in terms of being an interesting and enjoyable educational activity in which a diverse group of students could be involved?

The Solution

Offering community-based instruction to both nonhandicapped students and those with handicaps is undoubtedly beneficial. Observing a student in a grocery store can provide a wealth of information regarding whether the abstract concepts taught during lessons such as math or health can be understood and applied by the student in real-life situations. Traditional curricula artificially fragment the world into different "subject" areas; but the real world demands that the student integrate her or his knowledge. Occasional experience in community settings can afford the student an opportunity to integrate knowledge and skills in the presence of a teacher who can facilitate understanding and guide the student as needed.

Instruction in the community is consistent with several general principles of education, such as the importance of engaging the learner in an active manner with the subject material. "Participation, firsthand experiencing, realistic practice, and extensive learner activity enhance learning" (Shepherd & Ragan, 1982, p. 35). In addition to the planned educational goals of the community experience, an alert teacher will encounter many incidental opportunities for learning in the community. This type of experience also gives each student an additional opportunity to work cooperatively with a partner or small group, and engage in spontaneous problem solving in real-life as opposed to simulated situations.

With these thoughts in mind, the teacher at Ross Elementary School proceeded to create community-based learning opportunities that included students without handicaps. Although this type of instruction was not essential to their educational experience (as it certainly was for the students with severe handicaps), she was confident that with careful planning, there would be important educational gains made by all students. Two months later, the community-based instructional program at Ross looked much different—perhaps something like the following.

Going to the Grocery Store

Every Wednesday, fifth-grade students from Ms. Carmichael's class at Ross Elementary School received instruction on a variety of skills at the grocery store. Paula and John went every week, and other students went on a rotating basis. Cindy and Margie were scheduled to go on this particular day. They were working on division, decimals, and fractions during math instruction and this presented an opportunity for them to demonstrate to a teacher whether they understood the practical application of the math concepts they were studying in class. Paula was learning how to use a calculator to purchase several items. She was also learning to find items from a grocery list. John was learning how to maneuver his wheelchair down the store aisles, and reach for an item once someone helped him find the right section.

The store was about 3 blocks from school. Paula and Cindy were walking up ahead. There were three streets to cross on the way. Earlier in the year, Paula needed to be close to the teacher to receive instruction in crossing, but now she was able to cross lightly traveled side streets independently. Cindy was asking her about the science fair

coming up. Each had worked on a group project that would be on display.

Margie and the teacher took turns pushing John's wheelchair. He was able to wheel himself for short distances, and was pushed by others over long distances. Margie was talking to the teacher about an upcoming Halloween party. The teacher knew that this was a topic that John would be interested in, and included him in the conversation by asking whether he planned to go. She was not sure if he understood the question, but she knew he liked to be included in the conversation anyway. He usually smiled when someone—particularly another child—talked to him. After seeing what the teacher did, Margie also talked to John, even if John did not answer back.

After they got to the store, the teacher checked in with each student to make sure each knew what she or he was supposed to do. Cindy was supposed to make a list of three items priced on a multiple-item basis (e.g., concentrated orange juice —3/$1.19), and figure out approximately how much one of each item would cost. She and Paula were to work together and meet the rest of the group at the checkout counter in about 10 minutes. Paula needed to find the items on her list and use her calculator to figure out if she could buy them all for $2.00. Before leaving school, the teacher took Cindy aside and reminded her that it was best for Paula to find the items without any help unless she really needed it. If she did need help, the teacher suggested that Cindy just give her a clue —like showing her the right aisle.

The teacher brought John's attention to his list, which had a picture of hot dog rolls on it. John, Margie, and the teacher headed over to the bread aisle. Once there, John was expected to wheel himself down the aisle without bumping into items on display. With some instructional assistance, he was able to find the rolls and pull them from the shelf to his lap. Margie then pushed John to the canned food aisle. Her assignment was to find an item that comes in two sizes, list the prices and the number of ounces in each, and figure out for homework if a shopper saved money by buying a bigger size, and if so, how much would be saved. She asked John to hold her pack while she copied down the prices.

Everyone met at the checkout counter. The teacher checked Paula's calculations to make sure that she had made no errors, and took a look at Cindy's list to see if she had her three items. Then she asked Paula to go to the checkout counter. At first Paula started for a counter that was not "open," but realized her mistake before she put her items on the counter.

From the end of the counter, the teacher watched Paula check out. She was already thinking about next week. It would be important to teach Paula more directly next week since she had spent most of her time in the store with John and Cindy this week. She also needed to design a follow-up exercise for Cindy, who was still having some difficulty applying division skills to real-life problems.

Summary

Community-based instruction is an essential component of an educational program for students with severe handicaps, but it does not necessarily have to separate these students from others at school. This problem can be alleviated when both students with and without handicaps receive instruction together in the community. When a lot of students are involved in an activity, it loses its "specialness," and becomes just another part of what happens at school. This type of instructional arrangement not only reduces the stigma that may result from having a special, separate program for students with handicaps, but can also provide valuable learning experiences for all students involved.

Given that communities are rich with potential for presenting learning experiences, there is little reason that all students should not benefit from direct learning experiences in the community. For most students this would translate into an occasional outing, while for others, instruction will be a more frequent and fundamental aspect of their instructional program.

Redefining the "Self-Contained" Classroom

Karen Delaney, like so many of her fellow college graduates, had no difficulty landing her first teaching position. After all, she was graduated with honors, had an excellent student-teaching experience and held a degree in an area where significant teaching shortages existed. Karen is a special education teacher. For the past 2 years she has been teaching at Jefferson High School and is assigned to a "self-contained" classroom for students with severe handicaps. Currently, there are 7 students enrolled in her class in a school whose population easily exceeds 1,000.

The Challenge

One of Karen's primary objectives has been to enhance the level and quality of her students' integration into Jefferson High. She knows that if her students spend all day in a special class cut off from the rest of the student population, it is unlikely that they will become "a part of" the school and build meaningful relationships with other students.

During her first year at Jefferson, Karen structured the schedule so that her students would be out of the room as much as possible. As individuals, or in groups of two or three, her students could be observed passing through the hallways, in the cafeteria, in the library, and in a variety of other settings. Later that year and into her second year, she arranged for individual students to attend regular classes (e.g., industrial arts, music, physical education) with the support of instructional assistants. Indeed, these previously "contained" students were making their presence known in the school building.

Although Karen felt that these integration efforts were making a difference, she realized that her objective had only been partially addressed. When her students returned from various destinations they were the sole inhabiters of the room— giving the sense once again of being "contained." Was there a way to redefine the space such that it could also be used by nonhandicapped students for a common function?

The Solution

Redefining a secondary self-contained classroom is not a task that can be accomplished overnight. It requires thoughtful planning and consultation with the principal as well as other members of the school staff. Although the redefining process may involve considerable time and effort, there are many steps along the way that can produce immediate changes in the environment. Below are four guiding questions that teachers might pose as they plan for reconceptualizing space previously used for special classes.

Do the materials and the equipment in the classroom unnecessarily distinguish it from others? Stand back and take an objective look at the classroom. Notice how it appears in relation to other classrooms. Is there construction paper covering the window of the door? Is the door almost always closed? Do the classroom bulletin boards or walls contain images that nonhandicapped peers would consider unusual or age inappropriate? Is the room filled with "therapy" equipment and age-inappropriate toys or instructional materials? These were all things that Karen noticed about the classroom to which she was assigned upon her arrival at Jefferson High. Within days she was able to make significant changes. She took down the construction paper and routinely began to keep the classroom door open so that those passing in the hall could easily see into the room. She removed the Sesame Street figures from the walls and the bathroom-charting forms from the bulletin boards. The preschoolers' toys that lined the bookshelves were replaced with age-appropriate substitutes. And, instead of using computer software designed for younger children, she brought in software that was designed for teenagers yet could be adjusted for differing abilities. Each of these replacements were activities that would interest not only her students but might also interest their nonhandicapped peers. Finally, with the assistance of a physical therapist, Karen

sorted through the standing tables, mats, bolsters, wedges, large balls, balancing boards, and other "therapy" equipment that occupied the room. Only those items needed for positioning students remained in the room. The rest was moved to a storage room that could be accessed by the therapist.

How is the room used by the students with severe handicaps? The next task faced by Karen was to analyze how the room was being used by her students. After reviewing a typical daily schedule she was able to make the following observations. First, as previously noted, much of her students' time was spent outside the classroom in other areas of the school building (e.g., industrial arts room, library, gym) or in the community (e.g., grocery stores, restaurants, vocational training sites). Second, when the students returned to the room it was for periods of time lasting from 10 minutes to almost 1 hour. Third, rarely did all of her students return to the room at the same time. Usually no more than three or four students were in the room at any given time. Finally, the activities conducted in the room served several purposes: to teach recreation/leisure skills, to teach grooming skills, to prepare students for community outings, and to store and retrieve instructional materials.

Could any of the activities presently carried out in the self-contained classroom be moved to a less isolated setting within the school? An entire section of the classroom was referred to as the "grooming area." This was where the students kept many of their personal items (e.g., blow dryers, wash cloth, hairbrush) that they used at different times throughout the day such as after swim class, after lunch, or upon returning from outdoors. Karen felt that this area was particularly important for the students in wheelchairs. It seemed that the location and height of the mirrors and shelves in the bathrooms and locker rooms made it impossible for students to use them. Thus, a classroom grooming area was constructed with mirrors, shelves, and compartments at wheelchair height, making it possible for students to grasp and place their own materials and use the mirror effectively.

Because the grooming area of the room stood out as being distinctly different from other classrooms, and because grooming warrants some degree of privacy, Karen decided to reconsider this aspect of the room. Realizing that the logical place to perform grooming activities is in the bathroom and the gym locker room, she returned to those settings for another look. This time, instead of accepting their deficiencies, she spoke to the school principal and head custodian about making some modifications. They agreed to lower some mirrors and shelves in the bathrooms. The physical education teachers assigned strategically located gym lockers to the students in wheelchairs so they could adapt them with compartments and hooks, enabling greater access to their grooming materials. In addition, Karen was able to investigate other environments for recreational skills such as teaching the use of tape recorders in the media center and card and board games in the student lounge.

How could the space be redefined so that it would no longer be viewed as the "special ed" classroom, but a room used by various students involved in similar activities? As one strolls through the corridors of junior high and high school settings, one can usually tell at a glance how various classrooms are used. The books that line the shelves and the bulletin boards illustrate the subject matter taught (e.g., English, social studies, math). In some cases, the classroom arrangement and the equipment give additional clues as to the function of the classroom, such as a science lab, a home economics classroom, and a music room. The defining characteristics of a secondary school classroom tend to be tied directly to one particular subject area. Even after Karen made the modifications mentioned above, she realized that she was left with a room that continued to be used only by students with severe handicaps. Thus, her next step was to brainstorm ways to redefine the room such that

other students—students without handicaps—would have reason to use it also.

The Apprenticeship Center

A school improvement committee had been formed several years earlier in response to faculty, parent, and administration concerns regarding a range of school issues. Committee members reflected a cross-section of the different departments existing at Jefferson High School. It occurred to Karen that this might be an appropriate group with whom to discuss her ideas.

Since the main function of the special education room was to provide a space where students could go to prepare for community outings (i.e., gathering belongings for work, preparing money, preparing grocery lists), she and other committee members attempted to determine whether there were other students who shared a similar need for space. Karen expressed that the students who would share the space should be a highly valued group (both socially and academically) in order that the social image of the students with handicaps would be elevated by the association. (This reasoning is consistent with the principle of social role valorization as described by Wolfensberger [1983].) Or, conversely stated, she wanted to avoid placing the students with other members of the student body who were already suffering from a rather low social status within the school. Consider, for example, a school that has operated a "nondegree" vocational program out of several classrooms in the high school. Over the years, the students enrolled in this program had become regarded as nonachievers and were occasionally referred to in derogatory terms by their peers. Including students with handicaps in an existing program that has its own status problems was obviously not the solution to Karen's dilemma.

Jefferson High had just instituted an apprenticeship program in which many high-achieving students were enrolled. The purpose of the apprenticeship program was to link students with professionals from the community to enable them to work side-by-side with an individual and acquire firsthand knowledge of the roles and responsibilities assumed in a given profession. At the time, the apprenticeship program was functioning out of a small space in the guidance office. The committee decided to reallocate space so that both the apprenticeship program and the special education classroom would share one setting. The space would be called The Apprenticeship Center and would be utilized by both students involved in the formal apprenticeship program and students with severe handicaps who were receiving instruction in vocational and other community sites. Both groups of students would use this space as a stopping-off point between other classes and departure times for community activities. Students involved in apprenticeships would use this space for such activities as maintaining ongoing logs of their experiences, writing monthly reports, and meeting with advisors as well as other students regarding their experience. In this setting, Karen would be able to facilitate many types of relationships among the students.

Summary

Special spaces occupied solely by students with handicaps invariably stigmatize students. Some schools—particularly elementary schools—are avoiding this dilemma altogether by providing educational programs for students with severe handicaps in integrated regular education classes throughout the school day. Schools that have made use of a special class model for secondary students face considerable challenges given the departmentalized nature of the curriculum as well as the lecture format used in many classes. Some of these challenges have been addressed by ensuring that students start their days in integrated homerooms and then are scheduled into classes where the teaching methods are more experiential, such as art, physical education, music, science, drama, and home economics. Indeed, the description given above may be only a transitional stage for the teacher who is attempting to improve the de-

gree and quality of integration experienced by students with severe handicaps.

Although the evolution away from the use of special education classes may take many forms, it is guided by two major goals: 1) to restore the *individual* identity of each student with a severe handicap—that is, the student becomes known as a unique individual as opposed to assuming the group identity of being one of "the handicapped"; and 2) to facilitate a student's participation in the classes, activities, and school networks that define the life of the school. Furthermore, there is one ingredient that each planning effort must not overlook: the role of the regular education staff (and, perhaps students) in the problem-solving process. Redefining a self-contained classroom is not something a teacher can do alone. It will require substantial input and support from many other members of the staff and student body.

Extracurricular Activities

High school years are a memorable and enjoyable time for many young people—a period in a person's life that is relived long after graduation in the stories shared by former high school buddies and told anew to other friends. Many of those stories relate to daily classroom experiences (the junior high teacher who got his students to write and produce a film, the lab partner who fainted when dissecting frogs, the math teacher whose toupee fell off when he bent over); but just as many relate to

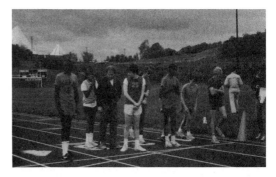

Extracurricular activities such as track and field can be options open to all students.

extracurricular experiences—candid shots for the yearbook, playing soccer, and going to dances.

The teenagers at Kingman High School will have many stories to tell about their involvement in extracurricular activities. Kingman offers various activities such as team sports (basketball, football, soccer, volleyball, cross-country), clubs, projects, and special events to enjoy after school and on weekends. While not all of the students take advantage of these activities, the wide range of choices should leave no one without *opportunities* to participate if they desire.

The Challenge

Although Marty enjoys sports, he did not spend much of his first year at Kingman participating in them. Actually, he spent most of his time after school watching TV, or walking around the backyard of his home. There was a basketball hoop on the garage, and sometimes he would use that. The only time he participated in sports activities (aside from physical education class) was once or twice a year with other teenagers who were also handicapped. He had a lot of extra time and plenty of interest, but not much to do.

The Solution

Things changed for Marty in his second year. He became involved with the Kingman cross-country team. In his opinion, school is okay, but cross-country is great. A typical practice day might look something like the following.

When the final bell of the day rang, Marty headed downstairs to the gym locker room. His was one of the few lockers that contained a key lock instead of a combination lock. Just as he turned the key, Jerry, one of his teammates, came in. Jerry greeted him with, "Hey, what's happenin'?" Marty smiled. He did not talk much, just a few words occasionally. Sometimes he used pictures to communicate—like at the restaurant or at other times when he needed them; but he did not need any for practice. He got along fine with a few words and gestures.

Marty headed out to the track and waited for the others. Most of the team sat on the grass on the inside of the track or just fooled around while they waited. When it was warm, Marty liked to lie down on the grass and catch some rays. The coach finally came out and started organizing the stretching exercises. Marty liked this part especially because it did not matter how fast you went. The stretches were really confusing for the first couple weeks of practice (and embarrassing when he made mistakes), but he kept watching the other guys and girls and he sort of picked them up after a while. If he kept doing a particular stretch after he was supposed to stop, somebody next to him usually said something, and then he looked at the others and saw what to do next. The first few times he did this, a few people laughed, but not anymore. Everybody was used to him being around, so it was not such a big deal that he made mistakes sometimes, or did the stretches in kind of a different way. If the coach thought he was not trying, he would yell at Marty just as he did at everybody else. (Yelling seemed to be one of the requirements for being a coach.) The first time that happened, Marty got upset and started hitting himself. A teammate he knew from homeroom had seen him do that before, and when it happened in homeroom, the students did not make a big deal about it. The teacher usually held his hands down for a moment and quietly asked him to relax. Then the teacher or another student got him involved in something interesting—something he could do with his hands. So the teammate told Marty to stop it and keep stretching, and he did.

Then it was time to run. They usually started out slow. Marty had a lot of energy and usually was in the lead for the first minute or so. The coach told him to slow down so he could run longer, but he had to get that energy out. After a few minutes, he would slow down and begin to have trouble keeping up with the others, and then he would walk for awhile. If he got too far behind, the coach would have someone walk with him. And since everybody took turns, nobody seemed to mind. John and Sandy did it a lot because they liked him.

There were other kids who had to walk after a while, too, so it was okay.

After practice, Marty got changed and put his running shoes in his locker up on the second floor. He had a ribbon he had won in the Special Olympics last year in his locker. That was fun, but it was not at all like practice and John and Sandy were not there. He did not get any ribbons from practice, but it did not seem to matter. What mattered was that practice was fun. Mostly, it felt great to run; he liked being part of the team, and he did it every day during the season. He was in the team picture for the yearbook, and his uncle talked about it every time he came over to the house because he had been on the cross-country team when he was in high school.

Ways to Get Students Involved in Extracurricular Activities

Marty's second year of high school was considerably different from his first due to his participation in the cross-country team. How did his involvement come about? What strategies can teachers, administrators, and friends use to facilitate the involvement of students with severe disabilities in extracurricular activities? Here are a few strategies to consider:

Investigate what opportunities are presently available at your school. Usually, those that are noncompetitive in nature are most conducive to incorporating students with severe handicaps. Of those activities that are competitive, attempt to determine to what degree competition is an essential element of involvement, and what creative alternatives might be pursued for the particular student.

Assist the student in determining what sort of activity interests her or him. Typically, students join organizations or activities for a number of reasons—not all of which are directly related to the nature of the activity. Does the student have friends or acquaintances who are already involved? This may be an important factor. If the student is unable to verbalize a preference

for a particular activity, it may be helpful to talk with family and friends to get a sense of what they think the person would like to do. The student might also begin an activity, and communicate by her or his actions whether it is a preferred activity.

Once an activity has been identified, assist the staff person (coach, faculty sponsor) in brainstorming ideas regarding the student's involvement, if necessary. A student does not need to be able to do all of an activity, or do it in the exact same way as the majority of the other students involved. Can the activity be modified? Can the student do part of the activity while a partner does the remainder? Do not underestimate other students' ability to adapt quickly to the student of concern, and to come up with brilliant ideas about how to include him or her.

Encourage or initiate the development of activities that are noncompetitive. As noted by Kohn (1986), an emphasis on competition in school activities can have destructive effects on many young people (including those with handicaps). He urges one to examine the goal of student activites. If the goal of sponsoring activities is to encourage widespread participation and enjoyment, then many after-school programs receiving the bulk of the resources and attention are running counter to this goal. Examples of noncompetitive or minimally competitive activities include those such as aerobic dancing, chorus, weight training, and "pep" club.

Determine what resources are available to include students who need a high level of assistance in order to participate in an activity. Often, it will not be possible for the teacher to provide this assistance. Consider whether it is possible for paraprofessionals to voluntarily shift their working hours on particular days in order to assist after school. Are there community volunteers who may be willing to assist, or a mature group of students willing to commit (possibly in pairs) to assist the student on a regular basis. Are any existing human services agencies involved in recreation or respite services that may be willing to provide assistance?

Summary

Unfortunately, many students with moderate and severe handicaps have not had the opportunity to enjoy the numerous afterschool activities that most public schools offer. Either as a result of segregated schooling, or limited involvement in the culture of the public school, the sense of belonging, accomplishment, and fun that accompanies these activities has generally not been an option for most of these students. Often, a young person with severe handicaps has fairly restricted choices when it comes to organized recreational activities. These usually take the form of episodic "handicapped-only" events. "Handicapped-only" programs once filled a vacuum for people who were without options for involvement in existing school or community activities. It is hoped that the reliance on these programs will wane in the future as students and adults with handicaps begin to demonstrate that, when given a choice and the support needed, separate "handicapped-only" activities are not necessarily where they want to be. The key element is choice. Most young people with handicaps have not had the experience upon which to base a choice.

The reasons for students with handicaps to participate in public school extracurricular activities are the same as those expressed for all students. In addition to being fun, these activities present the opportunity to enjoy and strengthen friendships that develop in classes or other school activities, and to develop new relationships. Membership becomes part of a student's identity—validates her or his place in the school community, and often gives family and friends outside of school a new perspective on the student and her or his abilities and interests. Extracurricular activities can provide students with a common bond, something they can talk about when they see each other during the school day. Furthermore, many of the activities to which students are introduced in school become lifelong recreational interests (e.g., swimming, softball, jogging).

Belonging to a school is much more than going to classes. What many people remember about high school is the bonfires, dances, proms, walkathons, basketball games, and their ongoing involvement in clubs or afterschool sports activities. Given support, students with severe handicaps can enjoy these same experiences and really become a part of "what's happening" at school.

Peer Networks

Next fall, Janice will be a newly enrolled 10th grader at Stratford High School. Achieving the status of a 10th grader did not come easily for Janice. Unlike her peers who followed the familiar path from elementary, to middle or junior high, and finally to high school, Janice was placed in a segregated school at age 5 where she was expected to remain until graduation. However, after years of negotiations with the local school district, Janice was enrolled in the district high school. Janice's parents argued that her development had suffered while attending the segregated school. Her teachers expected less of her, she lacked appropriate role models, and she was unprepared to enter the real world. The school district argued that Janice would become isolated in the high school. There were no other students functioning at her level and no existing programs to meet her needs. She would need a one-to-one teaching arrangement and the typical high school population would overwhelm her.

The Challenge

Although her parents found comfort in the fact that Janice had finally gained access to the regular school system, they were not without fears about her upcoming high school experience. Would Janice be accepted? Would she be able to make friends within these new and unfamiliar surroundings? For so many young people, the development of friendships requires little conscious effort, but in Janice's case there were many indicators that put her at risk of becoming isolated within the high school—of leading an existence without friends. First, because of school policies and practices that tend to separate out students with handicaps, the nonhandicapped students in the high school had limited exposure to peers with handicaps, particularly students with severe handicaps. Second, staff members were not fully committed to her participation within the school; indeed, many teachers became negatively predisposed to Janice's involvement in the school as a result of attention given to her parent's advocacy efforts and the misinformation transmitted from those professionals who argued against her enrollment in the high school. Also, it is important to note that the staff, like their students, had had limited exposure to students with severe handicaps. Third, as Janice's brother and two sisters were not yet of high school age, they would not be available to "watch out for her" or ease her transition into the high school. Fourth, Janice occasionally displayed some excessive behavior that tended to draw negative attention to her (although there was reason to believe it would decrease once she became familiar with her high school routine). Finally, she did not have a ready peer group. Since she had not been following the typical progression from middle to high school, she would see no familiar faces in the crowded hallways. Under circumstances such as these, it may not be in Janice's best interest simply to assume that she will be naturally absorbed into the flow of high school life. Instead, conscious efforts may be needed to prevent her from becoming isolated within Stratford High.

The Solution

The guidance counselor at Stratford High was acquainted with several peer support programs that had been developed in other high school settings. Although the programs varied from school to school and were applied differently to each individual student, they seemed to be based on several common premises. One premise is that all students, including students with the most severe handicaps, have both the need and the desire to build friendships and become part of a social group. Another premise is that school systems should be prepared to provide additional supports to students considered to be at risk of being iso-

lated from their peers. These peer support systems also function on the belief that, within any student body, there are individuals who will come forth to fulfill the role of a friend and/or ally when given the proper introduction and supports. Finally, the added supports offered through these programs are provided as long as the student and his or her peers need them, but with the ultimate goal of reaching a point where the support system no longer relies on external or unnatural interventions.

The McGill Action Planning System (MAPS) was the strategy eventually adopted to assist Janice in developing a peer network. It is a system designed by Marsha Forest and Judith Snow of the Canadian Association for Community Living that grew out of a need to support students, like Janice, whose situation was such that the forming of friendships could not be taken for granted (Snow & Forest, 1987). Using the MAPS framework, the teacher, guidance counselor, vice-principal, and Janice's parents devised the following plan.

Initial Orientation During the spring preceding Janice's high school enrollment, several orientation sessions will be held to acquaint her with the high school and to enable her to make contact with a new peer group. For the first session, Janice will visit the high school, tour the building, and be introduced to some of the students and teachers with whom she will have contact in the upcoming year. The second session will be used to elicit the involvement of Janice's nonhandicapped peer group. Meetings will be held with small groups of ninth graders. Each meeting will be conducted by the guidance counselor and the teacher who will be responsible for monitoring Janice's overall program. The meeting will serve a two-fold purpose: 1) to educate students about Janice's upcoming enrollment (Who is Janice? Why is this attention being drawn to her enrollment in the school? Where has she attended school in the past?), and 2) to generate interest in getting to know Janice and possibly becoming part of her social network. At the end of these meetings, students are asked to generate a list of ideas concerning Janice's involvement in the high school. Among the items that might be listed are:

Meeting Janice at the bus stop and riding with her to school

Sharing a locker with her

Telephoning her during the summer months to talk about school (This strategy was used with a student who was involved in MAPS. The student's parents reported that this was the first call their daughter had ever received. Although their daughter was not able to use words, she began to vocalize in the receiver each time her peer called [M. Forest, personal communication, June 12, 1987].)

Shopping together for school clothes and materials

Sitting next to Janice in homeroom and other classroom periods

Showing Janice how to use the cafeteria and inviting her to join the group for lunch

The meeting ends with the completion of the list. Students interested in engaging in one or more of the listed activities will be invited to remain and discuss their potential involvement with the teacher and guidance counselor. A third and final meeting will be held with those students who have indicated their desire to get involved with the activities. At this meeting, commitments will be firmed up as well as the procedures to use for communicating with the teacher and guidance counselor.

Getting Acquainted Throughout the summer months and into the first weeks of the fall semester, the students will engage in the activities to which they made commitments. While facilitating these and other interactions, the teacher will take note of the relationships that seem to be gaining strength and becoming mutually satisfying to the parties involved. Based on interest level and the relationship formed, approximately five or six of the nonhandicapped students will be invited to become involved in a more formalized peer group. MAPS refers to this peer group as a "team"; in

Janice's case, it will be referred to as a "peer network."

Establishing a Peer Network A small group of 10th graders will form Janice's peer network. They will meet regularly with the teacher for the purpose of reviewing Janice's involvement in the school and brainstorming new ways to enhance her participation. Some of these meetings will be attended by Janice, her parents, the guidance counselor, the vice-principal, and others interested in contributing to Janice's support system. The peers will be asked to play an active role in the planning process. Peers tend to bring a fresh perspective to the process—one that is unencumbered with past practices, policies, and concerns for other logistical constraints. Consider, for example, the peers' contribution to the following segment of a MAPS session conducted by Marsha Forest (1987a). At issue is the homeroom assignment of Jenny, another student with severe handicaps:

Marsha (facilitator): Everybody goes to homeroom. Where does Jenny go?
Peers: She goes here, in this room.
Principal: This is a homeroom, a legitimate homeroom. (The homeroom referred to is a room in which only handicapped students are assigned.)
Marsha: Anybody think she should go anywhere else?
Teacher: Maybe we could get her in a different homeroom.
Peer: Yeah, with more people her age that are . . . (pauses) well . . . integrated.
Marsha (to peers): Where do you go?
Peers: Different homerooms.
Teacher: It might be good to get her out of here; to get her in her own homeroom like everybody else.
Marsha (to peers): Would you be willing to invite Jenny?
Peers: Yes.
Peer #1: Yes. I would love to.
Marsha: What about your teachers?
Peer #1: There's empty spaces in our homeroom.
Marsha (to peer #1): Who is your teacher?
Peer #1: Mr. Humbolt. He wouldn't mind. He will get into anything.
Principal: There will be no problem at all with that.
(Forest, 1987a)

In this segment of the planning process, the peers advocated for an integrated homeroom and volunteered ways to support the student in this setting. The principal, who initially considered the segregated homeroom a "legitimate homeroom," reconsidered her position and later indicated that there would be "no problem" in reassigning the student with severe handicaps to a new homeroom.

Summary

It is highly likely that, at least initially, the members of a formalized peer network will see themselves as allies or advocates rather than friends —recognizing that this is a fine distinction. However, in time it is hoped that the relationships will evolve to the point that such distinctions no longer exist. When designing a structure for assisting students to develop social networks, it is important to be cognizant of the feelings and perceptions of the person with handicaps. It is one thing to become involved out of a genuine concern to include a fellow student who is at risk of becoming isolated in the school; it is quite another thing to become involved out of pity felt for that individual. No one wants a relationship that grows out of pity. It should also be noted that the authors are not completely comfortable with the formalization of what appears to occur naturally for many students; nor can they find comfort in knowing that some students face isolation. To avoid the loneliness that might occur for some students, a certain amount of formalization may be necessary, at least initially. Finally, one should not assume that every student with severe handicaps will need this degree of formalization in order to build meaningful relationships. The implementation of a MAPS program or a similar program should be based upon the unique needs of each *individual*.

FINAL REMARKS

Five examples of educational activities/innovations have been described that reflect the evolving meaning of integration as it refers to students with

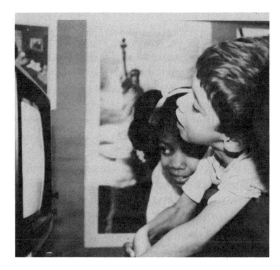

A computer exercise is one of many activities that can be designed to challenge a range of learners.

severe handicaps. These activities address the importance of adapting curriculum to reflect the needs of all students both in school and in the community, redefining educational space, involvement in afterschool activities, and the importance of friendships. While each activity offers a unique perspective on the movement toward greater integration, they share several common themes:

Schools provide a wealth of activities in which students with diverse learning characteristics can participate.

Furthering school integration will require conscious efforts on the part of students, parents, principals, district administrators, and others—teachers can create change, but they cannot be expected to do it alone.

Knowledge of specific educational techniques or practices is not enough; creativity and commitment are essential in moving forward with school integration.

The degree of student involvement in school programs and activities need *not* be determined by student ability, but rather by student interest, student need, and adult willingness to provide opportunities and support.

As noted by Bogdan and Taylor (1987), "being part of the community cannot be packaged" (p. 213); likewise, there is no recipe for assisting students with severe handicaps in becoming a part of a school. Integration is a social process, and the realization of activities such as those described here can be an important step forward in this process—a process driven by a vision of schools that welcome diversity among their members, and do what it takes to achieve growth and development for all.

STUDY QUESTIONS

1. Imagine that you will be preparing a unit in the area of math, science, or social studies. Propose a lesson plan that clearly demonstrates how you could meaningfully include a student with severe handicaps.
2. Discuss the limitations and problems associated with a self-contained classroom such as the one to which Karen Delaney was assigned.
3. Consider the following situation: A high school track club welcomes the participation of a student with severe handicaps—but limits her involvement to that of "assisting the equipment manager." You know that this student enjoys running but cannot compete at the level of her peers. As a person providing support to this student, what would you suggest?
4. JoAnn, a fifth-grade student who is not handicapped, receives instruction in a grocery store as part of her math curriculum. She is accompanied by several other students, one of whom has severe handicaps. JoAnn's parents have written a note requesting more information about this outing. Specifically, they want to know what she is gaining from the experience. As JoAnn's teacher, how would you explain how instruction in this context is relevant for JoAnn?
5. Assume that you are considering accepting a teaching position at a local school. You are given the opportunity to ask questions of the teachers and administrators during a visit to the school. What questions, if any, will you ask about the integration of students with severe handicaps? Explain.
6. Make a list of the people who play a significant role in your life. Do the same for someone you know with severe handicaps. What does this exercise reveal about the social network of the person with handicaps?

REFERENCES

Biklen, D. (1985). *Achieving the complete school: Strategies for effective mainstreaming*. New York: Teachers College Press.

Biklen, D., Ferguson, D., & Ford, A. (Eds.). (in press). *Schooling and disability* [Yearbook of the National Society for the Study of Education]. Chicago: University of Chicago Press.

Bogdan, R., & Taylor, S. (1987). The next wave. In S. Taylor, D. Biklen, & J. Knoll (Eds.), *Community integration for people with severe disabilities*. New York: Teachers College Press.

Forest, M. (Producer and Director). (1987a). *MAPS: McGill Action Planning System* [Videotape]. Downsview, Ontario: The G. Allan Roeher Institute.

Forest, M. (Ed.). (1987b). *More education/integration: A fur-ther collection of readings on the integration of children with mental handicaps into regular school systems*. Downsview, Ontario: The G. Allan Roeher Institute.

Kohn, A. (1986). *No contest: The case against competition*. Boston: Houghton Mifflin.

Shepherd, G.D., & Ragan, W.B. (1982). *Modern elementary curriculum*. New York: Holt, Rinehart & Winston.

Snow, J., & Forest, M. (1987). Circles. In M. Forest (Ed.), *More education/integration: A further collection of readings on the intregration of children with mental handicaps into regular school systems*. Downview, Ontario: The G. Allan Roeher Institute.

Stainback, W., & Stainback, S. (1984). A rationale for the merger of special and regular education. *Exceptional Children*, *51*(2), 102–111.

Strully, J., & Strully, C. (1985). Friendships and our children. *Journal of Persons with Severe Handicaps, 10*(4), 224–227.

Thousand, J., Fox, T., Reid, R., Godek, J., Williams, W., & Fox, W. (1986, September). *The Homecoming Model: Educating students who present intensive educational challenges within regular education environments.* (Available from The Homecoming Project, Center for Developmental Disabilities, 499c Waterman Building, University of Vermont, Burlington, VT 05405)

Wolfensberger, W. (1983). Social role valorization: A proposed new term for the principle of normalization. *Mental Retardation, 21* (6), 234–239.

CHAPTER 2

STUDENTS WITH LEARNING HANDICAPS

Donald H. Doorlag

Individuals with learnings handicaps can be found in almost all mainstream school and community settings. Examples of typical learning handicaps may be found in cases such as the third grader who has reading problems and has difficulty staying in his seat, the junior high student who has always struggled with his math assignments and can never quite understand the teacher's directions, or the high school student who is unable to keep up with his homework assignments and has difficulty relating to his peers. While these students are generally considered to have achievement potential that falls into the normal range, either their performance falls well below expectations or their behavior interferes with their own learning and/or the learning of others.

The limitations of learning handicapped individuals may affect them only in specific academic or social skills areas and the students' problems are not always readily apparent as their physical appearance and observable behavior is generally quite normal. They may experience problems in reading or in other academic areas, they may be overly active while in class or have problems attending to their assigned task or the directions provided by the teacher, or they may exhibit deficits in the social skills required to get along with others. Any of these may not become readily obvious to teachers or others until they have spent some time with the students. Many of these individuals will continue to experience similar problems when they leave school, problems reflected in areas such

as an inability to complete job applications, poor attendance record at work, difficulty following directions, difficulty reading written manuals, or continual problems relating to their peers. Professionals often use labels such as mildly handicapped, learning handicapped, or educationally handicapped for this group, yet there is no single widely accepted label or definition for this somewhat divergent group.

The learning handicapped (LH) category generally consists of individuals drawn from the groups traditionally labeled as: 1) having learning disabilities, 2) being educable (or educationally) mentally retarded, or 3) exhibiting behavior disorders (i.e., those students who exhibit behavioral disorders that are not severe enough to qualify them for programs for the person with serious emotional disturbances) (MacMillan, Keogh, & Jones, 1986). The professional literature (and often the educational programs in schools) tends to deal with these groups as separate entities, yet there is evidence that indicates that a great deal of commonality exists between these groups and that it is feasible to provide instruction and other services in a combined program designed to serve all the subgroups simultaneously (e.g., Hallahan & Kauffman, 1976; Hardman, Drew, & Egan, 1984).

During the past few years there has been an increasing number of learning handicapped students, especially those identified as learning disabled (e.g., Algozzine, Ysseldyke, & Christenson, 1983; Gerber, 1984). These increases can be related in part to the lack of a specific definition that is interpreted in a consistent fashion from setting to setting. As different individuals within each school may have different interpretations of who qualifies for service in programs for learning handicapped students, the prevalence figures and types of students found within different schools may vary significantly. In other cases regular class teachers may be unwilling (or lack the skills) to work effectively with students with learning problems and wish only to pass these students on to the special educator whom they consider as responsible for providing the educational program for these students. Prevalence estimates for this population vary widely, but the range of 3%–8% would be agreed upon by most professionals.

Learning handicapped students are most frequently identified by their regular classroom teachers. Many of their problems do not become apparent until they have entered school and are placed under the requirements of the classroom. Their academic and social performance can then be compared with that of their peers as their interactions with other students and with adults increases. When students initially exhibit a problem that concerns their teacher, alterations of their current educational program should be considered and attempted prior to considering the student for possible assessment for special education services. For example, a regular class teacher may have a concern about the performance of a student in the area of math. The teacher has the responsibility to exhaust the options available in her or his classroom prior to referring the student for special education. If these alternative approaches are not successful the teacher can then proceed in referring the student. If students are considered for special education, a battery of assessments are planned and administered (after the parents approve) to attempt to determine the current status of the student's abilities and/or performance, and this information is then used to plan the most appropriate educational intervention.

While in school the majority of these students are educated in mainstream settings with special education services provided by resource or itinerant teachers. The resource room program serves the largest percentage of these students. In this type of program the students spend the majority of their day in the regular classroom and leave the regular classroom daily for special instruction in the resource room. Some students with more severe learning handicaps are served in special classes or are provided additional assistance by counselors. Recently there has been an increased awareness of the need to develop programs designed to have the student spend the entire school day in the regular classroom with a consultant providing assistance to the student's regular teacher —not a total reliance on special educators to provide only direct assistance to the student (e.g., Stainback & Stainback, 1987; Stainback, Stainback, Courtnage, & Jaben, 1985; Will, 1986).

Various accounts have been provided to explain why individuals have learning handicaps. Some professionals believe that many of these students are affected by neurological deficiencies or psychological processing problems that interfere with their ability to process information or to form appropriate verbal or motor responses when they are required. There are also those who believe that the handicapping condition is the result of conditions such as heredity, nutrition, vitamin deficiencies, or other biogenic causes. Still others discuss poverty, family stability, or delinquency as causing the learning problems. A great number of professionals now consider that the problems experienced by persons with learning handicaps are a reflection of the fact that the individual has had inadequate exposure to the type of learning experiences needed to develop the skills required to perform effectively in academic, social, or work settings (e.g., Kauffman, 1985; Lewis & Doorlag, 1987; MacMillan et al., 1986). While it may be of interest to the teacher to know the specific cause of the student's problem, it is most often not possible to obtain this information. If the information is available, it frequently provides a very small contribution to assist educators in selecting or designing the most appropriate type of intervention needed for the student. The most important considerations involve identifying the specific skills the individual does or does not possess and then identifying the most appropriate way to directly teach those skills that are needed to function effectively in school and community situations.

EDUCATIONAL MODEL

During the past few years there has been a sizable change in the acceptance of various models advocated for educating students with learning handicaps. Educators have become increasingly aware of the importance of providing students with appropriate learning experiences and the teachers' use of effective instructional techniques with this group of students. They have also reduced their concern for the causes of the learning problems experienced by the students and have begun to consider that the most effective use of their time in school is to provide the students with high-quality instruction. These educators consider that the learning handicapped students are capable of learning the skills that will help them to function effectively in school if they are provided with effective instruction designed to directly teach these skills. No longer is instruction considered to apply only to the area of academics, but it is viewed as critical in improving the student's problem-solving skills, study skills, and social skills. In addition, recent research has determined that the use of effective instructional and classroom management practices can help reduce the likelihood that the learning and behavior problems will become apparent in the classroom (e.g., Englert, 1984).

Several years ago when educational programs for learning handicapped students were initiated in the schools there was a feeling on the part of the teachers that it was important to know the cause of the learning problem. Teachers considered this information important for it was used to design an educational program directed at removing or ameliorating the cause in order to remedy the problem experienced by the student. For example, if a student was experiencing a significant reading problem the student was tested in such areas as visual or auditory perception; if the student was found to function poorly in the skills related to these areas (e.g., tracing designs, repeating series of digits) remedial activities were selected that would work on improving these skills. In many cases there was little time spent on actually teaching reading skills, the area that was causing the student the problem in school. Recently, it has been found that working on the areas considered to be related to tasks such as reading (e.g., perceptual-motor) have little effect on improving the student's performance in the area of primary concern (e.g., Kavale & Mattson, 1983). This type of approach and others such as considering whether the student is minimally brain damaged or dyslexic serves only to remove the responsibility from the teacher and to place the onus of the problem on the student, and it provides a very small amount of useful information for planning an effective educational intervention.

Today, effective teachers of students with learning handicaps typically consider factors other than the cause of the problem as more important in designing and implementing an educational intervention. These teachers believe that the important factor is to regard the problem as one of instruction and feel it is their responsibility to determine the appropriate instructional strategy to resolve the problem. The instructional techniques used by the teacher can apply to the three areas in which problems normally occur: academic performance, study skills (e.g., notetaking, outlining, test taking), and social skills (i.e., ability to get along with peers and adults), as the skills needed by students in each of these areas can be taught.

An initial concern is to identify the specific skills demonstrated by the student. The teacher wants to know more than a grade-level score in an area such as reading; he or she needs to determine what specific skills the student possesses and what skills must be taught. The teacher may use the student's actual performance in class to conduct curriculum-based assessment, in which the student's performance is compared with that expected in the curriculum, or he or she may use criterion-referenced assessment, which assesses the student's ability to demonstrate certain skills specified in a set of objectives. The information derived from either of these techniques provides the teacher with data that relate directly to the educational needs of the student and that can be used to assist in designing and delivering an appropriate educational intervention.

Following the assessment to determine the student's current level of performance, if possible the student is grouped with others who require instruction in similar areas. Recently research has demonstrated that students are more successful in acquiring new skills if they are taught in groups (e.g., Englert, 1984; Lewis & Doorlag, 1987). Group instruction provides the students with a greater opportunity to benefit from the instruction provided by the teacher as it permits students to practice the skill under the direction of the teacher, who can assure that the skill is introduced appropriately, that it is modeled, that prompts are provided when students experience difficulty, that the lesson is appropriately paced, and that immediate feedback and reinstruction are provided when needed. Further, it is important that students can accurately perform the targeted skill more than 80% of the time, a situation that can be assured if they are closely monitored in a group setting.

While individual, or one-on-one, instruction was once considered to be the ideal instructional setting, it is now known to reduce the opportunities for teachers to continuously monitor and interact with a number of students while they are receiving instruction. One-on-one instruction reduces the amount of instructional time received by each student because only one student in the class is receiving the attention of the teacher and the remainder of the students are left to function (often flounder) without direct supervision. Individual or independent work should still be provided, but only when the student has demonstrated proficiency in the skill while receiving instruction in a group and uses this individual work to polish and complete the mastery of the skill.

Another area of primary concern to the teacher is the monitoring of student progress. This monitoring is most effective if it is conducted on a daily (or at least several times a week) basis. The data collected serve to provide the teacher with information on the effectiveness of the interventions (i.e., to determine whether to continue or to modify the instruction) and the student with knowledge of his or her progress. While many teachers are concerned about the total time this may take in a class session, it is possible to structure it in such a way that it consumes a minimal amount of time. For example, reading progress can be assessed by using 1-minute time samples in which the teacher records the number of words read and the percentage of the words read accurately. Time samples such as these could be used in other curriculum areas (e.g., math, spelling, writing) or other types of data-collection techniques could be used (e.g., number of assignments completed per day, number of talk-outs per day, number of minutes late to class each day) (see Figure 1 for an example). Peer tutors, other students, classroom aides, or the students themselves can be taught to collect and record the data. These data are most useful and effective if they are displayed in a graph that is easily interpreted by students, teachers, and parents.

Classroom management is another critical area of concern for teachers working with learning handicapped students. This area is the one that consistently concerns most teachers and it is the area that brings about the most negative attention to students. A student who experiences problems in his or her academic studies concerns teachers, but if this is combined with problems that appear in the areas of classroom behavior the likelihood of the student's being referred to special education is much greater. Competent teachers consider that this area is one that requires the same careful planning and instruction needed in providing academic instruction. Effective classroom management begins with the establishment of a carefully

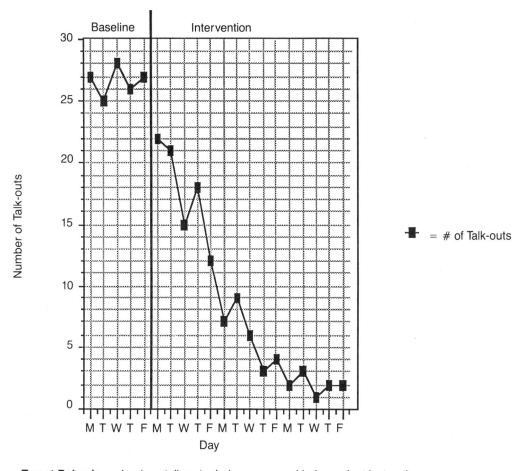

Target Behavior: In-class talk-outs during group and independent instruction

Intervention: Checkmark provided each time hand is raised during group instruction (and student waits to be called on) or for each consecutive 5 minutes of on-task behavior during independent instruction

Student: Lester

Figure 1.   Graph of baseline and intervention data regarding in-class talk-outs during group and independent instruction.

designed set of rules for the classroom. These rules must be stated in a positive manner (i.e., dos rather than don'ts), they must be carefully explained and taught to the students, the students must be provided with the opportunity to practice the rules, and the rules must be enforced (i.e., re-ward those who follow them and provide consequences for those who do not). This should be an ongoing activity in the class with the rules modified as needed and any new rules taught in the same fashion as those that were originally implemented. Often students who do not respond to the guidelines established in the regular class require more intensive use of reinforcements and negative consequences while in the regular class or they may need to develop the appropriate classroom behavior skills while being placed in a special setting. Following their acquisition of the appropriate skills, they should be returned to the regular class on a full-time basis.

Finally, one of the most critical concerns relating to the provision of appropriate educational programs for students with learning handicaps relates to the use of consultants. Typically the most effective use of these professionals is to serve as resources to regular classroom teachers. Their role is two-fold: They are concerned with assisting teachers in developing the skills needed to operate effective classrooms that serve a wide range of students with varying abilities (thereby reducing the number of students referred to special education) and they are concerned with helping teachers work with students who are returning to the regular classroom on a full-time basis after spending a portion of their day in a special education program.

Usually the consultant works with the teacher and does not provide direct service to the student with problems. The consultant is involved in providing the teacher with assistance, not in telling her or him how to deal with each specific problem that arises in the classroom. He or she may discuss particular problems with the teacher and assist in determining what may be contributing to the occurrence of these problems and in designing alternative strategies to reduce the possibility that they will occur again. In addition to discussing the problems, the consultant may observe in the classroom, collect data on student or teacher performance, provide resource materials to the teacher, provide instruction to the teacher, model teaching or classroom management techniques for the teacher, or provide other types of assistance directed at improving the skills of the teacher. The consultant will never be available on a daily basis throughout the school year and must provide the type of assistance that will improve the teacher's

ability to anticipate and handle the problems that occur in the classroom. The consultant should not assume the role of the "problem solver" who is always there to provide the solution to each problem experienced by the teacher, but should leave the teacher with improved skills in problem solving and delivering quality instruction related to the needs of the students.

INTEGRATION ACTIVITIES

Academic Instruction in a Resource Room

Rationale

Because the majority of students with learning handicaps are educated in programs in which they spend the bulk of their school day in the regular classroom and are provided special education services in a resource room setting, it is important to consider the components of a successful academic program serving these students. It is significant that students educated in this setting be considered as only temporary participants in the special education program, not long-term or permanent placements in the program, but individuals capable of acquiring the knowledge and skills necessary to function effectively alongside their peers in mainstream settings. The program is intended to be a highly efficient one that assists the students in the transition to function independently and successfully in the regular program by improving the rate of growth for the student above that achieved in the regular classroom.

Resource programs are established at all levels of the educational ladder. They serve students for short periods of time during the school day and attempt to provide minimal disruption to the student's regular classroom program. It is the purpose of the resource program to provide students with the experiences needed to develop the skills necessary to function in an independent manner in the regular classroom setting. In addition, the resource program should provide support for the regular classroom program in the form of supplementing the instruction provided there. The support needed to assure the coordination between the programs can only be accomplished when effective cooperation and communication are established and maintained between the teachers involved in both programs. This involves a two-way transfer of information that allows the parties involved to coordinate their efforts, to be informed of the progress of the student, and to exchange information regarding their findings related to effective instructional practices with the student.

Special educators have the advantage of specific professional training in working with this population of students and a lower caseload of students (typically 15 to 25). In addition, they normally have additional resources available (e.g., psychologists, consultants) who can assist them in designing specialized interventions to meet the special needs of the students. While these factors permit them to provide more intensive interventions than those already available in the regular classroom, there are other factors that add to the difficulty of operating their program. For example, these programs usually serve students from several grade levels (often during the same time period) and the range and types of difficulties are typically diverse (e.g., students with problems in reading, spelling, math, and social skills simultaneously placed in the program). The mix of students found in special class programs is generally similar to that found in the resource program with the difference being that the problems of the students placed in the special class are more severe. The resource program teacher is also restricted because of a time constraint, usually about 40–60 minutes per day, while the special class teacher has the student for the majority of the school day.

The interventions provided for students with learning handicaps by the competent teacher are directed at improving the skills required for the student to function effectively in a "regular" environment. These interventions focus on one of the three phases of learning information or skills:

acquisition (initial learning), maintenance (the recall of previously learned material), and generalization (applying learned material to similar problems and situations) (Lewis & Doorlag, 1987).

The effective resource program teacher provides a classroom setting that is under her or his direction and control and classroom activities have an academic focus directed at learning. These classroom activities are not directed primarily at affectively oriented goals (i.e., those that deal with the feelings and emotions of the students) because the teacher is concerned that the students acquire the knowledge and skills required to function effectively in mainstream settings. Improvement in affective areas such as self-concept will most appropriately be a result of the students' acquiring the necessary academic, social, and study skills through the instruction provided by the teacher in each of these areas. This instruction is provided in a manner that assures that learning takes place in a systematic, success-oriented manner (i.e., greater than 80% accuracy on responses or practice opportunities) that builds both the students' skills and confidence in their abilities. Furthermore, the students' growth in affective areas is highly difficult to develop in isolation; it most appropriately is the result of the positive learning experiences the students are provided in various educational, home, and community settings.

The resource program teacher holds high expectations for the students—for they are considered to be capable of learning. This is a different view than many educators have held, for they have often concentrated on viewing the students as having severe restrictions in their capabilities because of their being identified as learning handicapped. In addition, the students are held accountable for completing their assigned classwork. The teacher maintains a positive classroom environment that fosters cooperation rather than competition and he or she is responsible for assuring that the students are provided with success-oriented experiences and adequate amounts of corrective feedback and reinforcement for correct responses during all phases of the learning process. This success is assured by accurately placing them at an instructional level appropriate for their particular skills, providing them with high-quality instruction in groups, and pacing the instruction so that students move through the instruction at as rapid a pace as possible. Effective instruction (sometimes called "direct teaching" or "direct instruction") involves: explaining the purpose of lessons, introduction of skills and concepts, modeling the expected behavior, providing supervised practice (with prompts when needed), providing the students with the maximum opportunities to exhibit the behavior, and collecting performance data in order to assess the appropriateness of the instruction and to provide feedback to the students (Lewis, 1983). As a primary goal is to provide the opportunity for a high number of student responses, the instruction is considered to be individualized when students demonstrate a high proportion of correct responses (Stevens & Rosenshine, 1981).

Successful instructional programs that follow this model may be teacher designed, teacher adapted (using existing curriculum material), or commercially prepared. For example, a teacher working with a group of students with problems in the area of spelling may choose to use a commercially prepared program such as *Spelling Mastery* (Dixon, Engelmann, & Olen, 1981) as this program includes the components recommended for use in direct instruction. Students are placed within the program using a test that determines the current performance level of the student; scripted lessons are provided so the teacher does not have to design and develop the daily lessons; the students are provided with a sequential presentation of skills and concepts that builds in many practice opportunities; previously learned skills are reinforced throughout the program to provide for maintenance and generalization; and instructions for collecting and maintaining data on student performance are provided.

Participants and Setting

Albert is an 11-year-old student with learning handicaps (LH) who is currently in the fifth grade.

Albert has had difficulty in the area of math for some time and he has always been known to be "quite active" in the classroom. During the past year his teachers attempted a number of different instructional and classroom management strategies in his regular classroom, but these have not been successful in improving his behavior or his performance in math. Recently he has been identified as an LH student and is presently scheduled to spend 60 minutes per day in the resource room at his school to work on improving his math skills and his classroom behavior.

Intervention

Miss Collins, his resource teacher, has assessed Albert's math skills using an inventory that has provided her with a specific identification of the skill areas in which he is proficient and those in which he needs additional instruction. Armed with this information she has assigned him to an instructional group including other students with similar instructional needs. This group comprises students from the fourth, fifth, and sixth grades and the students all spend the same hour each day in the resource room. In scheduling the students Miss Collins has carefully avoided removing them from their regular classes at a time that they would miss instruction in other critical academic areas.

When Albert began attending the LH class he was introduced to the classroom rules. Each rule was carefully explained to him, students in the class modeled each of the appropriate behaviors expected in the class, and then several students were asked to demonstrate particular unacceptable behaviors. Of special concern for Albert were the rules regarding remaining in his seat during instructional times and respecting others and their possessions. These rules were practiced for a few minutes each day for the first week and the regular class teacher agreed to implement the same rules in her class. Because Albert enjoyed model cars he was able to earn new parts for his cars for following the rules in both the regular and special classrooms (his parents agreed to purchase these when notified by his teachers).

Miss Collins's class is operated in a way that permits very little wasted time. Changes in activities allow for a very short time period and the students are expected to go directly to their assigned seats and collect the materials for their instructional group at either the start of the class or when there are activity changes. A few minutes are provided at the start of the class for the students to check each others' homework assignments and for recording the scores. This is followed by a short review of the assignment and the provision of reteaching on any areas in which the students had problems.

The new lesson for the day is started with a short explanation of its purpose, followed by a demonstration of the skills to be taught that day. This demonstration is interspersed with questions to check the understanding of the students. Students are then provided with the opportunity for guided practice, which provides each of the students with many chances both to practice the skill with specific teacher feedback and to note the responses of others. Correct student responses that appear to be confidently expressed are followed by a brief teacher recognition of their correctness (e.g., "Good") and those correct responses that are tentative should be provided with process feedback (e.g., "Yes, Albert, that's right because . . . "). The amount of praise is kept at a moderate level in order both to maintain its value and to reduce the amount of time it takes away from instruction. The frequency of student errors indicates to Miss Collins the need for additional guided practice and feedback and it also determines when the students are ready for independent practice. This independent practice is directly related to the skills covered in their lessons and is designed to provide for overlearning of the material. Students are provided with independent work when they are capable of correctly responding at a 95%–100% level on this material; it is checked, and students are held accountable for its completion. Each week, and on a monthly basis, previously covered material is reviewed.

Miss Collins is most concerned that students are: 1) informed of what to expect, 2) provided with adequate information on how to perform the skill, 3) given many practice opportunities followed by immediate feedback, 4) provided with independent practice when they have acquired the skill, and 5) responsible for following and completing the assignments established in class. Her students develop a great deal of confidence because they are not expected to perform tasks they are not capable of successfully completing and they believe that she knows they can learn if they complete the activities provided in the class. In the case of Albert, he has improved significantly in his math skills and classroom behavior. In the past month his regular class teacher has visited Miss Collins's classroom and she has modified a number of her own classroom procedures because she was so impressed with the effect on Albert's progress in the resource room.

Teaching Secondary Students Learning Strategies

Rationale

While the general nature of learning and behavior problems is essentially similar for both elementary and secondary students, secondary students (and their teachers) experience some unique problems. Their primary problem is related to the demands of the secondary curriculum and the fact that the students no longer receive instruction in the basic skill areas. The curriculum is more complex and the instruction they do receive is centered on specific areas of knowledge (e.g., history, English, algebra) with the teachers assuming that the students possess the basic skills necessary to study the areas covered in class. Another problem relates to the teachers' "subject matter" orientation and their lack of interest (and often training) in providing students with instruction that they would regard as "remedial" as part of the class. The unique problems experienced by adolescents, especially those complicated by the many failures experienced by the learning handicapped student, tend to interfere with their performance in school. In addition, secondary students with learning handicaps have frequently participated in many types of specialized instruction during their school years (often unsuccessfully) and it is generally inappropriate to attempt further efforts at providing "traditional" remedial procedures that are not directed at providing them with skills that have direct application to their current school needs. This requires that educators explore interventions that have a more direct and realistic application to the students' current needs. It is important that this instruction be provided in such a manner that it is apparent to the students that the new focus of training will directly benefit their performance in school.

Deshler, Warner, Schumaker, and Alley (1983) advocate the use of the learning strategies model for adolescents. These strategies are basically a set of steps that the students are taught to work their way through a problem. This model concentrates the educational intervention primarily on the student, for the other factors involved (i.e., the school and teachers) are likely to undergo very little change. Deshler et al. believe that for secondary students the provision of basic-skill remediation alone will be inadequate to precipitate their "successful integration into the regular classroom and the world of work" (p. 266). These students can be taught both general and specific strategies that can be maintained and generalized across settings and time. Deshler et al. believe that it is possible to identify a set of learning strategies that can facilitate the functioning of the adolescent in various situations. While these strategies may assist many students, some may still require other interventions such as basic-skill remediation or career education.

Participants and Setting

Mr. Milligan is currently teaching in a resource room at the high school in the author's local community. He works with 18 students during the day for various amounts of time. Many of his students have had great difficulty in preparing written compositions required for their classes and this deficit has been noted in their Individualized Education Programs. The teachers in their classes do not feel that they can justify spending the time required to work on the basic composition skills needed by these students and they have appealed to Mr. Milligan to try to work with the students to improve their skills in this area.

Intervention

In searching for information on effective methods to teach composition, Mr. Milligan sought out the assistance of one of the district's special education consultants. He was referred to a textbook written by Alley and Deshler (1979), which included information on various learning strategies appropriate for adolescents. After reviewing this material, Mr. Milligan began teaching the students using a specific strategy originally developed by Kerrigan (1974) and detailed in the text. Alley and Deshler describe the method as follows:

> The goal of the method is to produce well-written themes characterized by the use of (1) a theme sentence that announces its point at once; (2) a topic sentence for each paragraph that is clearly and directly related to the theme sentence; (3) paragraphs that are clearly and directly related to their topic sentences and are well developed; (4) specific examples; and (5) the use of a transitional phrase in the second and third topic sentences to link them to the paragraphs preceding them. (p. 137)

Students in Mr. Milligan's class who were having difficulty in the area of composition were taught to complete the following steps in preparing a composition.

Step One: Write a short, simple, declarative sentence that makes one statement. This should be a sentence in which something else could be written about as it will serve as the basis for the following steps. A sentence such as "My dog's name is Max" would be more limiting in serving as a stimulus for further writing. An example of a good sentence would be: Traffic is becoming very congested in our city.

Step Two: Write three sentences about the sentence in Step One that are clearly and directly about the whole of that sentence, not just something in it. These sentences must be about the whole idea in the sentence, not just portions of it. It is suggested that the students will benefit if they start by first determining what questions a reader might ask about the first sentence. For example:

1. Traffic is becoming very congested in our city.
   a. The noise from the traffic is very disturbing.
   b. The congested traffic stops people from getting to places on time.
   c. The congested traffic creates many fumes and causes air pollution.

Step Three: Write four or five sentences about each of the three sentences in Step Two. These sentences must relate directly to the sentences written for Step Two and they should be written in a paragraph-type format with each of the sentences written for Step Two serving as the first sentence in a paragraph and the sentences written for Step Three serving as the remainder of the paragraph. For example:

1. Traffic is becoming very congested in our city.
   a. The noise from the traffic is very disturbing. Traffic noise seems to be everywhere. I can't hear the sounds of nature now. Traffic noise stops people's conversations. At some times during the day the noise is especially bad.
   b. The congested traffic stops people from getting to places on time. People limit their travel because of the time it takes. Being late because of traffic is always a problem. I can't go to as many places as I used to go. Family schedules are disrupted by traffic.
   c. The congested traffic creates many fumes and causes air pollution. The air

pollution can make my eyes burn. The smell of the traffic can make people sick. The air pollution can make it difficult to see. Air pollution can be bad for your health.

Step Four: Make the material in four or five sentences in Step Three as concrete and specific as possible. While the sentences in Step Three may be general or abstract, those written for Step Four are to be concrete and detailed. The student is expected to make the abstract words more concrete, thereby providing the student with practice in both writing and vocabulary development. For example, the following were developed by one student:

1. Traffic is becoming very congested in our city.
   a. The noise from the cars, trucks, and buses is very disturbing to me and to many other people. No matter whether I am inside or outside a building I cannot seem to get away from the noise of the traffic. When I used to take a walk I was able to listen to the birds and squirrels, but I cannot hear them now. The noise has become so bad that it is even difficult to hear my friends talk when we are walking to school (and some of them talk really loud). The noise is especially bad in the mornings when the big trucks are making their deliveries and everyone is in a hurry to get to work.
   b. The crowds of cars, buses, and trucks on the streets and freeways often make it difficult for people to get to work and to appointments on time. My parents don't want to go places now because it takes too long to get to many of the homes of our friends and relatives we used to visit. Because of traffic jams I have been late to my Little League practices seven times this year and the coach has not let me be on the starting team because he thinks I

am not interested in playing baseball. I have not seen a movie this year because my parents don't want to drive across town to the theater. We often don't eat until very late because it takes Dad so long to get home from work.

c. The cars, and especially the buses and trucks, create many fumes which are one of the major causes of air pollution. On some days the air pollution is so thick that it makes my eyes burn. The smoke from the buses and trucks often makes my friends sick to their stomachs when they are walking near the busy streets. On some days the air pollution is so thick that when I am coming home from school I cannot see my house until I am in the driveway. In science class we learned that the smog may cause lung damage and that we should take it easy and stay inside on days that there is thick smog.

Step Five: In the first sentence of the second paragraph and every paragraph following, insert a clear reference to the idea in the preceding paragraph. This provides a systematic way of introducing transitions into the theme by relating the paragraphs to each other. It is important that these transition sentences are clearly stated.

Step Six: Make sure every sentence in your theme is connected with, and makes clear reference to, the preceding sentence. It is possible to facilitate this by repeating a word used in the previous sentence, using a word in the sentence that is a synonym for a word in the previous sentence, or using a pronoun for the related noun in the previous sentence.

Conclusion

Mr. Milligan has found that these strategies provided his students a format with a structure that was flexible enough for them to state their own thoughts in a systematic fashion. The students have been provided with numerous opportunities to practice this set of strategies before they become proficient in its use. Several of his students have found that the use of a microcomputer and a word processor provides them with the opportunity to edit their material much faster and to use a spelling checker to correct their spelling errors. The teachers of their regular classes have noted improvements in the quality of the students' written work and have commented on the fact that the students no longer resist completing their writing assignments. Mr. Milligan has been impressed with the results of the use of the learning strategies and is now implementing others in the areas of reading, math, thinking, listening, and speaking.

Teaching Study Skills

Rationale

Many students with learning handicaps experience a great deal of difficulty in mainstream educational settings because they lack the study skills or critical school-related behaviors necessary for them to function comfortably (Alley & Deshler, 1979; Archer & Gleason, 1985; Lewis & Doorlag, 1987). These deficits may be exemplified by behaviors such as arriving late to class, never having all the materials needed for class, not listening to teacher directions, disregarding classroom rules, or not completing homework assignments. In many cases the students may possess the academic skills needed to achieve successfully in a class, but their lack of study skills interferes in their meeting the requirements for the class.

Educators cannot assume that the study skills needed by students will automatically develop as a result of their spending several years in school. Some students will acquire these skills with a minimal amount of instruction and/or by observing them being modeled by other students in their classes; this is often not the case with students with learning handicaps. The learning handicapped student commonly does not possess these skills and can best develop them by having the teacher directly teach the skills in a structured manner similar to that used in teaching other subject matter. In fact, many students in regular classes could benefit from such instruction in this area. This instruction would develop the skills much more rapidly than if they were presented in a more naturalistic manner involving minimal teacher direction and occasional observation of other students. In recent years a number of materials have been developed to assist teachers in providing the instruction needed for students to acquire and maintain these skills (e.g., Archer & Gleason, 1985).

Participants and Setting

When Mrs. Garcia was assigned to begin the following school year with a new fourth-grade class she had some concerns about her new assignment. While she has taught the upper elementary grades for the past 10 years, and she enjoys working with students of this age, there was some information about this particular class that made her think that this was not going to be her best year of teaching. She had heard from the principal (and other teachers in the school) that eight mainstreamed learning handicapped students were being placed in the class and that several other students in the class were known to have had problems achieving in the classes they attended during the past couple years.

Intervention

At the start of the summer Mrs. Garcia met with the school principal to discuss her concerns and to see if he had any ideas about how she could prepare for this assignment. While Mrs. Garcia had always been considered a good teacher who enjoyed working with children, she was known as somewhat of a "softy" who had had some problems with classroom control when she had difficult students; she also did not do very well with students who were not highly motivated and independent. The principal, being fully aware of the weakness of her skills in this area, suggested she attend a summer workshop the district was spon-

soring on methods for teaching study skills and appropriate school behaviors. He explained that this workshop involved instruction on the teaching of these important skill areas and the participants were also provided with specific materials they could use to teach the skills in their classroom. Feeling that she did not really like to give up part of her vacation, but considering that she needed help to get through the following year, Mrs. Garcia enrolled in the workshop.

In September Mrs. Garcia was ready and eager to start her new fourth grade class. She was very pleased with the information and skills she had gained in the summer workshop and felt that the time was well spent. She had received an instructor's guide and student workbooks for each of the students, materials developed by Archer and Gleason (1985). Because of the areas emphasized in the training she spent much more than her normal amount of time preparing for the start of the school year. For example, she developed a set of classroom rules to be implemented at the start of the school year. The training had emphasized that the teacher must set the tempo for the class immediately at the start of the school year, not wait for problems to occur and then attempt to implement rules that would respond to these problems. She was pleased to see that scripts are provided for introducing and conducting the lessons, for this reduced the amount of planning time she needed to spend to prepare for the school year. Also, the student workbooks correspond to the teacher materials and provide the students with material they can use in class and also share with their parents at home.

The student lessons involve teaching the students critical school behaviors, which included things they were to do "*before class* (e.g., arrive on time, bring their materials, get ready for class), *during class* (e.g., follow classroom rules, listen, ask for help when needed) and *after class* (e.g., take home materials, complete homework, return homework)" (Archer & Gleason, 1985, p. 2). The teacher materials outline the teacher practices that promoted the critical school behaviors and specific suggestions and scripts are provided for each of the lessons in the program.

The initial lesson introduces the guidelines for the students' before-class behavior. They are instructed to: 1) bring their materials to class (materials that Mrs. Garcia specified), 2) arrive before class begins, 3) enter the classroom in a pleasant manner, and 4) be seated and get ready for class. Each of these steps is carefully explained and the students are given the opportunity to provide reasons why these behaviors were important to the teacher, to other students, and to themselves. The lesson ends with a closed-book review of the guidelines and an indication that the students will be receiving points for following the rules. The following day the lesson covers the guidelines for the students' behavior during class, a review of the classroom rules, and the point system for following the guidelines is introduced. These are reinforced consistently during the following days of class and the students are gradually introduced to the expected behaviors in other areas. For example, the students are provided lessons on completing homework, organizing their desks and notebooks, maintaining assignment calendars, strategies for completing assignments, proofing strategies, gaining information from textbooks, and gaining information from classroom reference books.

After school had been in session for about 4 weeks, Mrs. Garcia again went to meet with the principal. This time her demeanor was much different, for she was very pleased with the results of the new techniques she was now using. The anticipated student problems has never occurred because she had prepared for the students and they were responding well to the specific instruction she was providing them on the critical school behaviors. The principal had not observed her class, but he had heard from other teachers that things were going well in her class and he knew that students were not being sent to the office from her class for discipline reasons. Several other teachers were interested in the program and Mrs. Garcia wanted to know if the principal could establish a

way for other interested teachers to receive the training and the materials for their classrooms. The principal asked if he could observe in her class and have an opportunity to review the materials before he proceeded with finding the resources for providing the training and the materials. Following his observations, and the review of the materials, he was able to obtain the needed training and materials and plans were made to implement the program on a school-wide basis.

Conclusion

Programs such as the one in which Mrs. Garcia was trained are becoming increasingly available to educators in regular and special education. Even when specific programs or materials are not readily available, educators have become increasingly aware of the need to provide definitive training for students in areas in which skills were once thought to be learned only through years of experience in an educational setting and outside the purview of instruction. It is especially important to consider that students with learning and behavior problems are much more likely to be in need of instruction in this area, as they have typically gained much less than their "normal" peers from unstructured learning situations.

Using Peer and Cross-Age Tutors

Rationale

Since the days of the one-room schoolhouse, educators have found ways of using other students to help those needing additional assistance in the classroom. In the one-room schoolhouse, one teacher was generally responsible for teaching students of quite different ages and ability levels; the students were expected to help teach others in the class. In today's schools, teachers are often assigned large groups of 25 to 35 students (or more) and while they may all be approximately the same age, they are often functioning at a very wide range of ability levels. The use of student tutors has often served to help teachers improve the quality of the instruction received by students in the class—often students with learning problems. Students can serve as tutors in several different ways. Peer tutoring occurs when a student is assigned to help another student about the same age; cross-age tutoring involves an older student (usually the tutor) working with a younger student.

The use of student tutors has been frequently advocated in the professional literature (e.g., Cooke, Heron, & Heward, 1983; Ehly & Larsen, 1980; Jenkins & Jenkins, 1985; Lewis & Doorlag, 1987; Maher, 1984; McCoy & Prehm, 1987; Strain, 1981), especially for students with learning problems. One of the points supporting the use of student tutors that is consistently mentioned is the research that has established that a positive relationship exists between the rate at which someone learns and the amount of time they have to practice the skill and the consistency with which specific feedback and reinstruction are provided when they are needed. Students can serve as tutors for those who have not mastered specific skills or areas of knowledge. They are readily available to the teacher, typically at no cost to the school. Student tutors have been shown to be effective in that both the tutors and tutees benefit academically and socially. While programs using students as tutors have received a great deal of support, they also tend to be only as effective as are the planning and tutor-training components developed for use with the program.

Participants and Setting

Jed Abel and Marti Schmidt are teachers in an urban middle school. Jed is a special education resource teacher and Marti teaches reading and social studies in the regular program. Both have been concerned about the progress of their students and the amount of time they can spend working with individual students who are having problems acquiring new skills and knowledge and lack the opportunity to practice the skills they have recently acquired. During the past 2 years both Jed and Marti have implemented programs that provide teacher-directed instruction and they have found that teaching the students in groups and providing a systematic method of instruction has been very helpful in improving the achievement of students in the classroom. Their concern now is with the few students whose level of achievement does not keep up with the other students in their groups. These students require additional individual instruction and opportunities to practice with someone who can provide them with feedback on the accuracy of their responses and provide the necessary corrections, reinstruction, and reinforcement for correct responses. While these are services Jed and Marti agree are needed, they cannot provide them with their current student and class load.

Intervention

Jed and Marti studied a number of options for providing the individual attention their students need. They found that there was no budget for hiring additional classroom aides and those who were already working in the school were scheduled for the entire day. Finding and recruiting parent volunteers was considered, but they soon determined that other teachers in the school who had tried obtaining volunteers failed because of the high percentage of parents in the neighborhood who work outside the home or are responsible for child care during the day. After a careful study of their options, they decided that the only viable alternative was to consider using students as tutors.

They found that there were many positive merits of using student tutors but that some potential problems could occur if the program was not carefully planned and administered. Both Jed and Marti spent many hours reading and studying materials on the use of peer and cross-age tutors; they also talked with several other teachers around the district about their experiences with such a program. After reviewing all of this information they identified components consistently found to be important in effective programs. The following paragraphs describe each of the components in the tutoring program they developed.

Identifying Tutors and Tutees   This component actually had two areas that Jed and Marti
wanted to consider: recruitment and selection. Tutors could come from their own classes, from
other classes within the school, or from the nearby
high school. Jed's learning handicapped students
could often be assigned tutors from classes in
which they are mainstreamed. They examined
whether students could get credit for the experience or possibly earn points toward the grade in
their current course. They determined that they
would select only tutors who could model the appropriate classroom behaviors as well as the academic skills needed for the job; and they would
consider the tutors' interest and level of responsibility in the job to be more important than their
specific skill in the academic area. Tutors were
matched carefully with tutees, with students with
the most difficult problems matched with the more
highly skilled or the older cross-age tutors whenever possible.

Training the Tutors   Jed and Marti designed
a training program that would teach the tutors how
to help the tutees acquire new skills. This program
also stresses information on the tutors' responsibilities and how they can best deliver the instruction and provide the tutees with appropriate reinforcement and corrective feedback. The teachers
are responsible for designing the daily lessons and
the tutors are trained to follow the format and
lesson content provided by the teacher. It is important that the tutors know how to deal with errors
made by the tutees and how to provide the teachers
with feedback on the progress of the students with
whom they were working. Table 1 provides an example of a program that uses students as tutors in
the area of spelling.

Collection of Performance Data   A system
of collecting data on the performance of the tutees
was designed for use by the tutors. This system
requires that the tutors collect daily data on the
percentage of correct responses and error rates
and that these data be presented on graphs that
provide feedback to the tutees and information for
the teachers on the effectiveness of the lessons

Table 1.   The use of peer tutors in spelling: An example

Peer tutors can provide instructional assistance for
teachers in a variety of academic areas. This example provides information on one method for using
peer tutors in a systematic fashion in the area of
spelling.

The steps included in this program are as follows:

1.   The tutor obtains a list of high-frequency spell-
     ing words (from the teacher) that provides
     words most often used at each grade level.

2.   The tutor administers a portion of the list to
     establish a list of 30 known and 30 unknown
     spelling words for the tutee(s). Words spelled
     on the pretest are considered to be known if
     they are spelled correctly on two consecutive
     trials.

3.   The teacher uses the test results (i.e., the
     group of known and unknown words) to de-
     velop an instructional list of 10 to 15 words
     that is composed of known words (60%) and
     unknown words (40%). This list constantly
     changes, for as the student masters the words
     (i.e., spells them correctly three consecutive
     times) a new unknown word is used to re-
     place the newly mastered word and at this
     time one of the known words is replaced by a
     new known word.

4.   The tutor or the teacher prepares 3 × 5 word
     cards, each of which has one of the instruc-
     tional words written clearly on one side of the
     card. The tutor uses the back of this card to
     record the date(s) that the word is used on the
     instructional list and notes whether the tutee
     spells the word correctly or incorrectly on
     each trial.

5.   An instruction period is scheduled for the tu-
     tee—approximately 10 minutes for younger
     students and 15 minutes for older students.
     Typically the tutor will try to get three passes
     through the entire instructional list.

6.   The tutor verbally presents each of the words
     in a word-sentence-word format. The tutor is
     expected to change the order of the words af-
     ter each pass through the instructional word
     list. For example:
     TUTOR: "Write dog" . . "I have a dog"
                    . . "dog."
     TUTEE: [Is expected to write "dog"]

7.   The tutor provides a verbal reinforcer after

(continued)

Table 1.   *(continued)*

each correct response. This is expected to be a short verbal statement, such as "Good," that is used consistently throughout the instruction. The purpose of this is to provide immediate feedback to the tutee, and it is presented in this concise way so that it does not consume inordinate amounts of the instructional period. In addition, the use of notably different verbal reinforcers may lead the tutee to consider that one of the written responses is superior to another because of the nature of the reinforcer presented (e.g., "Good" versus "That was really a terrific job"). With tutees who need a stronger reinforcer, the verbal reinforcer may be paired with a token that can be exchanged for a more meaningful reinforcer selected from a menu at a later time. Reinforcers are not presented after the tutee has corrected a word that was missed on the initial trial.

8. If the tutee spells the word incorrectly, the tutor uses one of two possible correction procedures that provides reinstruction on the word that was misspelled. The correction procedures for misspelled words are as follows:
    a. The word card for the misspelled word is placed next to the tutee's incorrect response.
    b. The tutor presents the word by saying, "That word was dog. Write it please."
    c. When the tutee writes the word correctly, the word card is removed. The tutor immediately presents the next word saying, "The next word is school" and follows the word-sentence-word format.
    d. If the student writes the word incorrectly, repeat Step b until the word is written correctly.

    The following is another method that may be used with tutees who do not respond to the initial correction procedure.
    a. The word card is placed next to the tutee's incorrect response (in this example the word is "school") and the tutor says, "This word is school."
    b. The tutor then says, "Look at it, please."
    c. The tutor then spells the word aloud saying, "Listen to me spell school. S-C-H-O-O-L."
    d. The tutor then asks the tutee to spell the word aloud with him or her saying, "You spell school with me. S-C-H-O-O-L."

    e. The tutor then asks the tutee to spell the word aloud by him or herself saying, "You spell school."
    f. The tutor then asks the tutee to write the word saying, "Write school."
    g. If the tutee writes the word correctly, the tutor says, "The next word is _____."
    h. If the tutee writes the word incorrectly, the tutor repeats the entire procedure.

9. The tutor is responsible for checking maintenance of the words the tutee has mastered by administering a test each week of the words that the tutee mastered at least 5 days prior to the test. If the tutee spells any of the words incorrectly, they should be considered for being returned to the instructional list.

10. The tutor is responsible for compiling accuracy (percentage of words spelled correctly) and rate (number of words spelled and number of correct words spelled per minute) data for each instructional session and for recording these data on a graph each day. In addition, they are responsible for keeping a record of the words the tutee has mastered and the date they were mastered.

Adapted from Doorlag and Lewis (1983).

they had designed. The tutors are responsible for calculating these percentages and rates and recording them on a separate graph for each student.

Supervision of the Tutors   Jed and Marti designed a schedule for supervising the performance of the tutors. They were concerned that the tutors receive feedback on their performance and correction of any errors they may be committing in their tutoring sessions. This supervision is much more intense at the start of the program (daily for the first 2 weeks) and it is then scheduled on a much less frequent basis after the tutors demonstrate effective tutoring skills. This also involves a careful monitoring of the data they collected on the tutees, and tutors are provided with retraining if problems are noted. Reinforcers such as awards, letters of appreciation from the principal, and special outings for the tutors are provided. In addition, the tutors are made aware of progress made by their tutees and are taught how they could gauge this from the records they are keeping. Regular seminars are scheduled for the tutors to review any questions they have concerning their responsibilities or problems that may be occurring in their tutoring sessions. It is also considered important that the tutees receive reinforcement for regularly attending their tutoring sessions and for following the directions provided by the tutor and the rules established for the tutoring sessions.

Management of Space and Materials Jed and Marti attempted to provide the tutors with a comfortable teaching station that was available for them on a regular basis. This area is one that permits both the tutor and tutee to concentrate on the instruction being provided and one that does not cause, or is not affected by, interference from the rest of the class. In addition, materials are placed in a storage area accessible to the tutors and arranged in such a way that they can obtain the directions on their lesson for the day, and the materials they need, without interfering with the ongoing instruction in the class.

Conclusion

The tutoring program introduced by Jed and Marti developed into a successful venture. They found that it was best to start only a small number of new tutors at a time so they could be provided with the type of supervision that would assure the success of both the tutors and the tutees. They did find that a few of the original group of tutors needed more training in dealing with inappropriate behaviors during the tutoring sessions, but the original training provided the tutors with a good basis for success in their work with other students. After the program had operated for two semesters Jed trained several of his learning handicapped students as tutors and they were able to provide tutoring to students in a remedial reading program at a local elementary school. Overall, Jed and Marti found that the program did require that they allocate portions of their time for the training, supervision, and development of materials, but that its success justified this time and provided their instructional program with an additional option that enhanced the achievement of their students.

SUMMARY

Four different types of activities for assisting learning handicapped students to gain the skills required in educational settings have been described in this chapter. These activities could be used in regular or special education settings and their presentation is intended to provide the reader with ideas that will assist in meeting the educational needs of students with learning and behavior problems. The application of these techniques is not limited to just those students who are identified as learning handicapped; they could also apply to low-performing students in regular classes or to students with other types of handicaps who exhibit similar types of problems in a school setting.

A basic premise of this chapter is that students who manifest learning and behavior problems are capable of acquiring and maintaining the skills needed to perform adequately in an educational setting. These students may not respond positively to traditional teaching methods and it is the responsibility of the teacher to explore alternative procedures to attempt to teach the knowledge and skills required of the students. Teachers can best determine the effectiveness of the instructional procedures by monitoring student progress and by making modifications in the instruction that have a positive effect on the student's performance. There is a growing body of research on the effectiveness of various instructional practices for teachers working with regular (e.g., Brophy & Good, 1986; Doyle, 1986; Rosenshine & Stevens, 1986) and special education (e.g., Englert, 1984; MacMillan et al., 1986; Morsink, Soar, Soar, & Thomas, 1986) students that should be reviewed by educators. These references outline practices found to be successful in improving the achievement of students and should be familiar to all teachers and educational administrators.

Other topics such as vocational integration, social skills instruction, and cooperative learning are important areas to be considered for use with the learning handicapped population. They have not been reviewed in this chapter, but they are covered more fully in Chapters 9, 10, and 11, respectively.

STUDY QUESTIONS

1. Describe how you would explain to another educator the reasons that it is feasible for students with learning disabilities, mild mental retardation, and behavior disorders to be provided with similar types of educational programs.

2. Explain how a consultant can assist classroom teachers working with students with learning handicaps by describing a regular classroom situation and how you would like to see a consultant help the teacher work with learning handicapped students who may be placed in his or her classroom.

3. Provide a definition of learning handicaps that would be meaningful to a group of parents. In addition, explain to this same group why it is important for these students to be considered for special education services. Be sure to eliminate educational jargon and to use terms that will be understood by the parents.

4. Explain why it is important for teachers working with learning handicapped students to have a high level of skill in the area of classroom management. Describe five specific classroom management skills that educators have found to be important for teachers to possess.

5. Describe what you consider to be important information to be obtained in the assessment of learning handicapped students. Cite examples of the types of information most useful to the classroom teacher working with the student and describe the most appropriate methods for obtaining this information.

6. Explain why cooperative learning programs have appeal for both regular and special educators. What role can these programs play in providing for the needs of learning handicapped students?

REFERENCES

Algozzine, B., Ysseldyke, J.E., & Christenson, S. (1983). An analysis of the incidence of special class placement: The masses are burgeoning. *Journal of Special Education, 17,* 141–147.

Alley, G., & Deshler, D. (1979). *Teaching the learning disabled adolescent: Strategies and methods.* Denver: Love Publishing.

Archer, A., & Gleason, M. (1985). *Skills for school success.* San Diego, CA: San Diego State University.

Brophy, J.E., & Good, T.L. (1986). Teacher behavior and student achievement. In M.C. Whittrock (Ed.), *Handbook of research on teaching* (3rd ed., pp. 328–375). New York: Macmillan.

Cooke, N.L., Heron, T.E., & Heward, W.L. (1983). *Peer tutoring: Implementing classwide programs in the primary grades.* Columbus, OH: Special Press.

Deshler, D., Warner, M., Schumaker, J., & Alley, G. (1983). Learning strategies intervention model: Key component and current status. In J. McKinney and L. Feagans (Eds.), *Current topics in learning disabilities* (Vol. 1, pp. 245–283). Norwood, NJ: Ablex Publishing.

Dixon, R., Engelmann, S., & Olen, L.G. (1981). *Spelling mastery: A direct instruction series.* Chicago: Science Research Associates.

Doorlag, D.H., & Lewis, R.B. (1983). *Trends in research and practice—Spelling: A direct instruction approach to spelling for special students.* Paper presented at the Council for Exceptional Children Conference, Detroit.

Doyle, W. (1986). Classroom organization and management. In M.C. Whittrock (Ed.), *Handbook of research on teaching* (3rd ed., pp. 392–431). New York: Macmillan.

Ehly, S.W., & Larsen, S.C. (1980). *Peer tutoring for individualized instruction.* Boston: Allyn & Bacon.

Englert, C.S. (1984). Measuring teacher effectiveness from the teacher's point of view. *Focus on Exceptional Children, 17*(2), 1–14.

Gerber, M.M. (1984). The Department of Education's Sixth Annual Report to Congress on P.L. 94-142: Is Congress getting the full story? *Exceptional Children, 51,* 209–224.

Hallahan, D.P., & Kauffman, J.M. (1976). *Introduction to learning disabilities: A psycho-behavioral approach.* Englewood Cliffs, NJ: Prentice-Hall.

Hardman, M.L., Drew, C.J., & Egan, M.W. (1984). *Human exceptionality: Society, school, and family.* Boston: Allyn & Bacon.

Jenkins, J., & Jenkins, L. (1985). Peer tutoring in elementary

and secondary programs. *Focus on Exceptional Children,*
17(6), 1–12.

Kauffman, J.M. (1985). *Characteristics of children's behavior
disorders* (3rd ed.). Columbus, OH: Charles E. Merrill.

Kavale, K., & Mattson, P.D. (1983). "One jumped off the balance beam": Meta-analysis of perceptual-motor training.
Annual Review of Learning Disabilities, 1, 118–126.

Kerrigan, W.J. (1974). *Writing to the point: Six basic steps.*
New York: Harcourt Brace Jovanovich.

Lewis, R.B. (1983). Learning disabilities and reading: Instructional recommendations from current research. *Exceptional Children, 50,* 230–240.

Lewis, R.B., & Doorlag, D.H. (1987). *Teaching special students in the mainstream* (2nd ed.). Columbus, OH: Charles
E. Merrill.

MacMillan, D.L., Keogh, B.K., & Jones, R.L. (1986). Special educational research on mildly handicapped learners. In
M.C. Whittrock (Ed.), *Handbook of research on teaching*
(3rd ed., pp. 686–724). New York: Macmillan.

Maher, C.A. (1984). Handicapped adolescents as cross-age tutors: Program description and evaluation. *Exceptional Children, 51,* 56–63.

McCoy, K.M., & Prehm, H.J. (1987). *Teaching mainstreamed
students: Methods and techniques.* Denver: Love
Publishing.

Morsink, C.V., Soar, R.S., Soar, R.M., & Thomas, R. (1986).
Research on teaching: Opening the door to special education
classrooms. *Exceptional Children, 53,* 32–40.

Rosenshine, B., & Stevens, R. (1986). Teaching functions. In
M.C. Whittrock (Ed.), *Handbook of research on teaching*
(3rd ed., pp. 376–391). New York: Macmillan.

Stainback, S., & Stainback, W. (1987). Integration versus
cooperation: A commentary on "Educating children with
learning problems: A shared responsibility." *Exceptional
Children, 54,* 66–68.

Stainback, W., Stainback, S., Courtnage, L., & Jaben, T.
(1985). Facilitating mainstreaming by modifying the mainstream. *Exceptional Children, 52,* 144–152.

Stevens, R., & Rosenshine, B. (1981). Advances in research
on teaching. *Exceptional Education Quarterly, 2*(1), 1–9.

Strain, P.S. (Ed.). (1981). *The utilization of classroom peers as
behavior change agents.* New York: Plenum.

Will, M.C. (1986). Educating children with learning problems: A shared responsibility. *Exceptional Children, 52,*
411–415.

CHAPTER 3

STUDENTS WITH PHYSICAL DISABILITIES

Philippa H. Campbell

Physical disabilities are common threads that tie together an often diverse group of students. Variance on dimensions of motor, intellectual, sensory, and social abilities is common. Some students may have impairments in neuromuscular, neurological, or orthopedic systems that result only in mild to severe limitations in posture and movement abilities. More common are multiple problems that may seriously influence abilities to learn and perform a wide variety of both academic and functional life skills (Bigge, 1982; Bleck & Nagel, 1982; Campbell, 1987b; Umbreit, 1983).

STUDENTS WITH DIVERSE DISABILITIES AND NEEDS

Categorization and labeling of students with physical disabilities frequently is confusing and nonuniform. Medical labeling, or diagnosis, relates specifically to the type of physical disability whereas educational labeling occurs on the basis of other characteristics that relate to learning needs. State education agencies categorize students still differently, using criteria that are dissimilar across states. Thus, students with physical disabilities are labeled as orthopedically impaired or handicapped, crippled and other health impaired, multiply handicapped, mentally retarded, developmentally disabled, or developmentally handicapped. In some states, students may be categorized as learning disabled, depending on the extent of physical disability accompanying the learning disorder.

Physical disabilities are also classified on the basis of severity. Labels such as mild, moderate, or severe may be used to describe the physical disability itself or to categorize the overall impairment in functional or life skills. A student with mild spastic diplegic cerebral palsy may be educationally labeled as nonhandicapped; or if the student has an additional problem, such as a perceptual disorder, he or she may be educationally classified as learning disabled. The same mildly physically disabled student with severe cognitive deficits may be labeled educationally as mentally retarded or developmentally handicapped. A student with cerebral palsy, spastic quadraplegia may be described as having severe spasticity (or severely increased postural tone) from a medical perspective and be labeled as severely handicapped from an educational perspective due to impaired performance of life skills.

Students with disorders in addition to a primary physical disability or orthopedic handicap often are labeled as multihandicapped from both educational and medical perspectives. Visual and/or hearing impairments may accompany some physical disabilities. Other students may have problems with cognition and learning or with communication and language. In most states, the term "multihandicapped" is used to describe students with deficit performance in more than one primary area. Thus, a student with a language disorder and a physical disability would be classified as multihandicapped. In other situations, students are described as multihandicapped when specialized educational, health, and therapy services are required. Students with multiple handicaps typically require adapted curricula to best compensate for physical and learning limitations, as well as a variety of related services to enable them to benefit from specialized educational programs.

Meeting Needs of Students with Physical Disabilities

A wide variety of physical disabilities are educationally labeled as orthopedically handicapped. Students may have congenital or acquired amputations, spina bifida, spinal cord injury, head trauma, cerebral palsy, muscular dystrophy, or musculoskeletal disorders. These students may not require extensive special education and related services. Some are able to participate in regular education with the support of related services. Students with mild to moderate physical disabilities alone are managed easily in regular education environments since their primary impairment mainly influences their ability to move around their environments. Federal legislation, such as the Education of the Handicapped Act (EHA) and the Rehabilitation Act, as well as changes in state and local public policy, parent preference, and social consciousness provide precedent for students with orthopedic handicaps to attend neighborhood schools and live and work in integrated environments.

However, historically and currently, the majority of students classified as orthopedically handicapped are educated in segregated classrooms or schools. A primary reason for maintaining segregated educational environments relates to ease in providing physical and occupational therapy and other related services necessary to maintain or improve physical functioning (Campbell, 1987a). A second reason is that segregating students restricts the number of schools that must be architecturally accessible. States reported that 50% of students classified as orthopedically handicapped and age 3–21 years were educated in separate classes or

schools and 8% were educated at home during the 1985–1986 school year (U.S. Department of Education, 1988). Comparisons of these percentages with data reported by states 10 years ago indicate little change in trends in educational placement across the past decade. Approximately 32% of school-age and 62% of preschool-age students classified as orthopedically handicapped were reported by states as educated in separate classes or school facilities during the 1976–1977 school year (U.S. Department of Health, Education, and Welfare, 1979). Recent state-reported data probably are more accurate than earlier data due to changes and refinements in the procedures and categories used to record data, resulting in data across this 10-year period that are not directly comparable. However, despite these changes in data recording, the current status of placement of students with orthopedic handicaps in segregated environments is indisputably clear.

One barrier to placement of students in neighborhood schools concerns mobility. Orthopedic handicaps may preclude easy movement around environments that are not architecturally accessible. School organization and practice, in combination with building characteristics, often inhibit attendance in regular schools (Orelove & Hanley, 1979). Students change classes, for example, in many upper elementary and middle school grades, often moving from floor to floor of a school. Even a student who is ambulatory with a walker or crutches may have difficulty navigating the required distance in a reasonable amount of time and/or may be judged as unsafe in halls with other students when classes are changing. While the same student may be able to go from class to class safely and in a reasonable amount of time using a wheelchair, this option may not be feasible due to the presence of steps and the absence of elevators. The student, thus, may be assigned to a special school or classroom for students with orthopedic handicaps due to difficulties with mobility and safety—not problems with learning.

Teachers of students with orthopedic handicaps must have knowledge about the origin(s) of the

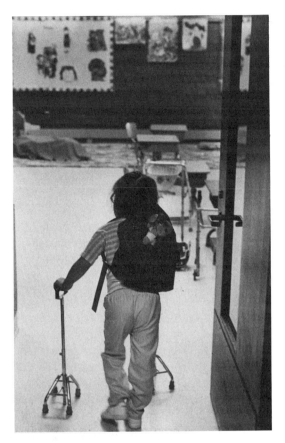

Architectural problems and safety issues may impede the successful integration of children with physical disabilities.

orthopedic problem, its impact on school performance, and any associated side-effects that may occur (Bigge, 1982; Campbell, 1987b). Skills in managing adaptive devices and in adapting school learning experiences to accommodate for a student's disability also are necessary. Regular education teachers are not likely to have had coursework or experiences sufficient to adequately educate and manage all students with physical disabilities. This general lack of knowledge is a second barrier to regular education placement. Fortunately, any teacher can easily learn about the physical disability of a particular student and its potential impact on the regular classroom routine.

Specialists, such as physical and occupational therapists, can provide on-the-job knowledge and training that builds on teachers' previous experiences of working with specialists who are part of regular education. Speech pathologists, school psychologists, home-school counselors, school nurses, remedial teachers, tutors, vocational instructors, and specialty teachers all work collaboratively to address learning and other needs of regular education students. These professionals constitute a team of specialists available to work with students with orthopedic handicaps at the elementary, middle, and secondary school levels. An informal plan or a formal individualized education program (IEP) defines the specific needs of a particular student. Such needs may include adaptive equipment; special devices, such as computers or augmentative communication aids; tutoring, or an attendant to assist with self-care skills, therapy services, or special transportation—services necessary for many students with physical disabilities to be maintained in a regular education environment. Historically, these services have been easier to deliver administratively when students are segregated into one classroom or one school than when they are dispersed throughout a district's schools. Particularly problematic is the delivery of therapy services that may be necessary to teach independence in self-care, mobility, and communication skills; prevent development of further disability; and remediate existing physical problems, such as muscle weakness or limitations in range of motion. The traditional one-on-one or small-group isolated-therapeutic-treatment model is not implemented easily when students are educated in neighborhood schools (Rainforth & York, 1987). Commitment to traditional ways of delivering needed services is therefore a third barrier to meeting student needs within neighborhood schools.

Of concern to many educators and school administrators is the capability to meet specialized health needs within the regular education environment (The Council for Exceptional Children, 1988). Most neighborhood schools do not have full-time school nurses, yet students with orthopedic handicaps may require periodic suctioning, specialized feeding techniques, medication, catheterization, or other procedures to adequately address health care needs. School health aides may be trained to provide needed procedures, visiting nurses may be used, or students may be taught to self-administer some procedures (Servis, 1988). That many health procedures appear complicated or the idea of administering them is frightening to individuals who are untrained is a fourth barrier to integration (Shelton, Jeppson, & Johnson, 1987). Most parents of children in need of ongoing procedures learn to administer them successfully with training by nursing personnel. A similar training approach can be used successfully with school personnel.

Meeting Needs of Students with Multiple Handicaps

Delivering services that address the needs of students with orthopedic impairments is less difficult than adequately meeting the often numerous and complex needs of students with multiple handicaps. Extensive intervention from specialists and therapists may be necessary for students to benefit from special education. Educational curricula may require significant adaptation in both content and teaching procedures to optimize student learning and compensate for motor, sensory, and other disabilities. Health needs may be substantial, with some students requiring several or more procedures on a daily basis. The needs of any one or two students with complex problems are easier to manage than are the needs of a group of students with multiple handicaps. Most often, however, these students are grouped in either segregated classrooms or schools to ensure the availability of expert personnel.

Students with multiple handicaps require opportunities for interaction with age-mates who are not handicapped even when educational needs are addressed best through the functional curricula and specialized teaching strategies necessary for preparation to live, work, and play in their communities. Location of classrooms and provision of related services within neighborhood schools pro-

vides students, with even the most severe and multiple disabilities, opportunities to make friends and develop a support network among age-peers.

Integrated programming teams comprising parents, therapists, teachers, and nurses (where necessary), ensure the expertise needed to provide education and related services for students with severe and multiple handicaps in home, school, work, and community settings (Campbell, 1987a). Achieving this goal requires a rethinking of service delivery organization and of applications of educational and therapeutic methodologies (Giangreco, 1986). Segregating students in isolated classrooms and schools with curricula that emphasize remediation of deficits rather than acquisition of functional life skills does not utilize existing resources in ways that result in greater independence in this group of students (Campbell, 1989). Opportunities for interaction among children with and without disabilities, within social and educational contexts, are difficult to promote when students with physical disabilities are educated in isolation from nondisabled peers. Reorganization of the structure and function of education and related services results in the capability to delivery needed interventions within age-appropriate educational and community environments.

INTEGRATION FOR STUDENTS WITH PHYSICAL DISABILITIES

Three general types of integration are important with students with physical disabilities: physical, social, and communicative. A first step is the physical integration of students in neighborhood schools. Without physical integration, the other types of integration are obviously more difficult to achieve. Social integration and communicative integration occur when students make friends and interact with students who are not disabled. Many students with physical disabilities can be integrated (or mainstreamed) for both instructional and noninstructional activities within the regular school curriculum, while the individual objectives for other students may be best addressed through specialized instructional curricular activities.

Team-Based Instruction

Essential to integration of students with physical disabilities is the team-based service delivery model used to support a student within regular education or to enable students to benefit from a variety of special educational placements (Campbell, 1987a; Giangreco, 1986; Rainforth & York, 1987). Teams share a common goal in each instance of placement in that their function, always, is to enable a student to participate in education. The members of teams vary dependent on the particular specialists necessary to meet each student's individual needs. The regular or special educator functions as a leader of the team, serving to coordinate the activities of all members in ways that best address individual student needs. Parents are key team members with input into programming decisions and responsibility for coordinating medical-educational linkages that may be necessary for their children.

Team structures are not always easy to establish and may be even more difficult to maintain. A number of typical difficulties include: 1) lack of administrative support for team activities; 2) insufficient time for and difficulty scheduling team meetings; and 3) discontinuity among team members in philosophical approach (*Integrated Services Project,* 1987). A team approach can provide assistance to the regular or special education teacher when school principals, district curriculum specialists, special education directors and supervisors, and related services supervisors adopt and sanction a team approach. Principals play a central role in educational teaming. Time can be provided for necessary team planning and review meetings through coordination of each member's schedule or through teacher release time when a principal values and supports the role of the team in addressing individual student needs.

Of primary importance to effective team functioning is a uniform philosophical approach among all team members toward education, in general, and the curriculum being used, in particular (Wetherbee & Campbell, 1987). The purpose of the team may be unclear when, for example, teachers focus on functional skills, therapists emphasize remediation of identified deficits, and nurses attend only to health-care needs. While each of these areas has importance with particular students, a central and unifying element must hold together what potentially are varied and conflicting approaches. The educational curriculum being used in the classroom(s) to which a student is assigned for the greatest amount of time provides this needed unification. The role of each team member is to deliver services that enable a student to participate in the adopted curriculum rather than provide traditional interventions that are isolated from the educational program. A model of integrated services where team members: 1) consult with the teacher to assist in enhancing a student's functioning in school, 2) teach and monitor therapy programs delivered through physical education classes and at home, and 3) delivery one-on-one direct therapy as necessary, allows sufficient flexibility to meet the needs of students in any educational environment (Dunn, in press).

Many students with physical disabilities are isolated from normal experiences in regular school environments when classrooms are located in separate wings or when activities for students with disabilities are organized separately from those for students without disabilities. Allowing students to eat lunch together, attend assemblies, or participate in nonacademic subjects such as music or art may be only "cosmetic" attempts at integration if teachers and other school personnel do not undertake activities designed to facilitate real interactions among students (Smith & Strain, 1988). This type of physical integration has been labeled as a neutral placement, in contrast to an integrated placement that includes daily and planned interactions among students with and without disabilities (Rostetter, Kowalski, & Hunter, 1984). When social interaction is included as an IEP goal, parents and professional team members can focus on incorporating interactions into daily instructional programs and designing strategies that will facilitate meaningful interactions among students with and without disabilities (Certo & Kohl, 1984). The needs of students with physical disabilities can be accommodated easily by using creative interactional strategies that compensate for deficits in areas such as mobility or communication.

Establishing Integrated Programs

An obvious first step in integration is to physically group together students with and without physical disabilities. School, home, community, and work environments provide integrated settings and contexts in which interactions naturally occur or can be facilitated. In this sense, neutral educational or work placements for students with physical disabilities are a starting point from which interactions can occur. Opportunities for interactions are limited in the absence of physical integration in school, work, home, and community environments.

There are numerous desired and expected outcomes to interactions among people with and without disabilities. Benefits include increased task learning when students with disabilities have opportunities to model the performance of people without disabilities, natural learning contexts provided through integrated options, and, perhaps most important, the opportunity to make friends and establish a support network of people without disabilities. Interactions among students are facilitated when goals are clear and strategies that enhance and support those interactions are used.

The following sections describe situations and strategies for facilitating interactions among students who are able-bodied and those with disabilities. Key roles played by teachers and related services personnel are discussed for each integration situation described. Strategies that are particularly helpful in each situation are outlined. While these strategies are presented with specific reference to a particular situation, most can be used across situations. Few of these strategies have

been described in the literature with specific application to students with physical disabilities. Some have resulted from modifications of strategies successfully used with students with severe handicaps. Indeed, perhaps the most significant implication of continued and widespread placement of students with orthopedic and other physical disabilities in segregated schools and classrooms is the lack of tested strategies for integration of these students in neighborhood schools, community environments, and work settings.

INTEGRATION ACTIVITIES

Student Placement in Neighborhood Schools

Activities that distribute students with physical disabilities across schools within a district are necessary when school districts operate centralized programs that segregate children with physical disabilities into separate schools or school wings. Ideally, all students attend neighborhood schools. However, in some districts, sufficient numbers of students with physical disabilities of particular grade levels may not live within the same neighborhood. Racial desegregation orders or other situations may prevent neighborhood school attendance in other districts. A second, but less ideal option, is a cluster-school approach where classrooms are located in particular schools throughout a district, enabling students with physical disabilities to attend schools near their homes but not necessarily the school that would be attended if they were not disabled.

Two major approaches may be taken to reassign students. The first is to ensure that all new students enrolling in a district's programs are placed in regular education classrooms or in special education classes that are distributed across schools while phasing out more segregated options that may be in place for older students. The already-enrolled students are redistributed across schools when the placement level (e.g., elementary, secondary) is changed, when families request regular school placement, or when other circumstances dictate change for one student or classroom. A second approach is to implement a district-wide redistribution or transition of all students at the same time. This approach requires the involvement of teachers, related services personnel, parents, regular education personnel, principals, and school administrators in both the planning and implementation phases. Planning must be carefully done, particularly in districts that enroll large numbers of students with orthopedic handicaps or other physical disabilities.

Planning for individual students is the basis for either a student-by-student or a district-wide redistribution plan. The individual capabilities and disabilities of each student and the methods that will be used to ensure physical and social integration within regular school and classroom environments are identified before placement is made or changed. Families and school personnel play important roles in this planning process.

Role of Teachers and Related Services Personnel

Special educators, related services personnel, and parents often work to keep students with physical disabilities isolated in segregated schools and classrooms. The disabilities of students are known best by their families and specialized professionals. Often, the focus is on identifying the reasons why a student may *not* be able to function in regular schools and classrooms rather than identifying strategies that facilitate participation in these environments.

Special education teachers and related services personnel who view all students as able to participate in activities outside of segregated environments are instrumental. Their skills and knowledge are essential in designing effective strategies that will facilitate physical and social integration. These personnel function as *senders* of students who are already segregated or who will be enrolled in receiving schools. Regular education principals, teachers, and other specialists are *receivers* in this process. Meetings and interactions among senders and receivers are the basis from which transitions from segregated to neighborhood schools or from preschool programs into schools are planned. Regular educators know what is required in a regular education classroom. Special educators, parents, and related services personnel have the knowledge of how these particular activities can be performed by a specific student. By applying concepts of transition from one environment to another to the process of placing students with physical disabilities in regular schools, parents and school personnel can collaborate to develop a plan for integration for each student (Edgar, 1987). This process is diagrammed in Figure 1 and can be followed for placing individuals or groups of students.

A Plan for Integration

A plan for the physical integration of each student with a physical disability is formulated by the family, team of professionals, and students themselves, where age appropriate. This individualized plan identifies the activities required in a particular school and classroom and lists the means to be used to enable a student's independent or assisted participation in these activities. Table 1 illustrates a plan developed for a 7-year-old boy with severe physical disabilities who was enrolled in a regular first-grade classroom. Some of the strategies used with this student involved administrative changes, some included minor changes in the regular education environment, and some focused on the student himself. More often than not, the types of strategies necessary to facilitate successful physical and social integration do not require changes in student abilities/disabilities, but instead are focused on methods that compensate for disabilities.

Enabling Participation in Regular Education Curriculum

The curriculum for a school district establishes expectations for both regular and special education students. Many students with physical disabilities are able to complete the regular education curricu-

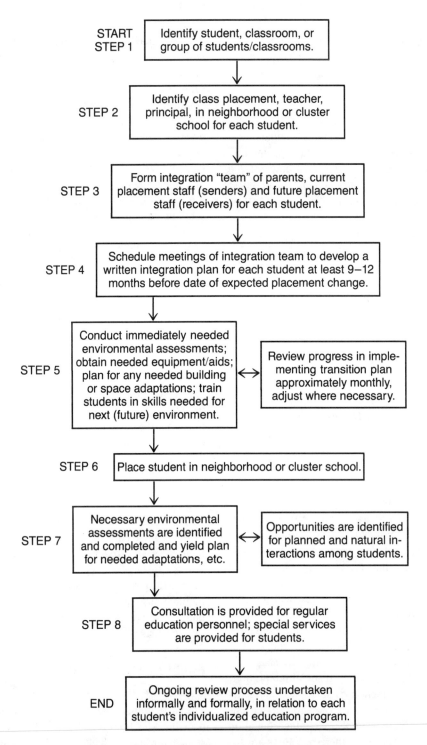

| START
STEP 1 | Identify student, classroom, or group of students/classrooms. |

| STEP 2 | Identify class placement, teacher, principal, in neighborhood or cluster school for each student. |

| STEP 3 | Form integration "team" of parents, current placement staff (senders) and future placement staff (receivers) for each student. |

| STEP 4 | Schedule meetings of integration team to develop a written integration plan for each student at least 9–12 months before date of expected placement change. |

| STEP 5 | Conduct immediately needed environmental assessments; obtain needed equipment/aids; plan for any needed building or space adaptations; train students in skills needed for next (future) environment. | ↔ | Review progress in implementing transition plan approximately monthly, adjust where necessary. |

| STEP 6 | Place student in neighborhood or cluster school. |

| STEP 7 | Necessary environmental assessments are identified and completed and yield plan for needed adaptations, etc. | ↔ | Opportunities are identified for planned and natural interactions among students. |

| STEP 8 | Consultation is provided for regular education personnel; special services are provided for students. |

| END | Ongoing review process undertaken informally and formally, in relation to each student's individualized education program. |

Figure 1.   Process for transition of students with physical disabilities into regular school.

Table 1. Illustration of an integration plan

Student's name: Thomas Roy   Placement: Special education kindergarten, Washington School

Date: March 2, 1988   Desired Placement: Regular first grade, Washington

Team: Special education teacher, PT, OT, ST, parent, regular education first grade teacher, school principal

When? September, 1988

Program area	Current status	Future requirements	Needed action, person(s), and dates
Communication	Good receptive; speech OK but not always understandable.	Must recite orally in reading and for class participation.	ST determine need for augmentative speech aid by 5/88.
Self-care/Eating	Can feed self independently if food placed in front; drinks from cup with straw.	Must go through cafeteria line or bring lunch; go to table area; open any containers; eat/drink; clean up tray; clean up self.	OT will do environmental assessment with first-grade class by 4/1/88. Determine areas of training to be provided in kindergarten class from 4/1/88 to 5/27/88; determine needed adaptations and obtain by 9/1/88. Mobility and manipulation are problem areas.
Self-care/ Clothing Management	Can remove coat; cannot do shoes or manage clothing for toileting.	Needs to change shoes for gym; manage clothing for toileting.	OT will teach shoes by 9/1/88 with Velcro adaptations and work on pants up/down during toileting.
Self-care/Toileting	Is independent but needs to be taken to bathroom, lifted on and off toilet; helped with clothing; can wash hands if water turned on/off; can dry hands.	Must get to bathroom by self at appointed time or request permission to use bathroom; must get on/off, flush toilet, do clean-up routine, return to classroom.	OT will do environmental assessment with first grade of whole toilet routine by 4/1/88; Determine areas of training in kindergarten class from 4/1/88 to 5/27/88. Obtain adaptations by 9/1/88. Mobility is problem area.
Mobility	Cannot move self; has adapted travel chair which requires pushing; cannot transfer into/out of chair to another chair, floor, toilet.	Must get around classroom and school by self; go from inside to outside by self (e.g., to/from bus; playground); get on/off playground equipment.	OT/PT will investigate possibility of motorized chair; determine type by 5/1/88; begin funding process to attain ASAP; PT will train transfer skills using regular wheelchair or chair; all trained by 6/1/88.
Gym	Does not have gym; goes to PT instead.	Needs to play games, do activities for physical fitness, etc. Adaptive physical education not available at Washington.	OT/PT will meet with first-grade gym teacher by 5/1/88 to discuss needed task adaptations; will provide written suggestions by 6/1/88; Tom will have gym one time per week, PT other times class has gym.

(continued)

61

Table 1. *(continued)*

Student's name: Thomas Roy   Placement: Special education kindergarten, Washington School

Date: March 2, 1988   Desired Placement: Regular first grade, Washington

Team: Special education teacher, PT, OT, ST, parent, regular education first grade teacher, school principal

When? September, 1988

Program area	Current status	Future requirements	Needed action, person(s), and dates
Library	Does not currently have—but has similar activity in classroom.	Needs to go to library one time per week; select books; listen to story; can also use computer.	OT/PT will provide suggestions to librarian about location of books for selection and use of computer by 9/1/88; can already listen to story and use adapted computer.
Classroom Activities (Academics)	Participates in "readiness" kindergarten activities with adapted materials and with computer.	Needs pencil/crayon use for worksheets; movement around classroom to learning areas; follow group instructions; read; manipulate materials.	OT will consult with teacher to locate software programs by 9/1/88—adapted writing aid can be continued; detailed environmental assessment may be needed in 9/88.

SUMMARY PLAN:

NEEDED EQUIPMENT: Wheelchair and motorized chair.
Adapted computer for full-time use (one is currently available to him only part time and is for kindergarten only).
May need speech aid.
First-grade bathroom may need adaptations (e.g., grab bars).

ENVIRONMENTAL ASSESSMENTS NEEDED IMMEDIATELY Cafeteria/eating (4/1/88).
Toilet routine (4/1/88).

SKILLS TO BE TRAINED:
1. Shoes on/off (OT/teacher/parent)
2. Pants up/down (OT/teacher/parent)
3. Transfer skills (PT/teacher/parent)

SERVICES NEEDED IN NEW ENVIRONMENT
1. Information to regular education staff through ongoing PT/OT consultation.
2. Environmental assessment in classroom by OT or PT or special education teacher.
3. Direct PT one time per week for stretching and exercise.

PT = physical therapist/physical therapy.
OT = occupational therapist.
ST = speech therapist.

lum, with or without minor adaptations. Special devices facilitate a student's ability to respond to educational instruction. Adapted writing instruments or equipment, such as computers or augmentative communication devices, enable some students to complete written work or to do so within reasonable time limits. Other students require adaptations to curriculum content or special assistance, such as tutoring, to master particular content areas. Students with more severe or multiple disabilities require extensive adaptations and altered curriculum content in order to be successful in school.

Role of Teachers and Related Services Personnel

Regular educators may have expectations that require children with physical disabilities to complete work in the same way and as quickly as children without disabilities. The *product* and the *concept(s)* that are being taught may become merged. One typical kindergarten activity, for example, teaches children color concepts through worksheets where partiular shapes are drawn or colored in with specific colors. A child with a physical disability may know the correct colors but may be unable to hold the crayon and, therefore, would be unable to complete the activity. Regular educators may not know how to devise alternate ways to teach or assess color concept knowledge and thus may judge that the child does not know colors.

Special educators and other team members, such as occupational therapists, are knowledgeable about instructional adaptations and content modifications that facilitate a student's participation in the work required in a classroom. When team members have a focus on *maintaining* the students in the regular classroom, emphasis is placed on generating ideas that support and enhance student participation. Working together with the regular education teacher and the family, team members can experiment with adaptations and instructional methods until successful modifications are found. In this instance, special edu-

cation has as a goal to support student participation and integration in regular education.

Environmental-Based Assessment: A Method for Problem Solving

Both instructional and noninstructional activities occur within regular education environments, including classrooms, cafeteria, hallways, bathrooms, and special instruction areas. Each activity may have numerous response requirements for successful completion. Many students with physical disabilities may be successful in all but one or two parts of an activity while others may be able only to partially complete some steps. Effective adaptations to and modifications of expectations for student performance are more likely when team members are knowledgeable about a student's participation in specific parts of an activity.

A plan for analysis of activity requirements is illustrated in Table 2. This format was modified from a more detailed assessment protocol devised by Baumgart and others (1982). This approach assesses a student's performance of all parts of a particular activity and helps identify those specific parts in which a student is discrepant from other students in a classroom. Both the mother and the teacher of the 7-year-old student, whose integration plan was described previously in Table 1, were concerned about his lack of independence in getting to the classroom and in participating in the initial activities of the classroom day, which frequently were less structured than other classroom activities. Table 2 illustrates the assessment process used to identify an instructional plan to facilitate more independent performance of these activities. Team members then collaborated on the basis of this assessment information to develop adaptations, provide planned assistance, and implement appropriate training strategies to facilitate student participation.

Collecting assessment information may seem time-consuming in the beginning as, ideally, one team member observes either all the activities in a classroom and other educational environments on

Table 2. Illustration of an environmental assessment

Student's name: Thomas Roy   Placement: First grade, Washington School
Person(s) Requesting Assessment: Mom, teacher
Person(s) Completing Assessment: Physical Therapist   Date: 9/9/86

What are the steps that a person without disabilities uses?	What adaptations or assistance might help?	What works best when these are tried?	What skills can be performed without adaptations or assistance?
I. Enters classroom			
1. Goes to locker	Adult currently pushes chair to locker; motorized chair might work	Peer can currently push; make application for funds for new chair	Can be independent with motorized chair
2. Opens locker	Cannot reach locker to open; place cord through handle to pull up	Cord does not work; peer can assist when Tommy requests	
3. Removes coat	Some adult help needed for tight sleeves	Raglan sleeves or poncho	Can remove coat if sleeves are raglan or if poncho
4. Hangs coat	Can do if positioned sideways to locker	Peer will position chair	Hang coat
5. Closes locker	Can do door but not latch	Peer will latch	Close door of locker
6. Goes into classroom	Currently pushed	Peer will push	Can be independent with motorized chair
7. Sits at desk	Adult adjusts chair to desk	Peer will push chair under desk	Can be independent with motorized chair
II. Opening activity			
1. Listens to announcements	None	Not applicable	Can listen
2. Stands for pledge	Can do hands and say pledge; not stand	Allow Tom to sit during pledge	Place arm correctly and say pledge
3. Sits at desk	Not applicable	Not applicable	Not applicable
4. Listens to and follows teacher instructions	Tom sits quietly but cannot execute more than one direction without adult assistance; cue cards with pictures might help	Use cue cards to illustrate next activity, where located, and what to bring or what materials are needed	Fade cues to allow independence with normal teacher instruction
5. Goes to area of classroom for reading (next activity)	Adult currently pushes	Peer will push when Tommy requests	Can be independent with motorized chair

a given day or, minimally, the ones that have been identified as problematic. The process yields valuable information that is not available through any other means and increases team efficiency in generating solutions that are likely to work. Effective solutions and accurate judgments about student ability are not likely when student performance is assessed in isolation from classroom expectations (Campbell, 1987b).

Implementing Planned Participation

Adaptations that appear useful are validated in the setting(s) where planned for use. Three questions are important: 1) Does the person who will use the adaptation with a student have the necessary training or expertise? 2) Does use of the adaptation physically or socially isolate the student from other students in the classroom? and 3) To what extent is the student a full or partial participant in the adapted classroom activity? Many well-designed adaptations fail when personnel who are responsible for using the adaptation are not trained in its use. Some adaptations are quite simple and require limited if any training while others, such as computers or augmentative communication devices, may be quite complex or subject to frequent malfunction. The team member who designs or selects a particular adaptation also provides training to all individuals with whom a student is expected to use the adaptation.

Some adaptations inadvertently isolate a student from other students. A student, for example, who is positioned in equipment such as a prone stander to work independently at a computer while other students are participating in a reading group may be completing the necessary work but is doing so in both physical and social isolation from other students. Minimizing the types and degree of isolation that may occur is important. A major purpose in educating students with physical disabilities in regular environments is to facilitate social and communicative interactions with students without disabilities. Implementing instructional activities to include the student with physical disabilities is one strategy to minimize isolation.

Positioning the student with physical disabilities in a chair with the computer during reading group allows physical integration with other students in the group. Incorporating the computer into the activity for all children further reduces the type and degree of isolation imposed by adaptations in this example. In another example, a student who is placed with age-mates in a fifth-grade classroom but who is reading on a first-grade level can complete reading activities individually through computer instruction. Less physical isolation from regular students occurs when such instruction is maintained in the classroom than when the student is removed for special tutoring or remedial activities.

Not all students, however, will be able to participate fully or easily in instructional activities in a regular classroom even with response or content adaptations. Curricular content may require significant modifications that cannot be addressed through regular instruction and additional assistance, such as tutoring. Family priorities for a child may include areas that are nontraditional in regular classroom instruction. A family, for example, may want a child to be able to play with other children in the neighborhood, use the community library, or eat meals with other family members. Individualized training provided by special education personnel, such as teachers, community trainers, or job coaches, may be necessary to best meet instructional priorities for particular students. Integrated instruction occurs when teaching is provided in a variety of academic and functional skill areas with students based in regular education classrooms but removed for specialized instruction in targeted priority areas.

Facilitating Integration through Combined Regular Education and Special Education Curricula

Special education curricula can be described as *remedial* or *functional*. The traditional diagnostic-prescriptive approach uses a variety of assessment procedures to determine student strengths and weaknesses. The result of the assessment process is an individual program of instruction and remediation to enhance strengths and minimize weaknesses. The remedial focus in this special education emphasis is on "fixing" the targeted students through specialized instructional methods and techniques (Campbell, in press–a). In contrast, life skills are taught when a functional and integrated approach is taken toward a student's education. The purpose of this curricular emphasis in special education is to prepare students to live, work, and play in communities as adults. Both the remedial and functional emphases in special education share commonalities with and distinct differences from purposes of regular education. (e.g., Sailor & Guess, 1983; Snell, 1987). A combined approach is essential when integrating students with physical disabilities who receive both regular and special instructional curricula.

Students with severe or multiple disabilities are more likely to require a combined curricular approach than are those with physical disabilities alone. Such an approach allows joint focus on both the social and instructional needs of students. The IEP provides a vehicle for combining the goals and purposes of both regular education and special education around individual needs. The result is a comprehensive package of services that addresses individual needs without removing a student unnecessarily from regular education environments.

Role of Teachers and Related Services Personnel

Educators and related services personnel who understand the purpose and use of remedial, functional, and regular education curricula, and the roles and functions of personnel within each approach, can design individual programs that are responsive to each student's unique needs. In this way, a student is based in a regular classroom but receives a combined program that includes needed instruction and social integration within appropriate settings.

Integrating regular and special education curricula requires careful planning to ensure that individual student needs are addressed through individualized instruction and related services. Educational activities are viewed in terms of opportunities for both integration and instruction when this approach is used. Key members of the programming team are parents, regular educators, and special educational personnel, who may include community instructors, transition specialists, or job coaches. Each student's individualized program is designed and implemented by team members and evaluated to ensure maximal opportunities for instruction and integration. An example of this approach is presented in Table 3, which illustrates the individual program planned for a 13-year-old student with severe and multiple handicaps who attended a neighborhood middle school.

Facilitating Social and Communicative Interactions

A primary purpose in integrating students with and without disabilities is to provide opportunities for interactions among students. While interactions may occur naturally among students in physical proximity to each other, most interactions require some sort of facilitation by adults. Interactions among students who are grouped together in noninstructional settings, such as the cafeteria or playground, are facilitated through environmental arrangements as well as through more specific mechanisms. For example, in most elementary schools, children from each classroom sit together, often at staggered, scheduled times. When children with physical disabilities who are members of regular education classrooms are receiving specialized instruction and related services, natural noninstructional interactions occur more easily.

These natural interactions can be increased by specific facilitations. For example, having children without disabilities assist those with disabilities to manage activities in the cafeteria, rather than having these needs met by the teacher or an

Table 3. Example of process to provide opportunities for planned and natural interactions

Student's name: <u>James Rafall</u>

Placement: <u>SMH, Gibson Junior High</u>

Daily morning schedule	Planned interactions	Possible natural interactions
Entering school	Bill will get Jim off bus, into school, and to his locker.	Students may interact with Bill and Jim in hallways and locker area.
Going to classroom Locker area and classroom	Will help at locker area and push Jim into classroom (special friend approach)	
Homeroom activities	Teacher facilitates interaction through planned activities among students.	Students may interact with each other in getting organized for the school day.
Transition to art	Tom will push Jim to art room.	Regular class change; students may interact in hallways.
Art	Jim is placed in regular art class with a peer tutor to ensure participation.	Other students may interact to provide assistance in and generally around the art activity.
Community Training Travel and restaurant	Jim is learning to use special transportation for wheelchair needs. Bill has elected a study hall to help Jim and the community trainer. Peer tutor provides planned interactions.	Individuals in local fast-food restaurant—personnel and customers—will interact; bus driver will interact to learn where Jim wants to go.

attendant, establishes a basis through which children can develop friendships and understandings of one another. A child without a disability can assist in selecting books in the library, setting up materials for art and other noninstructional subjects, or wheeling the chair of the child who is not yet indepedent in mobility. Children with physical disabilities who require total assistance to perform a particular activity may be given a nonparticipant role in this activity. For example, an older student may be responsible for equipment for a sports team when unable to participate in the actual sport.

Natural acceptance of students with disabilities occurs more readily when children are grouped together beginning at preschool and kindergarten age. Younger students are not as concerned with differences as are older students. Informational programs such as *Kids on the Block* (The Council for Exceptional Children, 1976) can be helpful in providing accurate information about various disabilities. More important, however, is the support given to interactions by adults. The attitudes and values of teachers, administrators, therapists, and parents are communicated, both verbally and nonverbally, to children in school settings. Even natural interactions among children may be inhibited when adults have inaccurate information about disabilities, are unsure about how to manage a child's physical and instructional needs, or do not support integration. Team members play a major role in providing information for adults involved in supporting social interactions. Additional formal inservice training provides adults with the information and skills needed to integrate children successfully and facilitate interactions among all children.

Facilitating Integration within Special Education

Students with significant needs for functional skill training spend a majority of their time in special education and related services activities. These activities occur in any number of settings, including school, home, community, or work environments. Instruction is often provided by specialized teachers such as community trainers, transition specialists, job coaches, or related services personnel. Opportunities for interaction with individuals who are not disabled occur in each of the environments where training is provided. Interactions with adults increase as students move through high school and into community and work settings. Examples of the types of environments in which instruction and related services are provided are listed in Table 4 by approximate age level. Included are listings of individuals with whom interactions may occur. Social and supportive interactions may require facilitation although

Table 4. Examples of special education instructional environments

Age level	Environments	Interactions
Infancy (birth–3 years)	Home	Family-siblings, extended family, friends of family
	Day care	Other children, personnel
	Center school	Other children, teachers, therapists
Preschool	Home	Family-siblings, extended family, friends of family
	Day care	Other children, personnel
	Community preschool	Other children, teachers, therapists
Elementary school	Regular classroom	Students, teachers, therapists
	Special class—art, music, gym	Students, teachers
	Tutoring classroom	Teachers
	Other—hall, cafeteria, bathroom, playground	Students, school personnel
	Community—stores, etc.	Community environment employees—store clerks, children, adults
Middle school	Homeroom, regular classes, special classes	Students, teachers, therapists
	Tutoring classroom	Teachers
	Other school environments	Students, school personnel
	Community—transportation, stores, etc.	Bus drivers, clerks, children, adults
	Work environments—school office, etc.	Adults, students
High school and postschool	Homeroom, regular classes	Students, teachers, therapists
	Other school environments	Students, school personnel
	Community—stores, recreation, service, transportation	Bus drivers, clerks, children, adults
	Work environments—community settings, stores, etc.	Other workers, job coaches
	Group homes, supported living arrangements	Attendants, support personnel
	Postschool educational settings—colleges, community colleges, technical schools	Teachers, other students

natural interactions may occur on the basis of physical proximity.

Role of Teachers and Related Services Personnel

A critical function of special education personnel is to facilitate appropriate interactions between students with disabilities and other typical individuals in their lives. A wide range of typical individuals with whom a student may interact is provided when special education programs teach functional life skills in nonschool environments. Educational and related services personnel use instructional methods to teach appropriate interactions as well as to train students to perform desired skills. An essential skill for students with physical disabilities is communication sufficient to request assistance in areas in which they remain totally or partially dependent even with training and use of adaptive devices. Students who are unable to communicate in some form will have difficulty requesting assistance in physical activities for which they are not independent (e.g., opening doors of buildings) or using community resources such as stores, movie theaters, or dry cleaners. Social in-

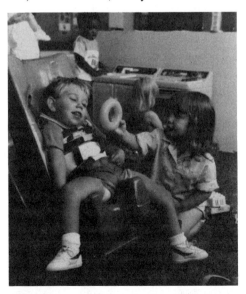

Young children interact easily and naturally together.

teraction and communication often are linked in adult interactions and are directly related to a student's capacity to communicate independently with others (Certo & Kohl, 1984).

Facilitating Communication

Many students with severe and multiple disabilities communicate using means that are unconventional and, therefore, not easily understood by individuals who are not familiar with the student (Campbell & Wilcox, 1985; Wilcox & Campbell, in press). Others may communicate verbally but unintelligibly or through communication devices that may be laborious for the "listener" and "speaker" alike. Still others use gestures or sign language or various eclectic approaches that combine verbal and nonverbal modes of expression. Any of these means of expression may not be easily understood by an average individual who is not handicapped, due to unfamiliarity with expressive modes that are alternatives to speech.

Initiation versus Response Students may use alternate modes of communication to respond to other individuals but may not *initiate* interaction or communication with other individuals. Often, physical and other needs of these students are addressed automatically by the adults in their environments, eliminating situations that might require a student to initiate interactions. Students who are taught to spontaneously use expressive communication modes to initiate interactions with other students or adults are less helpless and dependent on adults than are students who use communicative modes to *respond* to interactions only when prompted. For example, a teacher who asks a student if she or he needs to use the bathroom and waits for the student to point to a communication symbol for "bathroom" or sign or gesture for "bathroom" is prompting use of this communicative expression. The student is not independent in requesting his or her need to use the bathroom until the student spontaneously (and without prompts) indicates this need when the bathroom is required and does not initiate this request when the bathroom is not needed. Teachers and related services personnel train functional (spontaneous) use of communicative interactions by: 1) structuring school and nonschool environments to provide maximal opportunities for initiation of communicative interactions, including expressions of requests, needs, ideas, or feelings (e.g., McDonald & Gillette, 1986); and 2) using specific strategies to train initiation (Reichle & Keogh, 1986).

Selecting Expressive Communicative Modes
Any number of guidelines are available for selecting modes by which students may communicate ideas, feelings, needs, or wants (e.g., Blackstone, 1986; Halle, 1982; Nietupski & Hamre-Nietupski, 1986; Reichle & Karlan, 1985). While some students may use a communication board or device, others may use some form of gesture or sign. Most students with physical disabilities, however, will use a combination of expressive modes including gesture or body movement, vocalization, and communication boards or devices. The particular system developed and used for communicative purposes will depend on a student's physical abilities and the situations in which a student will need to communicate (Cohen, 1986). Equally important, however, is a consideration of the "listener," the person with whom a student may be communicating. Designing communication systems that resemble conventional speech and that, therefore, are more easily understood by a listener facilitates a student's ability both to communicate and to be understood. Augmentative communication devices that "speak" through synthesized speech are easier, for example, for listeners than is the process of looking at and interpreting Blissymbolics or other forms of picture/symbol expression.

Many speech-language pathologists have additional training in augmentative communication and provide valuable information to the team that can be used to: 1) select expressive communication modes; and 2) design appropriate training strategies for their use. Augmentative communication is rapidly becoming an area of specialty not only for speech-language pathologists but also for teachers and occupational therapists (Blackstone, 1986). Team members, whatever their discipline,

need to have knowledge not only of the variety of devices and systems that have been used but also of training strategies that are effective in teaching students to use communicative modes across home, school, and community environments. Assessment of communicative expressions needed and used across environments is an important component in selecting appropriate communicative modes. Effective decisions about modes cannot be made separate from the environments in which communication will be used (Campbell & Wilcox, 1985; Cohen, 1986).

Facilitating Social Interactions

Many students with severe disabilities may communicate in ways that are not easily understood by others and may have difficulty interacting with others using conventional types of behavior. For example, a student with severe physical disabilities may not be able to attract someone else's attention using typical means such as calling out to or touching another person. Students may not be able physically to engage in typical social interactions that involve turn taking; sharing, such as in joint recreation or leisure activities; engaging in conversations; or performing appropriate behavior in the presence of other individuals. Instead, students with severe physical disabilities may become isolated if specific programming attempts are not undertaken to facilitate social interactions.

When goals are established for social interaction for each student in a classroom, opportunities for students to learn these skills are available more readily (Schutz, Williams, Iverson, & Duncan, 1984). Teachers and other program personnel cannot simply place students in situations where social interactions are required, but must specifically guide, facilitate, and train these interactions (e.g., Campbell, 1989; Odom & McEvoy, 1988.) Information about training social interactions with students of a variety of disabilities suggests that one strategy that can be used is to train typical peer models or students with less severe disabilities to socially interact with students with more severe disabilities (e.g., Stainback, Stainback, & Hatcher,

1983). Other strategies include: 1) prompting a student with severe disabilities through interactions with another student; and 2) using systematic environmental engineering to ensure interactions among two or more students (Certo & Kohl, 1984). For example, a teacher might physically prompt a student to move to another student, physically touch that student, and initiate an interaction through some sort of communicative greeting. Or, a teacher might select a particular activity in which two or more students may have essential roles. For example, one student might turn on a blender after another student has put in ice cream and milk to make a milkshake. Interactions among students result when the environment is engineered so that the demands of the activity ensure that each student has an essential and interactional role in a "final product." A student with a physical disability may be able to activate a blender using a microswitch but may not be able to scoop ice cream. The routine of activities such as these ensure that students with more severe disabilities have an essential role and one that will facilitate interactions with other students.

STRATEGIES TO ENHANCE INTEGRATION

Students with severe physical disabilities do not initiate behavior frequently, may have significantly limited and restricted behavioral repertoires, and may be grouped with other like students—thereby reducing opportunities to initiate behavior and learn ranges of appropriate behavior (Orelove & Sobsey, 1987). The severe nature of the disabilities of this group of students may isolate them from other students (with or without disabilities) even when these students are placed in integrated environments. Systematic programs that train or facilitate other students to initiate interactions with these students who are severely disabled are necessary to prevent the social isolation that occurs as a result of the severity of the disability. A number of different options have

been used to ensure social integration with students with severe disabilities. In general, strategies focus on training typical peer models to perform specific functions with children with disabilities. Included here are: 1) peer tutoring or training; 2) social prompting; 3) peer modeling; and 4) special friends programs.

Peer Tutoring or Training

In a peer-tutoring approach, children without disabilities are taught how to provide tutoring or special training for students with severe disabilities (e.g., Kohl, Moses, & Stettner-Eaton, 1983, 1984; Odom & McEvoy, 1988; Stainback, Stainback, & Hatcher, 1983; Voeltz & Evans, 1983). This strategy has been applied successfully across a number of instructional tasks with students from preschool through high school ages. In essence, children without disabilities are taught to provide necessary and systematic instructional antecedents and reinforcers that would normally be provided by a teacher for particular children with disabilities around specific tasks or activities. Typical children have been successful in teaching children with severe disabilities any number of tasks ranging from playing with toys, to eating in the cafeteria, to performing specific academic or instructional tasks. This is a formal approach that uses students who are typical or who have less severe handicaps to provide specific instruction for students with disabilities. While such an approach allows for interactions among students, those that occur may be more instructional than social and may inhibit the development of more friendly social interactions between both students if not appropriately implemented.

Social Prompting or Peer-Initiation Strategies

The strategies of social prompting or peer initiation are a less formal derivative of the peer-tutoring approach in that students who are not handicapped are trained to initiate interactions with those with more severe disabilities. This approach has been used in early childhood settings, in particular, around recreation-leisure activities such as free play. Children without disabilities initiate interactions by socially directing children with more severe disabilities to engage in appropriate behavior. For example, a child may initiate an interaction around a toy by going over to the child with more severe disabilities, getting a toy, and saying "Let's play," or he or she may direct a child to follow the routines of a classroom through initiation/verbal direction (e.g., Strain & Kohler, 1988.) This approach does not use specific training and may be easily facilitated by a teacher suggesting to a child, for example, "Help Billy get his mat for circle time." This approach facilitates social interactions among children by guiding their interactions around specific activities rather than giving the child without disabilities a direct instructional role with a child with disabilities.

Peer Modeling

Children without disabilities naturally model appropriate behavior for children with disabilities when skill levels among children are not too discrepant. A student with severe physical disabilities, for example, will not learn to walk by following the model established by a mobile student. However, a student who is able to wheel a wheelchair, operate a motorized chair, or walk using a walker may learn to do so with a normal rate and within reasonable time limits by following the models of more mobile students. Similarly, students who vocalize but do not speak may learn to do so by following models of speaking students, but a student who uses a communication board or some form of gestured or signed speech will not learn to talk by following the model of a speaking student. In a most general sense, students without disabilities provide incentives and establish "normal" environmental expectations for students with disabilities. When students are grouped by disability levels, no student in the group may be mobile or speaking. This type of grouping eliminates peer modeling of any sort and establishes expectations for limited behavior from students with

severe disabilities. When teachers and other personnel group students together to allow natural modeling to occur, less able students can model the behavior and skills of more able students.

Use of a peer-modeling approach frequently includes more systematic guidance by teachers than just grouping students together so that natural modeling can occur. Students without disabilities have been taught to cue those with disabilities by, for example, directing the student with disabilities to "Watch me" or "Do it like I do." Even more systematic applications of this approach resemble peer tutoring in that students are taught how to model procedures that are appropriate for the student with disabilities (e.g., Apolloni, Cooke, & Cooke, 1977; Guralnick, 1976). The more structured the application of a peer-modeling approach the less natural are the interactions that occur among students.

A common denominator in both natural and structured peer modeling is that students with disabilities must be able to imitate the behavior being modeled by more able students. Two factors are involved in the ability to imitate. One is that the student must be able to produce some approximation of the model's behavior. The second is that the student must demonstrate imitation skills. Teachers can enhance the capacity of a student with disabilities to follow a model by teaching imitation skills. This training may be systematic or may be carried out in a natural setting or context. Formal imitation training occurs when students are systematically taught to imitate either motor ("Raise Hands") or verbal ("Say 'spoon' ") models in what are often quite contrived training situations. Students, for example, may be trained to imitate a fixed set of models using a fixed number of training trials using a least-to-most prompting sequence for training (e.g., Bricker & Bricker, 1976; Guess, Sailor, & Baer, 1977). Teachers and parents may also prompt imitation skills in naturally occurring contexts by verbally directing or physically cueing or guiding students to imitate the model being produced by another student. Verbal cues such as "Do what John is doing" or physically guiding a child to reproduce modeled behavior can assist students to learn imitation skills.

Special Friends Programs

Friendships are an important part of the lives of all individuals. Friends provide support and assistance, someone to do something with, and the simple enjoyment of interacting with another individual. Able-bodied friends provide a support network for individuals with physical disabilities by providing assistance with tasks or activities that may not be able to be accomplished independently by the person with disabilities. Most people, with or without disabilities, need periodic assistance and support from friends, family members, or paid individuals to manage various aspects of their lives. Students with physical disabilities are no different in these needs. Some students need assistance in the cafeteria, the bathroom, or during specific activities, such as fire drills. Others need assistance in changing classes, carrying books, or completing specific assignments. A typical public school response to these needs is to provide special education in segregated classrooms or schools with paid attendants or classroom assistants.

Many of these needs can be managed by able-bodied students when students with physical disabilities are educated in regular classrooms or regular schools. Some programs facilitate friendships among students with and without disabilities through special training programs while other approaches rely on more naturally occurring interactions and instruction. Most students without disabilities will require some sort of instruction to manage the physical needs of students with disabilities. Parents and teachers can provide this instruction by showing more able-bodied students how to perform caregiving routines such as lifting, carrying or transfer, feeding, and clothing management, and how to understand the communications of a child who is disabled. In addition, showing students how to manage and use any adaptive equipment or devices increases competence in managing and understanding the needs of the student with disabilities.

These types of information may be provided through formal instruction programs where students from a particular school, for example, volunteer to participate in a special program to interact with children with disabilities (Voeltz & Evans, 1983) and often are assigned specific tasks or activities that provide a context in which friendships may develop. Parents and teachers may also provide information within the contexts in which information may be needed (Haring, Breen, Pitts-Conway, Lee, & Gaylord-Ross, 1987; Strully & Strully, 1985). For example, children in a Girl Scout troop may need to know that it is acceptable and not hurtful to move a child's arm or hand in a particular way to help the child complete an activity, or they may be assisted by demonstrations of the best ways to help a child move. More natural interactions among children occur when information can be provided on an as-needed basis. In these situations, more able-bodied children generate solutions for interacting with a child, and these solutions are verified or modified by knowledgeable adults who use nonintrusive strategies. For example, reinforcing a child who is interacting with a child with disabilities by saying "That is a nice way of helping Susan hold the paint brush" increases natural interactions and reinforces friendships among children to a greater extent than does first showing a child the "correct way" to provide assistance.

No one method is the only and best way for allowing friendships to occur among children with and without disabilities. Reinforcing natural interactions is the least intrusive or structured method. Providing information within the context of an activity is a more formal way of facilitating interactions. Teaching children without disabilities the general skills needed to interact with children with disabilities is a more structured method. Group training programs for children without disabilities are the most structured method for developing interactions and friendships among children. Each of these methods is appropriate given the circumstances surrounding and the context in which expected interactions may take place. Teachers, parents, and other adults who are sensitive to the needs and concerns of both the children with and without disabilities can use methods that range in degree of intrusiveness to facilitate interactions.

SUMMARY

Children with physical disabilities traditionally have been placed in special education classrooms and settings due to limited architectural accessibility of many public school buildings, centralized models of therapy services, needs for a variety of specialized adaptive devices, and attitudes concerning the needs of students with physical disabilities. Interactions among these students and students who are more able bodied cannot occur when students with physical disabilities are placed in segregated schools, orthopedic "wings" of schools, or segregated classrooms. An initial step, therefore, is to use strategies that ensure the physical integration of students in regular schools. Ideally, placements support participation in the regular education curriculum, in a combined regular education–special education program, or in a special education curriculum with regular and planned interactions with able-bodied students. Facilitating interactions among students is enhanced when students with severe disabilities are taught to communicate and to interact socially with other students. Interactions are further increased through the use of methods that teach students without disabilities to interact with those who are disabled. Most important, true friendships among students develop when teachers and parents learn and use strategies that facilitate and support naturally occurring interactions among students.

STUDY QUESTIONS

1. Describe two approaches to obtain physical integration of students with orthopedic impairments and with severe and multiple handicaps.
2. Differentiate between peer-tutoring and peer-modeling approaches toward facilitating interactions among students.
3. List several methods that can be used to manage the special health care needs of students with physical disabilities in regular education settings.
4. Conduct an environmental assessment for a student with physical disabilities who is being integrated into a regular education placement.
5. Describe three approaches that a teacher might use to facilitate friendship among students with and without disabilities. Differentiate among the levels of structure required in each approach.
6. Provide a rationale for maintaining students with physical disabilities in segregated schools and contrast this with a rationale for integrating all students with orthopedic handicaps only, in regular classrooms and schools.

REFERENCES

Apolloni, T., Cooke, S.A., & Cooke, T.P. (1977). Establishing a normal peer as a behavioral model for developmentally delayed toddlers. *Perceptual and Motor Skills, 44*, 231–241.

Baumgart, D., Brown, L., Pumpian, I., Nisbet, J., Ford, A., Sweet, M., Mesina, R., & Schroeder, J. (1982). Principle of partial participation and individualized adaptations in education programs for severely handicapped students. *The Journal of the Association for the Severely Handicapped, 7*(2), 17–27.

Bigge, J.L. (1982). *Teaching individuals with physical and multiple disabilities.* Columbus, OH: Charles E. Merrill.

Blackstone, S.W. (Ed.). (1986). *Augmentative communication: An introduction.* Rockville, MD: American Speech-Hearing-Language Association.

Bleck, E., & Nagel, D.A. (1982). *Physically handicapped children: A medical atlas for teachers* (2nd ed.). New York: Grune & Stratton.

Bricker, W.A., & Bricker, D.D. (1976). An early language

training strategy. In R. Schiefelbusch & L. Lloyd (Eds.), *Language perspectives: Acquisition, retardation and intervention* (pp. 118–136). Baltimore: University Park Press.

Campbell, P.H. (1987a). The integrated programming team: An approach for coordinating professionals of various disciplines in programs for students with severe and multiple handicaps. *Journal of the Association for Persons with Severe Handicaps, 12*(2), 107–116.

Campbell, P.H. (1987b). Programming for students with dysfunction in posture and movement. In M. Snell (Ed.), *Systematic instruction of students with moderate and severe handicaps* (3rd ed.). Columbus, OH: Charles E. Merrill.

Campbell, P.H. (1989). Dysfunction in posture and movement in individuals with profound disabilities: Issues and practices. In F. Brown & D. Lehr (Eds.), *Persons with profound disabilities: Issues and practices.* Baltimore: Paul H. Brookes Publishing Co.

Campbell, P.H. (in press). An essay on preschool integration. In L. Meyer, C. Peck, & L. Brown (Eds.), *Critical issues in the lives of people with severe disabilities.*

Campbell, P.H., & Wilcox, M.J. (1985). *Communication effectiveness of movement patterns used by non-vocal children with severe handicaps.* Paper presented at Fourth Annual ISAAC Convention, Cardiff, Wales, U.K.

Certo, N., & Kohl, F. (1984). Strategies for developing interpersonal interaction instructional content for severely handicapped students. In N. Certo, N. Haring, & R. York (Eds.), *Public school integration of severely handicapped students: Rational issues and progressive alternatives* (pp. 221–244). Baltimore: Paul H. Brookes Publishing Co.

Cohen, C.G. (1986). Total habilitation and life-long management. In S.W. Blackstone (Ed.), *Augmentative communication: An introduction* (pp. 447–469). Rockville, MD: American Speech-Language-Hearing Association.

The Council for Exceptional Children. (1988). *Final report: CEC ad hoc committee on medically fragile students.* Reston, VA: Author.

The Council for Exceptional Children. (1976). *Kids on the block.* Reston, VA: Author.

Dunn, W. (in press). *The pediatric service delivery process.* Thorofare, NJ: SLACK.

Edgar, E. (1987). Secondary programs in special education: Are many of them justifiable? *Exceptional Children, 53*(6), 555–561.

Giangreco, M.F. (1986). Effects of integrated therapy: A pilot study. *The Journal of the Association for Persons with Severe Handicaps, 11*(3), 205–215.

Guidelines for the practice of occupational therapy in public schools. (1986). Rockville, MD: American Occupational Therapy Association.

Guralnick, M.J. (1976). The value of integrating handicapped and nonhandicapped preschool children. *American Journal of Orthopsychiatry, 46,* 236–244.

Guess, D., Sailor, W., & Baer, D. (1977). A behavioral-remedial approach to language training for the severely handicapped. In E. Sontag, N. Certo, & J. Smith (Eds.), *Educational programming for the severely and profoundly handicapped* (pp. 360–377). Reston, VA: Council for Exceptional Children.

Halle, J.W. (1982). Teaching functional language to the handicapped: An integrative model of natural environment teaching techniques. *Journal of the Association for Persons with Severe Handicaps, 7*(4), 29–37.

Haring, T.G., Breen, C., Pitts-Conway, V., Lee, M., & Gaylord-Ross, R. (1987). Adolescent peer tutoring and special friend experiences. *Journal of the Association for Persons with Severe Handicaps, 12*(4), 280–286.

Integrated services project: Coordinating special education services through integrated programming. (1987). Akron: Mid-Eastern Ohio Special Education Regional Resource Center and Children's Hospital Medical Center of Akron, Family Child Learning Center.

Kohl, F.L., Moses, L.G., & Stettner-Eaton, B. (1983). The results of teaching fifth and sixth graders to be instructional trainers with students who are severely handicapped. *Journal of the Association for Persons with Severe Handicaps, 8*(4), 32–40.

Kohl, F.L., Moses, L.G., & Stettner-Eaton, B.A. (1984). A systematic training program for teaching nonhandicapped students to be instructional trainers of severely handicapped schoolmates. In N. Certo, N. Haring, & R. York (Eds.), *Public school integration of severely handicapped students: Rational issues and progressive alternatives* (pp. 185–196). Baltimore: Paul H. Brookes Publishing Co.

McDonald, J., & Gillette, Y. (1986). Communicating with persons with severe handicaps: Roles of parents and professionals. *Journal of the Association for Persons with Severe Handicaps, 11*(4), 255–265.

Nietupski, J., & Hamre-Nietupski, S. (1986). Guidelines for making simulation an effective adjunct to in vivo community instruction. *Journal of the Association for Persons with severe Handicaps, 1*(11), 12–18.

Odom, S.L., & McEvoy, M.A. (1988). Integration of young children with handicaps and normally developing children. In S.L. Odom & M.B. Karnes (Eds.), *Early intervention for infants and children with handicaps: An empirical base,* (pp. 241–267). Baltimore: Paul H. Brookes Publishing Co.

Orelove, F.P., & Hanley, C.D. (1979). Modifying school buildings for the severely handicapped: A school accessibility survey. *AAESPH Review, 4*(3), 219–236.

Orelove, F.P., & Sobsey, D. (1987). *Educating children with multiple disabilities: A transdisciplinary approach.* Baltimore: Paul H. Brookes Publishing Co.

Rainforth, B., & York, J. (1987). Integrating related services in community instruction. *The Journal of The Association for Persons with Severe Handicaps, 12*(3), 190–198.

Reichle, J., & Karlan, G. (1985). The selection of an augmentative system in communication intervention: A critique of decision rules. *Journal of the Association for Persons with Severe Handicaps, 10*(3), 146–156.

Reichle, J., & Keogh, W.J. (1986). Communication instruction for learners with severe handicaps: Some unresolved issues. In R.H. Horner, L.H. Meyer, & H.D.B. Fredericks (Eds.), *Education of learners with severe handicaps: Exemplary service strategies* (pp. 189–220). Baltimore: Paul H. Brookes Publishing Co.

Rostetter, D., Kowalski, R., & Hunter, D. (1984). Implementing the integration principle of P.L. 94-142. In N. Certo,

N. Haring, & R. York, (Eds.) *Public school integration of severely handicapped students: Rational issues and progressive alternatives* (pp. 293–320). Baltimore: Paul H. Brookes Publishing Co.

Sailor, W., & Guess, D. (1983). Severely handicapped preschoolers. *Topics in Early Childhood Special Education, 4*(3), 47–72.

Schutz, R.P., Williams, W., Iverson, G.S., & Duncan, D. (1984). Social integration of severely handicapped students. In N. Certo, N. Haring, & R. York, (Eds.), *Public school integration of severely handicapped students: Rational issues and progressive alternatives* (pp. 15–42). Baltimore: Paul H. Brookes Publishing Co.

Servis, B. (1988). Students with special health care needs. *Teaching Exceptional Children, 20*(4), 40–44.

Shelton, T.L., Jeppson, E.S., & Johnson, B.H. (1987). *Family centered care for children with special health care needs.* Washington, DC: Association for the Care of Children's Health.

Smith, B.J., & Strain, P.S. (1988, Spring). Implementing and expanding P.L. 99-457. *Topics in Early Childhood Special Education, 8*(1), 37–47.

Snell, M. (Ed.). (1987). *Systematic instruction of students with moderate and severe handicaps* (3rd ed.). Columbus, OH: Charles E. Merrill.

Stainback, S.B., Stainback, W.C., & Hatcher, C.W. (1983). Nonhandicapped peer involvement in the education of severely handicapped students. *Journal of the Association for Persons with Severe Handicaps, 8*(1), 39–42.

Strain, P.S., & Kohler, F.W. (1988). Social skills intervention with young children with handicaps: Some new conceptualizations and directions. In S.L. Odom & M.B. Karnes (Eds.), *Early intervention for infants and children with handicaps: An empirical base* (pp 129–143). Baltimore: Paul H. Brookes Publishing Co.

Strully, J., & Strully, C. (1985). Friendship and our children. *Journal of the Association for Persons with Severe Handicaps, 10*(4), 224–227.

Umbreit, J. (1983). *Physical disabilities and health impairments: An introduction.* Columbus, OH: Charles E. Merrill.

U.S. Department of Education. (1988). *10th annual report to Congress on the implementation of the Education of the Handicapped Act.* Washington, DC: Author.

U.S. Department of Health, Education, and Welfare. (1979). *Progress toward a free appropriate public education* (A report to Congress on the implementation of Public Law 94-142: The Education for All Handicapped Children Act. Prepared by the State Program Implementation Studies Branch of the Bureau of Education for the Handicapped). Washington, DC: Author, Office of Education.

Voeltz, L., & Evans, I. (1983). Educational validity: Procedures to evaluate outcomes in programs for severely handicapped learners. *Journal of the Association for Persons with Severe Handicapps, 8*(1), 3–15.

Wetherbee, R., & Campbell, P.H. (1987). *The effects of integrated team planning on the instructional programs of students with orthopedic and multiple handicaps.* Manuscript submitted for publication.

Wilcox, M.J., & Campbell, P.H. (in press). *Communication programming from birth to three: A handbook for public school professionals.* San Diego: College Hill Press.

York, J., & Rainforth, B. (1986). Developing instructional adaptations. In F.P. Orelove & D. Sobsey, *Educating children with multiple disabilities: A transdisciplinary approach* (pp. 183–217). Baltimore: Paul H. Brookes Publishing Co.

CHAPTER 4

MAXIMIZING SOCIAL INTEGRATION FOR STUDENTS WITH VISUAL HANDICAPS

Sharon Zell Sacks and Maureen P. Reardon

One of the major precepts of mainstreaming is that interaction between nondisabled and disabled peers would yield benefits for both groups. Proponents of such a perspective believed that such placement would enhance spontaneous interaction and influence the development of positive social relationships. Although blind and visually handicapped (VH) children have been mainstreamed into regular educational placements for over 50 years, there is recent concern regarding their social competence and their ability to interact effectively with peers.

The effect of blindness or visual impairment in children limits their ability to acquire a repertoire of social behaviors that allows for the development of autonomy and independence. Perhaps of all the developmental processes, socialization is most strongly affected by vision. How children perceive their environment and initiate interactions with others (parents, siblings, and peers) is related to the ability to use effectively the visual system to obtain information regarding appropriate social behavior. In addition, when children have no sense of visual imagery, or have a limited conceptualization of the world around them, their ability to grasp abstract ideas such as values or judgments may be limited or strongly influenced by the adult world. More important, how others react to and interact with the visually impaired child can di-

rectly affect the child's ability to develop a positive self-concept, a sense of independent functioning in later life, and a variety of opportunities to enhance social competence throughout childhood and adolescence. Scott (1969) suggests that:

> without vision the adolescent is cut off from a larger segment of the physical and social environment to which he must adapt. He cannot easily relate to the environment; he can only infer; and therefore misses meanings and intentions which are created when words are combined with the rich vocabulary of expressive gestures. (p. 1025)

Richardson (1969) also contends that "absence of accurate feedback makes it difficult for the person who is handicapped to learn appropriate behaviors and therefore makes it more difficult for him to develop skills and to learn what others think of him" (p. 1058). Given such limitations, the social development of the visually impaired child may not follow the same developmental stages as his or her sighted counterpart. As a result, the acquisition of social conventions (Turiel, 1978) through environmental experiences or allegiance with social groups may not occur, or may develop in a different manner.

Hartup (1977) proposed that children are developmentally "at risk" when they do not experience encounters with peers. Other evidence has indicated that socially isolated children have problems acquiring appropriate language, behaviors, moral values, and acceptable methods of expressing one's emotions and feelings (Harlow & Harlow; 1962; Piaget, 1932; Strain, Cooke, & Apolloni, 1976). Such a thesis seems logical since much of a child's social experiences are with agemates in school settings. Yet investigations that have examined the effects of social interactions between disabled and nondisabled children have demonstrated that without structured training, simple social proximity between groups is not effective and in fact may be counterproductive (Asher & Gottman, 1981; Asher, Oden, & Gottman, 1977; Cowen, Peterson, Babigian, Izzo, & Trost, 1973; Fredericks et al., 1978; Gotlieb & Budoff, 1973). Gresham (1983) asserts that "placement of handicapped children into regular classrooms without providing them with social skills which are critical to peer acceptance may result in increased social isolation and a more restrictive environment" (p. 140). Such has been the case for visually impaired children in mainstreamed and self-contained settings alike.

Recent research has indicated that visually impaired individuals are socially isolated (Eaglestein, 1975; Hoben & Lindstrom, 1979; Van Hasselt, 1983), they tend to interact with peers whose social skills are deficient (Centers & Centers, 1963), and their physical appearance and social physique influence successful interaction with nondisabled students (Dion, 1972; Scott, 1969). Furthermore, professionals in the field of visual impairment and blindness have come to recognize that many youngsters exhibit additional lags in concept development, sensory development, abstract thinking, language acquisition, self-perception, and social functioning (Santin & Nesker Simon, 1977). Despite such findings, the trend within educational service delivery models for blind and visually impaired students continues to place a high priority on the attainment of academic skills within the most integrated setting possible, with little attention directed toward the implementation of skills that promote social competence and independence in preparation for adult life.

Given such a thesis, one must begin to examine the characteristics of such a diverse population, as well as understand the impact of a visual disability on the social development and successful integration of visually impaired persons into the sighted environment. Further, it is important to understand how trends in education of visually handicapped persons have helped shape the development of existing program models and educational philosophies. With such perspectives in place, it is the purpose of this chapter to present creative and practical strategies to enhance and encourage the social integration of visually handicapped students into school, home, and community environments.

PERSONS WITH VISUAL HANDICAPS

The heterogeneity that exists among visually impaired persons makes it difficult to develop programs and to implement curricular strategies that can be useful with a wide variety of students. Traditionally, distinctions were made between those students who were "partially sighted." Such classifications created discrepancies in placement and instructional implementation. As a result, many children were misplaced and taught in a mode that was inconsistent with their appropriate learning style. For example, many children were taught Braille even though they demonstrated high levels of visual ability. However, many programs for visually handicapped students have adopted a more functional definition of visual disability that integrates the medical-rehabilitative definition along with a more functionally based framework. Such a perspective may encourage the use of residual vision for independent living tasks, but recognizes the importance of using auditory and tactile skills for academic endeavors.

Definitions

Legally blind (Jose, 1984) means a visual acuity for distance vision of 20/200 (Snellen notation) or less in the better eye, with best correction; or visual acuity of more than 20/200 if the widest diameter of field of vision subtends an angle no greater than 20 degrees (visual field deficit). The 20/200 notation refers to a fractional equivalent that provides the evaluator (eye-care specialist or educator) with a comparative measure of visual acuity. In other words, if an object is viewed at 200 feet by an individual with average visual ability or visual functioning that has been corrected within average limits and if another individual is only able to view a similar object at 20 feet with best visual correction, then that person is considered "legally blind."

Partially sighted means a visual acuity greater than 20/200 but not greater than 20/70 in the better eye with best correction.

Low vision (Corn, 1980) refers to one who is still severely visually impaired after correction, but who may increase visual functioning through optical aids, nonoptical aids, or environmental modifications and/or techniques.

Functionally blind (Hatlen, 1980) is used to define one who uses a combination of auditory and tactile input for interpretation of written language.

It is also important to consider the differences between those individuals who have *congenital* visual impairments (a vision loss that is present at birth or manifests itself in early childhood) and those who have an *adventitious* visual loss (a visual loss that usually occurs later in life—adolescence or adulthood). Most visually impaired children and youth have congenital losses, or have lost their vision at an early age. The simple presence of some vision, or having a sense of visual imagery, makes a difference in conceptual development, organization of the environment, and understanding of abstract ideas such as understanding of personal space or appropriate physical appearance. In addition, the nature of the visual disability may affect daily functioning. Illumination, environmental obstacles, general physical health, tolerance to visual fatigue, and emotional stability may be influenced by specific visual etiologies.

Multihandicapped visually impaired persons constitute another group that requires some discussion. Perhaps of all the visually handicapped students who are served, this group is understood the least. There are a growing number of students with visual impairments and other anomalies. Their diversity of needs and program services is complex. The mere absence of vision makes it increasingly more difficult to teach fundamental concepts and tasks. However, a clear decision needs to be made as to whether the visual impairment is the primary obstacle to learning. Educators with expertise in visual disability need to work alongside specialists who have extensive training in behavior management, functional skills, positioning, and environmental adaptations so that optimal learning will occur.

PROGRAM MODELS

Educating blind and visually impaired children within public school settings initially began in the early 1900s. The prevailing philosophy among educators was, and to some degree still is, that given the appropriate nurturing, educational placement, and training, the blind or visually impaired child would develop just as his or her sighted peers except without sight or with limited visual ability. Although there was a great thrust forward to integrate visually impaired students into local school programs, the structure of the programs was highly restrictive, separating the blind students into their own classes on public school sites (Huebner, 1985). Despite such trends, most blind and visually impaired students continued to receive their educational training in residential school programs until the mid-1950s.

Residential School Programs

As in integrated programs, residential school programs emphasize the attainment of academic skills, while teaching adaptive tasks such as Braille, typing, abacus, and slate and stylus. The residential school also provides a social network for blind persons. Many schools provide lifelong support including vocational training and permanent residence. More recently, the role and function of residential schools has shifted to meet the functional needs of a more multihandicapped population or to provide short-term intensive training for students who are mainstreamed, yet are unable to receive specialized educational services such as orientation and mobility, daily living skills, or utilization of technological devices.

Hierarchy of Integrated School Programs for Visually Handicapped Students

The Pinebrook Report (American Foundation for the Blind, 1954) expanded the perspectives set forth earlier, and designed a framework for educating blind and visually impaired children in the "least restrictive environment." Participants at Pinebrook believed that "a blind child is a child first with the same needs and potentialities that all children possess" (American Foundation for the Blind, 1954, p. 13). This philosophy permeated the educational structure and established the role of the teacher of visually handicapped students (VH teacher) as one who provided equipment, materials, and specialized training to facilitate academic success in the regular classroom. Educators measured successful integration by the amount of time the child spent in the regular education setting. Three education models were presented, and still exist today; the appropriate placement is determined by the severity of the student's visual impairment, other educational needs, the home environment, and the structure and quality of services provided by the community.

Self-Contained VH Classroom The self-contained VH classroom provides a specialized program for visually handicapped students who have additional disabilities or who may require intense support in a structured classroom environment. Students who exhibit physical, emotional, behavioral, or other sensory impairments may be served in such a program. Often such classes are housed on public school sites, which can allow for opportunities to promote socialization with non-handicapped peers. Such programs can also be provided in a special school facility. The emphasis in programming is highly dependent upon the philosophical perspective and the educational training of the VH educator. However, there is a trend to incorporate a more functionally based approach into the structure of the daily curriculum.

VH Resource Room The VH resource room provides blind and visually handicapped students with a less restrictive educational program. It is housed on a public school campus and staffed by a VH teacher, and students are mainstreamed into regular education classes depending on their level of academic independence. A wide range of student abilities and needs is served within a resource room program. Many students use the resource room as a facility to receive training and assistance in adapting materials and learning to use assistive equipment and devices. The resource room program also lends itself to helping students acquire a set of essential nonacademic skills such as activities of daily living, career education, and social skills training. However, most of the students served in a resource room program must travel to one central geographic location instead of attending their neighborhood school program.

VH Itinerant Model The VH itinerant model allows blind and visually handicapped students to attend their neighborhood school, while receiving services from a teacher of visually handicapped persons. Usually the students are mainstreamed into the regular classroom setting for most of the school day. The VH teacher comes to the students' school and provides direct service on the school site. The amount and intensity of services are contingent upon the students' academic and nonacademic needs. The VH teacher also acts as a consultant to classroom teachers, program administrators, and specialized service personnel. Often itinerant services are provided to students who exhibit disabilities in addition to vision. Direct as well as consultative services may be provided depending on the individual needs of the students.

PHILOSOPHICAL STATEMENT

Given the variety of program models, the particularized needs of visually impaired students, and the "low prevalence" nature of this disability group, a philosophy that addresses the educational needs of an entire population of school-age children best finds its roots in its history. As stated earlier, visually handicapped students made up the first disability group to be mainstreamed into regular educational placements. In order to assure the success of such integration, the VH teacher has been called upon to provide a wide range of instructional services. These include: instruction in the use of the Braille code for reading, mathematics, music, and foreign language; teaching the use of electronic and computer technology; assistance in the acquisition of compensatory reading skills, tutoring of academic subjects; and provision of materials transcribed into appropriate media. The VH teacher has also been called upon to provide accurate assessment of academics, functional low vision, and developmental processes. In addition, the VH teacher has been the central "manager" of services—working with classroom teachers, orientation and mobility instructors, private service providers, and families to coordinate successful program endeavors. Increasingly, the field has recognized the need for intervention in the areas of daily living skills, community-based instruction, and prevocational skills and experiences. Finally, teachers have recognized the importance of social skills intervention as an underlying component of personal and academic success.

Providing an adequate and appropriate level of service can be a real challenge; one can be tempted to provide the media, the tutoring, and the coordination of services, and rightfully call it a day. The difficulty has been that often there are academically competent students who are socially isolated, and who are in critical need of socialization skill training. Yet the overriding educational priority for the teacher, the family, and the student continues to focus on the attainment of age-equivalent academic skills. Conversely, there are students with a multiplicity of physical, cognitive, and visual challenges whose family and teachers need the assistance of a specialist in visual impairment to interpret and to implement educational programming that fosters the acquisition of functional skills, and for whom traditional instructional academic models of Braille or large print do not apply.

However, there is a growing recognition among educators of visually handicapped students that the inclusion of nonacademic skills into the regular educational context is important. Bishop (1986), in her research dealing with the components that address successful mainstreaming of visually handicapped students, concludes that peer acceptance and interaction, adequate social skills, and a positive self-image have an impact on successful integration. Social skills are the foundation for much of what constitutes academic success. For example, the visually impaired child who can read but cannot wait his or her turn or can work appropriately in class but cannot engage in interactive play with a sighted peer is reaping only part of the benefits of an integrated program, and is building only part of the skill base for success outside of the school environment. The educator's challenge, then, is to search for ways to provide social skills instruction within the model provided to the visually handicapped student.

Each of the program models described present specialized opportunities for social skills instruction. First, the VH teacher must recognize the need for social skills instruction, and work with the family and the student in creating or supporting expectations of socially appropriate behavior in all educational and community environments. Second, within each of the service delivery models, each teacher can learn to recognize or create opportunities for social skills instruction for both special education and regular education students. Finally, the role of the teacher requires flexibility. Parents, educational supervisors, and school personnel can utilize the teacher of the visually impaired students best when traditional expectations are evaluated in light of the students' needs and long-term potentials. In fact, the needs of many visually impaired students classified by staff as "higher" functioning may be quite similar to those of a student exhibiting multiple disabilities. Each pupil needs to demonstrate a set of socially requisite behaviors in order to achieve acceptance by adults and peers alike.

To the visually impaired child, who lives in a world of social interactions that are largely visually cued and expressed in a nonverbal manner, social skills acquisitions is vital. When one assists students to acquire skills, to learn behaviors, and to compensate for some of the visual, observable interactions most people take for granted, one will have furthered integration at its most basic level. The ability to function socially underlies every classroom or program placement, and affects the quality of the student's interactions at large in the community. No philosophy of services for visually handicapped persons is complete if it encompasses only academic needs. The functional needs, particularly the social needs, of the visually impaired child must be addressed in every setting, by all of the people involved in the child's daily program.

SOCIAL INTEGRATION ACTIVITIES

The activities that follow address social skills instruction in a wide variety of settings. The authors have used the activities successfully, offering them in a variety of program models. In addition to these activities, the authors have found that many materials developed commercially or by local school districts lend themselves to adaptation for use with visually impaired students. They can also provide a springboard from which instructional programs can begin. For example, "Project Esteem" (Santa Clara Unified School District) contains a series of award certificates and behavior management materials that can easily be enlarged or Brailled to meet the needs of visually impaired children. *Developing an Understanding of Self and Others (DUSO)* (Dinkmeyer, 1970), *Magic*

Circle (Ball, 1974), and the "ungame" (The Ungame Co., 1975) provide meaningful ways to facilitate social interactions in group situations, either within a special day class setting using "reverse mainstreaming" techniques, or in a mainstreamed classroom environment where sighted and visually impaired students can learn more about one another. In addition, the Sex and Disability Unit of the Department of Psychiatry, Medical Center, University of California, San Francisco provided an initial foundation for the development of many social skills activities implemented by the authors.

It is important to note that the opportunities for social skill instruction are not limited by the program model, or by what is readily available, but rather by the ability of teachers and parents and later by the students themselves, to identify goals based on realistic expectations. Where teachers are given the flexibility and support to create such instruction, creative and meaningful strategies can occur. Presented within the following pages are six different instructional activities to help promote and maximize social integration for visually handicapped students.

The Kitchen Curriculum

The development of competent social behavior in visually handicapped children is a partnership between the home and school environments. Further, the development of such skills is highly dependent upon experiential learning and consistent expectations for appropriate social behavior. In studies of early language development of visually handicapped children, Anderson, Dunlea, and Kekelis (1984) demonstrated that the blind children in their study tended to be self-centered; they failed to acknowledge the interests and perspectives of others and they were unresponsive to the language and behaviors of others. Further, they asked many questions and made numerous demands on adults and peers to facilitate collaborative interactions. In a recent qualitative study examining young visually handicapped childrens' (5- to 7-year-olds) social interactions with sighted age-mates in a school setting, Kekelis and Sacks (1988) observed similar characteristics and noted that the students' imaginative play behaviors with peers were very restrictive and concrete. The children had difficulty with expansion and elaboration of real-life experiences. Their language mimicked that of an adult or caregiver in their daily environment.

In order to facilitate greater exposure and experience for the young visually handicapped child, Naughton and Sacks (1977) designed a curriculum to help parents create activities that foster social competence, responsibility, and independence; and to help parents enhance cognitive and language skills through experiential learning. Naughton and Sacks proposed that much of a family's interaction may occur within the kitchen during meal preparation, mealtime, and during clean-up. They also hypothesized that the kitchen with all its gadgets creates an environment where exploration and early social development can take place.

The "kitchen curriculum" provides suggestions for parents, and can be used by educators to promote social interaction while teaching basic living skills. The curriculum begins with general guidelines for introducing the child to touch, taste, sound, and smell. These are basic to growing and learning. Then suggestions are provided for helping the child to develop skills in performing daily tasks, survival cooking, and clean-up so that the child becomes a contributing member of the family unit. The ultimate goal of this outline is to ensure that the visually impaired student has an equal opportunity to share in the pleasure and fulfillment of developing a sense of independence and self-worth. Although the kitchen environment may pose some initial danger, protecting the child from such experiences can be just as dangerous. A child who is deprived of experience does not continue to seek new experiences. Curiosity, especially for the blind child, may decrease, and the motivation for learning new concepts and ideas may diminish. The opposite occurs when the child is encouraged to participate in new experiences.

The skills and suggestions provided in the curriculum are arranged according to chronological age, but the authors recognize that the individual development of each visually impaired child is different, and that the activities outlined for each age range are only guidelines for implementation. Most of the activities presented in the kitchen curriculum are specifically designed for preschool and elementary-age visually handicapped students, but are not exclusive of older students.

Intervention

Each activity is designed to develop a close working relationship between the parent or caregiver and the child. Many of the activities focus on the importance of appropriate social behavior, or the acquisition of a specific social skill such as eye contact. Through the acquisition of such skills, the child begins to develop a sense of self-worth and social competence. For example, the activities for 2–3-year-olds (see Table 1) encourage independence and a sense of responsibility while promoting interactive communication skills.

Allowing the child to perform specific household chores provides opportunities for him or her to develop a sense of self-sufficiency, to learn a natural means of asking for assistance in initiating or completing a task, and to expand and enhance expressive language through adult facilitation. Parents can encourage discussion of the shape, form, texture, and size of items used for particular chores around the kitchen by making open-ended statements such as, "Tell me all about this napkin" or, "Tell me some ways you can use the napkin." While talking with the child, the parent or caregiver can also provide positive cues regarding appropriate direction of gaze or body posture. Such information will help the child to recognize what is expected of her or him within appropriate social contexts. Several illustrations of activities are presented in Table 1. (If the reader is interested in obtaining the entire kitchen curriculum, contact: Franczeska Naughton, South Metropolitan Association for Low Incidence Handicapped Children, 800 Governors Highway, Flossmore, IL.)

Table 1.   Kitchen curriculum activities

2–3 Years

1. Allow child to experience function of movable parts. For example: spray plants, squirt detergent in bowl, open cans, assist in scooping ice cream.
2. Begin household chores.
   a. Carry napkins to table.
   b. If samples of food are available, such as carrot stick from salad, say "Bring to Daddy, sister, brother . . . "
   c. Place frequently used utensils where child can reach and ask child to give you: the pan, the measuring cup, serving spoon, and so forth.
3. Increase exposure to different textures and tastes. Include child in one or more steps of cooking and baking. Example: softness of flour, grittiness of sugar, moistness of butter, sliminess of eggs, feel of dough. Taste raw dough, mold like clay. Then experience taste and temperature of newly baked product.

3–4 Years

1. Assist in household chores.
   a. Teach child to fold napkins
   b. Bring utensils to table.
   c. Return dishes to kitchen table.
   d. Push food scraps off plates into wastebasket (or sink if there is a disposal). This is good early training for search-exploring techniques essential to a wide range of activities.
2. Assist in cooking:
   a. Stir batter, salads, vegetables, and so forth.
   b. Shred lettuce.
   c. Mix powder with liquid, such as chocolate milk, pudding. Child will need to check progress of mixing with fingers. Fingers are a most efficient tool and a blind child learns to substitute touch for sight. The wise parent quickly accepts what might appear to be messy and unsavory as an essential learning step. During the child's third year he or she is also gaining independence in washing his or her hands. Helping in the kitchen provides many opportunities to clean hands, too!
3. Use cooking and baking activities to become aware of time.
   a. Baking cookies.
   b. Cooling pudding.
   c. Freezing ice cubes.

Using a kitchen timer to alert child to time period. Adapt timer for visual impairment by raising dots or enlarging minute signs with nail polish or glue.

4–5 Years

1. Assist in household chores:
   a. Learn correct table placement and help set table.
   b. Put cheese on crackers; meat on bread.
   c. Spoon out jelly on bread. (This will probably be messy but will prepare the child for later tasks and is a tasty job.)
2. Use left and right side orientation skills. Knife goes on right side of plate. Fork goes on left side. Cup goes in front of knife. Chair goes behind plate.
3. Set standards of appropriate table behavior. Because of the importance of practice, the family of the visually impaired child will benefit if everyone regularly eats together and high standards of behavior are maintained. Learning good manners is important for later socialization away from home. *Socially acceptable eating habits and manners are the right of every blind child.* They don't come naturally. Good habits are taught.
   a. Use "please" and "thank you" regularly.
   b. Pass food around table rather than always serving child. For example: teach child to *take* one roll—not to *feel* every roll.
   c. Wait for child to ask for help—don't anticipate every need.
4. Introduce fork. Use of spoon is now well established. In teaching use of fork, identify and maintain appropriate use. For example, insist that fork is used for meats and pancakes. Do not let child revert to fingers. A stabbing motion (enjoyable) is used until child is comfortable. With greater practice, child should be encouraged to use a slower, smoother, rhythmic movement. At this age child will use one hand to locate bite-size food and the other to pierce food.

5–6 Years

1. Assist in household chores.
   a. Increase independence in completing previous tasks.
   b. Fill glasses with assistance. (During early years buy quart containers or transfer from larger containers to pitcher.)

(continued)

Table 1. *(continued)*

c. Spread butter, peanut butter, jelly.
2. Add to table manners.
  a. Serve own food at table. Practice appropriate amount on spoon.
  b. Discourage use of hands to eat. Use spoon and fork. Don't rush. Allow extra time at family meals. Make the dinner hour a pleasant family sharing time allowing plenty of time for child to carry through
	good manners. (Blind child needs time for eating. An extra 15 minutes built into each mealtime really pays off.)
	3. Supplement cooking tasks by discussing the different textures of foods through changing conditions. Example: cookies changing from soft to hard through baking-cooling process; renew and review touching, molding, smelling, tasting with more emphasis on change.

Adapted from Naughton and Sacks (1977).

Peer-Mediated Social Skills Training

Description and Rationale

Social skills research that has investigated the social competence of visually handicapped students within the mainstream is limited. Previous studies have provided valuable information about how visually impaired individuals acquire and maintain a set of appropriate social skills. Unfortunately, the training procedures that have been implemented have been weak in their methodological approach and replicability. Also, many of the investigations used adults as training confederates in artificial settings. While some short-term, positive results were yielded from such studies, more recent research has examined the efficacy of using competent age-mates as social skills trainers with a variety of disabled children. Strain and his colleagues

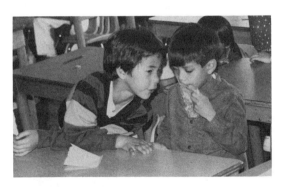

Friendships are developed between blind and sighted children when effective peer training occurs in natural contexts.

were the first to employ such strategies with emotionally disturbed and autistic children (Hendrickson, Strain, Tremblay, & Shores, 1982; Ragland, Kerr, & Strain, 1981; Strain, 1977; Strain, Shores, & Timm, 1977). Voeltz (1982) expanded the peer-mediated approach in a more naturalistic manner. Instead of an adult or teacher directing the training, nonhandicapped peers and their disabled counterparts mutually determined play and training activities. In her *Special Friends* studies with elementary-age severely handicapped students and their nonhandicapped age-mates, Voeltz observed the development of genuine friendships, as well as the attainment and maintenance of socially appropriate behaviors among the severely handicapped students. Similar effects were obtained with severely handicapped and autistic high school students in a mainstreamed school environment (Chin-Perez et al., 1986; Gaylord-Ross, Haring, Breen, & Pitts-Conway, 1984).

Sisson, Van Hasselt, Hersen, and Strain (1985) initiated a peer-mediated social skills training intervention with young (9–11-year-old) multihandicapped, visually handicapped students in a residential school setting. They employed nonhandicapped (NH) peers from a local elementary school to become peer trainers. The NH peers received instruction that helped them to facilitate greater interaction and responses from their VH counterparts. Results of a multiple baseline design across subjects indicated substantial gains in positive social initiations and appropriate play behavior, with moderate generalization of skill acquisition to other settings and children on a 3-month follow-up probe.

Most recently, Sacks (1987) initiated a peer-mediated social skills training procedure with elementary-age (7–12-year-old) visually handicapped students within a mainstreamed school environment. Grounded within a social learning framework, Sacks hypothesized that the impact of peer modeling and reinforcement (Bandura, 1977; Bandura & Walters, 1963; Corsaro, 1985; Gaylord-Ross & Pitts-Conway, 1984; Mischel, 1966) would provide a powerful tool to initiate and maintain positive social behavior among visually handicapped students. The information that peers provide to one another helps them develop skills to gain entry into groups, to maintain their activities, and to generate new interests. The power of peer input and honest feedback also provides a basis for the development of genuine relationships. In other words, peers will maintain and generalize appropriate social behavior learned through peer direction because they want to be accepted and liked by others. Sacks recognized, however, that in order for such training to yield successful results, the nonhandicapped peers needed to receive inservice training and consistent feedback from an adult facilitator (teacher or social skills trainer). Using a multiple baseline across behaviors design, Sacks clearly demonstrated the efficacy of such an approach. Increases for each targeted behavior were observed from baseline to training. More important, the students demonstrated even stronger effects on each targeted behavior during generalization probes, with some maintenance of behaviors on 1-month follow-up probes. Figure 1 illustrates the social gains that were observed for Anna.

Program Model

Although the peer-mediated intervention employed in the Sacks (1987) study utilized only elementary-age visually handicapped students, similar procedures could be initiated with other age groups, particularly adolescent and secondary-level students. The training strategies themselves seem to be most effective when performed in a re-

source room or special day class environment. The structure and consistency of such settings provides the visually handicapped and the non-handicapped students with a variety of alternatives for play and relaxed interactions.

Intervention

In the Sacks (1987) study each visually impaired student selected for the peer-mediated social skills training intervention agreed to participate in the training before its onset. The visually handicapped students were informed that nonhandicapped peers from their mainstreamed classrooms would be invited to participate as peer trainers in a brief in-class presentation. Every effort was made to make sure that the VH peers recognized that their relationship with their NH peer counterparts was one of equality and was mutually beneficial for both groups.

The visually handicapped students were invited to attend the in-class presentations. The presentation itself emphasized the importance of developing friendships among disabled and nondisabled students. The teacher or social skills trainer pointed out that without vision or with limited vision, learning specific social behaviors such as making eye contact or joining a group may be particularly difficult for VH peers. The presentor outlined the specific time requirements of the program: the number of training days per week (3 per week); the training time per session (30-minute training session); a weekly inservice training session to enhance specific intervention strategies, to give an explanation of where training can occur (resource room or playground), and to provide examples of activities to encourage social interaction among both groups of students. The NH students were encouraged to ask questions. After the presentation the nonhandicapped students volunteered for participation in the program.

The mainstreamed classroom teacher along with the VH teacher or social skills trainers selected the nonhandicapped peers. It has been the experience of the first author of the chapter that selection of same-sex dyads (one VH and one NH peer) or same-sex triads (one VH peer and two NH peers) seems to be most effective. Also, choosing high-status nonhandicapped students (students with above-average academic skills, and an ability to demonstrate positive social behaviors in acquiring and maintaining friendships with a group of peers) has helped to facilitate more positive effects. It should be noted, however, that other peer-mediated strategies could be initiated depending on the school environment. For example, utilizing the skills of older, socially competent visually handicapped students may be an effective alternative.

Before the actual social skills training begins, specific social behaviors need to be targeted for training. Generally, the VH teacher with student input determines which behaviors will be targeted for training. It is also interesting to ask the non-handicapped peer trainers to observe their visually handicapped age-mates in natural social contexts, and have them target specific social behaviors that they feel justify training. Some initial baseline data should be taken to determine pretraining levels of performance in structured (classroom) and unstructured (playground, cafeteria) environments.

At the onset of training for each program week, the nonhandicapped peers should meet with the adult social skill trainer. The inservice training should last approximately 30 minutes and should focus on training one specific social behavior. Initially the adult facilitator should introduce and clearly define the social behavior being trained. Then, the NH students should be encouraged to think of ways they could learn the targeted behavior without vision. Next, modeling of specific training strategies is presented to the peers. They are then asked to role play being the visually impaired student and the peer trainer. Verbal feedback and physical modeling from the adult trainer provides immediate reinforcement to enhance later training strategies. Examples of the inservice training protocols are provided in Table 2. (For a complete set of the inservice training strategies employed during the peer-mediated social skills training sequence, contact: Sharon Zell Sacks,

Department of Special Education, San Francisco State University, 1600 Holloway Avenue, San Francisco, CA 94132.)

Before the onset of each training session, the adult trainer briefly met with the nonhandicapped peer trainers to review the specific strategies for training a targeted social behavior. Then the VH peers and their sighted counterparts met in the resource room to select a mutually determined activity. Initially, the peer groups needed some prompting to facilitate the initial play process. The social skills instruction given to the visually handicapped peers was somewhat more unstructured and relaxed than the typical behavior training sequence (instruction, modeling, role play, rehearsal, feedback). Much of the instruction took place within the context of play. Those visually handicapped students who had useful vision began to physically model the behavior of their peers. Other students with very limited visual ability received feedback from their peers regarding facial expressions, body stance, and physical positioning within groups. The VH students also began to use age-appropriate initiations and elaborations in conversations with peers. At the end of each training sequence, positive feedback and suggestions to improve the training were provided to the nonhandicapped students. Table 3 provides a list of activities and responses initiated by both groups of peers during the peer-mediated approach.

Behavioral Contracts

Description and Rationale

Along with a structured social skills training procedure, visually handicapped students can benefit from behavioral contracts that reinforce appropriate social behavior in a variety of educational and community settings. Such strategies can employ self-monitoring techniques where the reminder of a tangible cue (written contract on desk) can stimulate appropriate social behavior. Such strategies are particularly beneficial for students who are preparing for an integrated classroom experience.

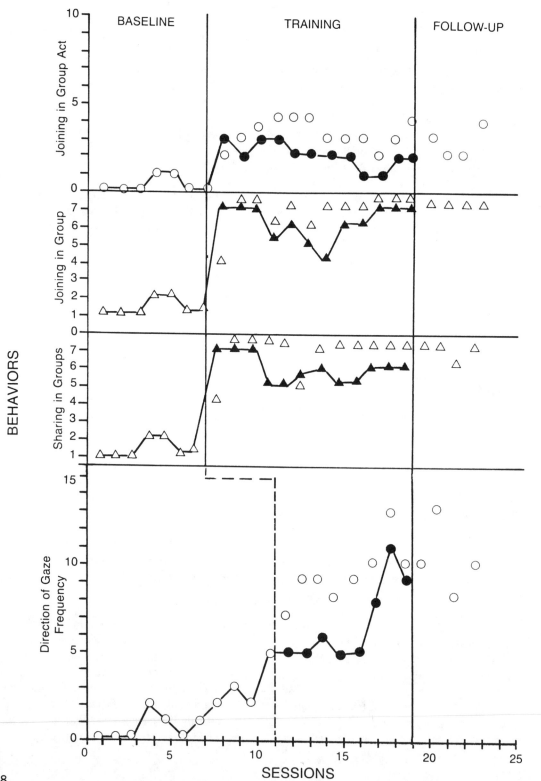

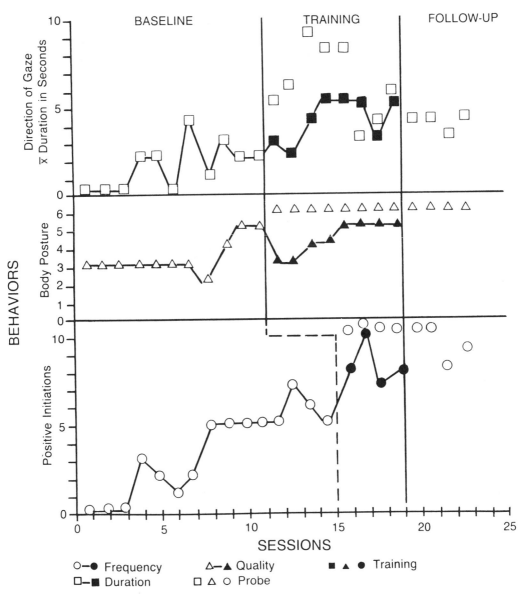

Figure 1. Effects of peer-mediated social skills training for Anna.

Initially, many of these students have some difficulty working independently or interacting effectively in a group environment.

Participants

The population included students who had a range of vision from moderate loss to total blindness. Some students had additional challenges that included moderate to severe hearing impairments, learning disabilities, behavioral disorders, neurological involvements, language delays or disorders, and/or developmental delays.

Program Model

The authors have used behavior contracts in special day classes at regular education sites and at a

Table 2.   Inservice training protocols for nonhandicapped (NH) peer trainers

Behavior Trained

Introduction to the visually handicapped (VH) student and a description of his or her visual impairment.

Procedure

Investigator names and describes specific visual disability. Simulation of visual impairment may be employed to help the NH peers understand the adaptations and limitations incurred by the VH student. Discussion of the ways VH students can adapt and participate in activities within school and community each session. The sequence of training follows that of the peer-mediated approach and targeted behaviors are randomly selected for training. Environment without the use of optimal vision is encouraged.

Answer questions and clarify any preconceived notions about how visually impaired individuals perform tasks.

Outcomes

The nonhandicapped peer trainers will develop heightened awareness of and sensitivity toward their visually handicapped peers' abilities and limitations. They will also develop more realistic expectations for their VH counterpart.

Behavior Trained

Direction of gaze (eye contact) and body posture (Trained simultaneously).

Procedure

Name and define behavior being trained.

Discuss the importance of using appropriate eye contact and body posture in social situations.

Have NH peers identify the elements of acceptable eye contact and body posture.

Ask the students to interpret the meaning of specific behaviors being modeled by the investigator (e.g., investigator talks to students, but does not look at them, or investigator keeps head down while engaged in a conversation).

Ask the students how they would change the behaviors modeled. If the students do not respond, provide specific prompting procedures such as verbal phrases (look up) or physical prompts (tap on shoulder).

Provide role play scenarios where the NH peers must employ corrective feedback or praise. Encourage the peers to praise their VH counterparts, but also to give honest feedback. Use role plays that reflect experiences that both peers have encountered.

Have the NH peers practice corrective and praise responses through the role-play scenes until the desired responses are used with 80% proficiency.

Outcomes

The VH student will improve his or her ability to initiate and to maintain appropriate gaze and posture in a variety of social contexts.

The incidence of mannerisms (rocking, head or hand waving) will be reduced to enhance acceptable body posture.

Behavior Trained

Positive social initiations.

Procedure

Name and define behavior being trained.

Discuss with NH peers the way they greet friends, topics of conversation, games and activities they particularly like to play.

Have the NH students role play a typical social interaction or greeting.

Ask the students to analyze the good and bad parts of the interaction. Emphasize that interactions or initiations have a beginning, a middle, and an end. Ask the peers to think about what part of an initiation might be particularly difficult for a VH student. If the students have difficulty responding, the investigator might prompt some thoughts (e.g., If you cannot see another person standing nearby, how do you know the person's identity, or that there is a peer in proximity?). Encourage solutions such as providing verbal feedback, using auditory cues, or sensation cues (changes in temperature or shadowing).

Provide role plays where the investigator assumes the role of the VH student. Provide situations for peers where the VH student will not initiate a conversation, where the VH student is overly verbal, or where the VH student is overly aggressive and uses hostile phrases to engage in social interactions.

Provide verbal feedback (praise or prompts) for each NH peer response. Model specific responses or initiators to specific situations (e.g., If the VH student is overly verbal [talks about the same topic or self] have the NH peer use phrases such as, "You always talk about that. How about changing the subject?" or, "Gee! I really like you, but I can't get a word in. You're always talking.").

Encourage NH students to train VH students to

(continued)

Table 2. *(continued)*

use complimentary statements about others (e.g., "Good shot" or "That's neat").

Have NH peers practice phrases and statements that will prompt the VH student to use initiators ("Hi, How ya doin?" or "I like what you're wearing today."), icebreakers ("Wanna have lunch together?" or "Hey, did you watch *Cosby* last night?"), or engaging statements ("You were great in class today." or "I have that transformer."). Practice role plays until prompts and feedback responses are used with 80% proficiency.

Answer questions and encourage discussion.

Outcomes

The visually handicapped student will demonstrate increases in positive initiations with peers, expanded conversations, and greater use of complimentary statements.

Behavior Trained

Joining in group activities (trained simultaneously with sharing in group activities).

Procedure

Name and define behavior being trained.

Have NH students describe how they join a group on the playground at recess, in the cafeteria at lunch, or in the classroom during a free-time activity.

Explain or reinforce how the effect of limited vision or no vision may influence independent joining.

Blindfold or use vision simulators on NH students. Have the students practice joining a group engaged in play while under simulation.

Have NH peers provide impressions and discuss ways to facilitate joining.

If the NH students do not provide solutions, provide several suggestions (e.g., meeting a friend at a designated spot, having the VH student practice asking for assistance to find a friend or a particular game on the playground).

Have NH peers practice phrases that will help VH peers gain entry into groups in a positive manner (e.g., "Gee, can I play?" or "How about playing, _____?"). Use role plays and actual practice in

natural settings until phrases and prompts are used with 80% proficiency.

Outcomes

The visually handicapped student will enter into group activities in an independent manner. If assistance is needed, the visually handicapped student will use statements that generate positive responses from peers.

Behavior Trained

Sharing in group activities (trained simultaneously with joining in group activities—an extension of joining).

Procedure

Name and define behavior being trained.

Ask NH peers to describe positive sharing techniques

Ask peers to describe techniques that are negative.

Help NH peers to understand that without sight or with limited vision, the VH peer may need help with turn taking in game playing or not interrupting in actual conversations.

Teach peers phrases or statements to help the VH student become aware of turn-taking techniques (e.g., "Hey, _____, just wait a minute." or "Wait for your turn." or "You're interrupting me, wait a minute, okay?").

Have NH peers teach games to VH peers that will facilitate sharing and turn taking (e.g., board games, outdoor games, sharing snacks, trading toys, sharing a special toy.)

Have NH peers practice phrases that will help the VH peers to understand good sportsmanship (e.g., "It's just a game." or "You don't always have to win." or "Don't get so upset, it's only a game.").

Provide role-play situations where the NH peers can practice corrective responses and honest feedback with 80% proficiency.

Outcomes

The visually handicapped student will increase his or her ability to share in a variety of group situations using turn-taking techniques and asserting rights in a positive manner.

state school where some of the students were in residence and others were day students. The contracts were modified to include mainstream experiences as they developed for individual students.

Intervention

1. Attach a written statement to the student's desk in either large print or Braille, which includes:

Table 3. Peer-mediated training activities, interactions, and responses from nonhandicapped (NH) peers to visually handicapped (VH) participants for each targeted behavior

Behavior	Activities	Nonhandicapped peer input	Visually handicapped peer responses
Direction of gaze and body posture	*Board games* Checkers, Simon, Sorry, Connect Four, Monopoly, Fish, 21, Othello, computer games *Outdoor games* Playing on equipment (play structures), hand claps, finger plays	*Phrases used* Hey! Sit up. ____, when you talk to me, how about looking at me? ____ (pause) ____, you look really neat. ____, please stop that.	*Verbal responses* Okay, I forgot. Thanks for reminding me. Ya, I'll stop. Ya, I know I do. *Nonverbal responses* VH student sits or stands with appropriate posture and longer gaze
Positive initiations	Drawing on blackboard Playing with dolls, with a doll house Playing with transformers or action figures, sharing a snack or toy, talking about school, talking about boys	Gee, you did a good job. What do you want to play? You decide. Hi! What's new? What did you watch last night?, Hey, did you see *ALF* last night?, So what's happening? It would sure be neat if you could come over after school. Hey, did you hear about ____? He likes ____.	Ya, thanks, it's a ____. How about dolls or a game? Hi, how ya doin?, Hey, did you see *ALF* last night? I'd like that, but I have to ask my mom, and figure a way home. No, what happened? He's cute.
Joining in group activities and sharing in group activities	Playing on play equipment (dramatic play), kickball, wallball, basketball, chase, jump rope Dramatic play with action figures, waiting in line for food in the cafeteria, eating lunch on the grass (small group), hanging out on a bench (conversing), walking around the play area. *Indoor activities* Cooking projects, computer games, puzzles, hangman, board games, art projects.	Okay, ____ let's meet and then we can play ____. Wanta play kickball? (peer runs off). Okay, ____ it's your turn. Just wait, ____. It's ____ turn. First you'll have a turn, and then me.	I'll meet you at the drinking fountain. Ya, wait for me. Thanks, but where do I stand? I'll go after you, all right? That sounds great.

a.   A statement of the time period involved (e.g., by Friday afternoon; or, every day this week; or, from the beginning of the day until first recess).

b.   A statement of the goal to be achieved (e.g., I will earn [set a number] of [note the markers given]) that will be attached to the contract so the student can monitor his or her progress.

The authors found the following to be successful for younger students:

1) Scratch-and-Sniff stickers.
2) Brightly colored stickers.

For middle elementary and older students:

1) File "flag" dots.
2) Holes made with a paper punch.

c.   The behaviors to be achieved (e.g., raising my hand for help, waiting my turn, working at my desk).

d.   The reward to be gained at the end for the period (e.g., a free-time certificate to be "spent" for time at a favorite activity, selection of something from the "prize box").

2.   Review the document with the student on a regular schedule; the authors began with short time periods, then extended the time over which the behaviors sought were noted. Be consistent with rewarding the behavior; the authors attached a paper punch to their belts, or carried dots in their pockets at all times. A "runner's" watch was useful, because they could set it either to remind themselves that a period of time had passed requiring the teacher to monitor behavior, or to beep softly as a reminder to students that an agreed-upon, limited time was passing.

3.   Identify with students specific behaviors that are expected. The authors held a conference with each student on Monday morning to review the general contract, and to identify something special he or she was working on. The conferences gave the authors an opportunity to talk about why rocking, eye poking, or heading turning was targeted. In addition, it gave them an idea of how the student was responding; in one case, they discovered that the student, who had a severe hearing impairment, knew only the signs for "angry" and "happy." The authors added new signs for emotions and responses, and included their appropriate use in contract goals.

4.   For younger students, stickers can themselves be the goal, and they will want to take them at the end of each period of monitoring. When the period becomes extended, the authors added free-time tokens or certificates; time at favorite activities; and the "prize box," which contained tangible rewards related to grooming, recreation, or personal organization. Prizes included perfume and after-shave samples, hand-lotion samples, combs, toothbrushes, make-up samples, key rings, wallets, inexpensive book bags or totes, inexpensive athletic totes, lip glosses or Chapsticks, shampoo samples, toothpaste samples, deodorant samples, heavy paper folders, signature guides, small binders for Braille notes, Braille erasers, inexpensive cassette tapes— each of which cost between 59¢ and $2.00. Using the "prize box" also gave the authors an opportunity to teach the use of the items selected.

5.   The authors ultimately extended the contract to the mainstream setting. Where the student was traveling to another classroom or school, independence at travel, bringing and delivering homework, participating in extracurricular activities, and so forth became goals. The authors dropped the contracts when the student was participating in the mainstream environment not only academically, but socially as well.

Figure 2 provides an example of a behavioral contract for a visually handicapped student. The contract was developed for a younger student who had particular difficulty with group skills. Although having very low vision, the student wrote

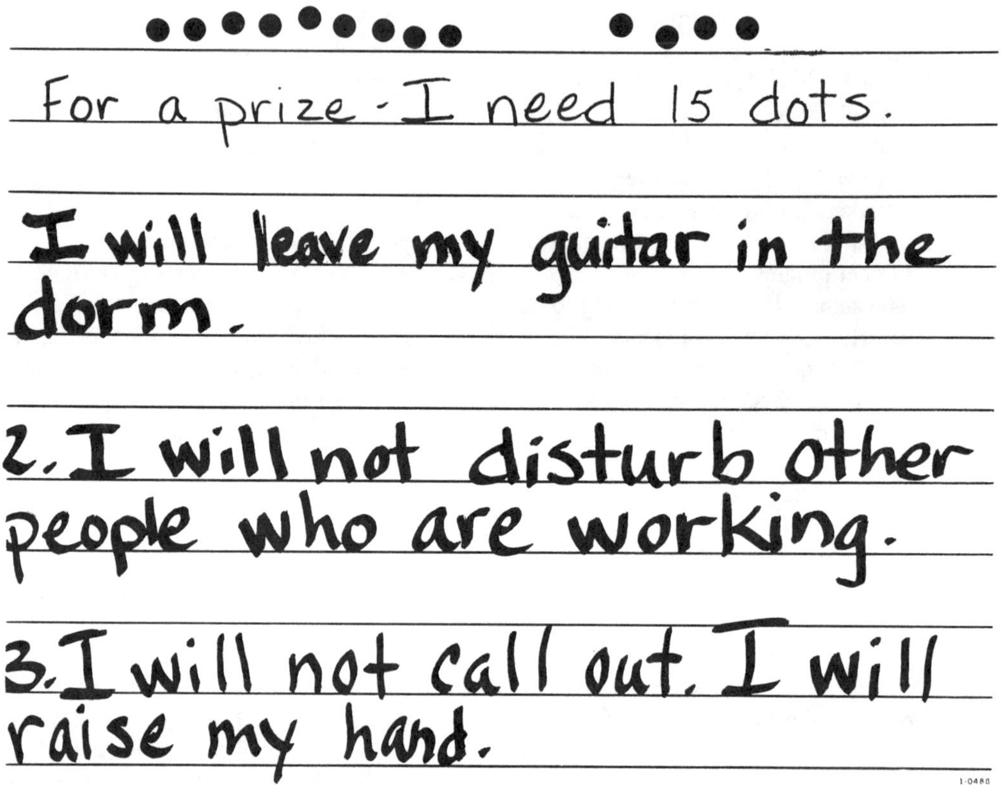

● ● ● ● ● ● ● ● ● ●   ● ● ● ●

For a prize. I need 15 dots.

I will leave my guitar in the dorm.

2. I will not disturb other people who are working.

3. I will not call out. I will raise my hand.

Figure 2.   Example of a behavioral contract written by a student with difficulty with group skills.

out his own contract with assistance from the VH teacher.

Training Physical Skills

Description and Rationale

Many social interactions are learned visually through imitation and modeling. Appropriate social behaviors that are taken for granted are learned incidentally at a very young age. For example, persons who are sighted know that there is a field of "personal space" that varies from person to person and culture to culture, that people face one another while conversing, and that postures or gestures can be "statements" in and of themselves or can affect the impact of verbal statements. Fur-

ther, much of this knowledge is not consciously considered when engaging in social interactions. For the visually impaired child, however, learning these common assumptions about the utilization of appropriate physical behavior requires direct intervention.

Program Models

The development of such skills is critical to the interactive ability of visually handicapped students and can be incorporated into a variety of program models. Training of such physical skills can easily be infused into group discussions in special day classes or resource room programs. It is not uncommon for a VH teacher to work individually with an itinerant student on increasing or decreasing a targeted social behavior. In addition, many of these skills can be easily implemented in a group format.

Participants

The intervention strategies outlined in this section can be used with a wide range of severely visually handicapped students. Many of the techniques and examples employed were used with multi-handicapped/visually handicapped students, deaf-blind students, and students who were considered functionally blind.

Intervention

Several specific examples of physical behaviors requiring training are presented both for individual and group instruction. When developing intervention strategies for visually handicapped students in a mainstream, vocational, or community-based program, some general guidelines need to be addressed. These include:

1. The student should be prepared for the intervention. Many children and adolescents are at once concerned about their appearance and defensive about direct approaches to changes in their appearance or behavior. An approach that stresses the rewards of changed appearance from the outset has distinct advantages.
2. Target the items you and the student will work on. Identify the strategies you will use, and preface the need for changes by providing information on how posture, body movement, gesture, and body position communicate to persons who are sighted.
3. Use positive reinforcement strategies, and ensure that others involved (parents, support staff, siblings) use the same positive approach.

For students with a multiplicity of challenges, behavior management strategies are useful. Target the behavior sought, and ensure that adequate baseline data are obtained. Use reinforcement techniques that are known to be successful with the student.

Eye Contact The concept of eye contact has numerous implications for a blind child. It is difficult to convey the importance of a skill that is virtually impossible to perform for the child who has no vision, who may have a cosmetic problem, or whose vision is so limited that "gaze" is meaningless. The authors have found it helpful to use alternative descriptions of what is needed:

1. "People face each other when speaking."
2. "If you face me, I know that you're paying attention."
3. "When your face is pointed to the floor (or to the desk top, or your ear is turned to me) I don't know whether you are talking with me or someone else."

For the child who has multiple disabilities, visual and/or auditory stimulation can accomplish the same goal:

1. Use a bright toy (a pinwheel, a battery-operated toy, a tape recorder) and pair it with gaze. Reinforce the head turn and keep the object close to the face. Fade the toy, and continue to reinforce head turns toward the face of the speaker.
2. Pair a handshake with a light touch to the face, turning the child's face to the speaker. Reinforce with a statement or an extra handshake.

Gestures All students can be taught gestures in one setting or another. For one child, simply learning to extend a hand as a good-bye and a hello is a significant increase in communication. For another child, learning to wave a car past, to shake hands, to "flag" a waitress, or to raise a hand to an oncoming bus means independence and improved communication.

1. Determine the level of gesture communication appropriate to the student. Use commu-

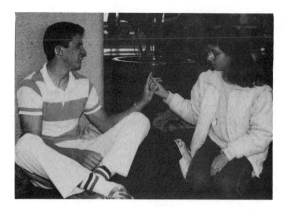

Adaptive communication enhances positive social interaction.

nity-based activities where possible, as the reinforcement comes quickly from peers and the public rather than from staff members and/or family members alone.

2. Most severely visually impaired students will need some motor prompting or motor support to learn gestures. Where appropriate, give a verbal cue along with motor support.

3. For the student who signs, careful observation of gestures used should be made. Manual communication may occur only within the field of the student's vision, and much information about other gestures may be missing.

4. Rehearse gestures either by consistent motor support intervention sequences or through instruction and practice.

5. Prompt or support the student in using the gestures on the playground, at the bus stop, and so forth.

6. Encourage independent expression by gesture through wider use of gestures in the environment.

Body Language   It is important to master some posture, gaze turn, and gesture skills before beginning with body language. Therefore, the skills discussed here should be used by students who have mastered some physical communication skills. Social skills groups are useful for these activities.

1. Using motor support, assist students in making a fist, then shaking it. Discuss the possible messages inherent in doing this to another person. Have the students lean forward, coming very close to another, and have them speak loudly. Discuss the physical messages here.

2. Describe some of the basic body language messages (any text or work on the subject will provide the information), then assist the students in demonstrating them.

    The authors found it useful to relate this to passive/aggressive/assertive stances. They used relaxation exercises (deep breathing, head rolls, shoulder lifts) to prepare the students for movement. Then, they practiced hunched shoulders and clenched fists, followed by dropped heads and loose arms, then erect posture and comfortable arm and leg stances.

3. Use role playing between students and peers, student and staff, to practice.

4. Introduce the concept of the "double message"—an assertive request with an aggressive stance, an aggressive statement with a passive stance, and so forth. Students who had limited vision and a hearing impairment found these activities generally useful in improving their communication skills.

5. Have the students demonstrate their body language skills to family, peers, and staff (particularly the orientation and mobility staff), and support their use of appropriate body language in community activities.

Inappropriate Movement   One of the most common concerns about visually impaired students among staff, family, and peers is behavior such as rocking, "flicking," eye poking, head rolling, and repetitive hand gestures that appear meaningless to sighted persons.

1. Determine where the behaviors occur, and ensure through a physical or occupational therapist (PT/OT) that the behavior can and

should be addressed by family and staff without the assistance of a PT/OT.

2. Use behavior modification techniques to determine baseline, goals, and intervention strategies.

3. Some students will respond to a stimulus that reminds them that they are moving. (One student wore a small bell in the rubber band holding her pony tail; she preferred to self-correct without reinforcement from someone else.)

4. Other students preferred to choose a setting in which they worked on diminishing a behavior while remaining free to demonstrate it elsewhere. The authors used this as an introduction to the idea of privacy and private place, helping the student to distinguish rocking on public transportation from rocking while relaxing in the privacy of his or her room.

NOTE: Facial expression can be taught with difficulty. The authors generally worked to assist students to reduce inappropriate expressions (such as smiling while relating sad news), and included some general information while working on body language.

In addition to the examples provided thus far, Table 4 provides some specific curricular strategies for training physical behaviors in a structured group format. Attainment of each targeted physical behavior is written in terms of a behavioral goal and objective. Then specific methods and evaluation procedures are presented to help facilitate acquisition of the target skill.

Assertiveness Training

Description and Rationale

Once visually handicapped students have developed a set of socially competent behaviors, it is important to apply such behaviors in assertive interactions with peers, adults, co-workers, and potential employers. One concern among educators and rehabilitation personnel working with visually handicapped students is that the behavior exhibited by their clients seemed passive or aggressive, rather than assertive (Rickelman & Blaylock, 1983). Van Hasselt, Hersen, and Kazdin (1984), for example, observed that on initial social skills assessments of visually handicapped adolescents, use of hostile tone, lack of positive statements toward others, and lack of eye contact and appropriate body posture were apparent. Harrell and Strauss (1986) provide several suggestions to facilitate assertive behavior among visually handicapped persons. In their work with visually handicapped students within a classroom setting, they have successfully used journal writing, sentence-completion exercises, role playing, and self-help groups to promote assertion skills. They have also found that interaction with competent visually handicapped individuals fosters assertive behavior and provides a positive vehicle for students to share experiences unique to the visually impaired person.

Program Model

Assertion training seems to be most effective in a group format where the students have similar cognitive or functional abilities. It is also helpful to develop a program where video and audio equipment is readily available. The authors found self-monitoring techniques to be extremely useful in developing assertive behavior in the students they served.

Participants

Because assertive behavior involves higher order skills and techniques, such strategies were implemented with secondary-level students. The students were functionally blind or had low vision, and had good communication skills. Many of the students involved in the training were deaf-blind, but demonstrated good signing techniques. The authors also found it effective to invite nonhandicapped peers to participate in the assertiveness training sessions. These students provided another dimension to the overall success of the training.

Table 4.   Training physical behaviors in a structured group format

Physical Skills: Introductory Unit

Goal: The student will be able to define body language, and describe it as communication. The student will demonstrate the ability to show a change in posture, use a gesture, and display a functional knowledge of body language.

Curriculum Item	Instructions to teachers	Pupil behavior/evaluation	Assessment criterion
The student will define body language as communication.	Introduce student to concept of body language through discussion. Discuss the various things communicated by posture, gesture, personal space. Add body language to list of items describing communication.	The class will define body language as a communication device. The class will be able to name at least one item expressed through body language.	90% class accuracy. 90% class accuracy.
The student will develop a repertoire of behaviors that demonstrate the use of body language.	The student will discuss various body communications: touching, leaning forward or back, and so forth, and will practice them in class. The students will demonstrate the ability to display body language on cue.	The class will demonstrate the ability to display a rehearsed body communication on cue from the instructor.	80% class accuracy.

Goals: The student will define a mannerism as an inappropriate form of body language or behavior, and will reduce the display of a selected mannerism on cue.

Curriculum Item	Instructions to teacher	Pupil behavior/evaluation	Assessment criterion
The student will identify various behaviors as "mannerisms."	In class discussion, the students will name rocking, eye poking, hand waving, and so forth as mannerisms.	The student will be able to identify at least two behaviors as mannerisms.	90% individual or class accuracy.
The student will be able to cite reasons for discontinuing mannerisms.	Name negative consequences in class discussion (poor response from strangers, friends, cosmetic changes).	The class will be able to identify at least three negative results of mannerisms.	90% class accuracy.
The student will identify settings where the expression of mannerisms is acceptable.	Review definitions of public and private. Identify private areas where students may choose to express mannerisms.	The class will be able to identify that such behaviors may be performed in private, and name at least two appropriate private places that might be used.	90% class accuracy.
The student(s) will respond to an agreed-upon teacher cue for the reduction of mannerisms in the social skills class setting.	Identify behaviors the instructor wishes to alter. Identify the cue statement or activity. Practice response to cue. Establish reward for class response to cue.	The class will respond to an established cue by diminishing identified behavior.	

The activities described below incorporate the utilization of assertive behavior in real-life experiences so that the students were able to apply the skills learned during training to travel experiences, shopping encounters, dating experiences, and interactions with co-workers or supervisors. The activities are most successful for students with intact communication skills, and can include students who sign.

Intervention

1. Demonstrate passive, assertive, and aggressive responses. ("If I wanted help at the store, I could . . . ")
2. Have the student demonstrate responses in given situations ("If you wanted information on the telephone [assistance at a bus or rapid transit station, directions on the street, etc.], show me a passive [or aggressive or assertive] way of asking.")
3. Identify with the student which response they like to receive or hear.
4. Videotape or voice record the sessions, and play them back to the students.
5. Identify with the students the connotations of the styles they have demonstrated:
   a. Aggression = anger, threat, rudeness
   b. Passivity = fear, an "I don't matter" attitude
   c. Assertion = confidence, ability, independence
6. Associate posture, gestures, and personal space with communication (see "Training Physical Skills" section).
   a. Aggression = fist shaking, foot stomping
   b. Passivity = head down, exhibition of mannerisms with silence
   c. Assertion = erect posture, facial gaze to others
7. Record sessions emphasizing voice, tonal qualities.
   a. Aggression = shouting, demanding tone

   b. Passivity = silence, whispering, long pauses before requests or statements
   c. Assertion = audible voice, clear statements/requests, use of courtesies
8. Practice behaviors in actual settings. Each student should:
   a. Make a telephone call to a store or business for information
   b. Request information or assistance on public transportation
   c. Request assistance or directions while shopping
   d. Identify the person or place in a grocery store where assistance can be obtained (e.g., the checkout stand, the manager's station)

The student should develop a repertoire of opening statements:
a. "I would like assistance with my shopping today. Please let me know when a clerk is available."
b. "Please let me know when we reach Main Street—I will need to make my transfer there."
c. Other statements as needed.

For students using alternative communication skills:
a. For a teletouch for deaf/blind students: A clearly visible statement on the cover. For example: "Hello. This is a teletouch, which I need to communicate with you. Please use it as you would a regular typewriter." The student should learn to take the teletouch to a counter or checkout stand (requires orientation to the shopping area), place the teletouch on the counter, and say "May I have assistance when someone is available?"
b. For the nonspeaking student, learning to present a list (made independently or with assistance) is similar, except that the list is presented without a statement.
c. For the low-vision student with some

typing ability who is hearing or verbally impaired, a hand-held communicator that prints what is typed in can be useful.

9. Identify situations in which passive or aggressive behaviors are both useful and appropriate:

    a. When touched by a stranger on public transportation, a loud request to be left alone is indicated.

    b. For the visually impaired person who cannot tell the source or cause of a disturbance while traveling, simply moving closer to a checkout stand, a taxi stand, the bus driver, the office location in a store, and so forth to request help is preferable to trying to ascertain what is happening.

    c. Have the student add to this list, and discuss responses that will assure safety or assistance.

10. Have the students carry a tape recorder with them into the community, and help them review the interactions they have experienced. Rehearse possible variations of encounters prior to going out again, and use a series of tapes to help the students identify their own success.

Table 5 provides additional social skills activities that help the instructor to promote and facilitate assertive behavior for his or her students. The activities are criterion referenced so that each activity relates to a specific goal and set of program objectives. Furthermore, each objective provides guidelines and suggestions to the instructor for successful implementation.

SUMMARY

The activities and strategies presented within the context of this chapter have provided a foundation for the development of social competence within integrated school and community environments for visually handicapped students. However, the interventions suggested are only a framework for further investigation and implementation. Practitioners in the field of blindness and visual impairment recognize the critical need for the inclusion of such skills, and must begin to gain the cooperation and support from program administrators, parents, and the students themselves. Further, the task of infusing social skills interventions into a traditional educational context requires creativity, flexibility, and a commitment to initiate such practices on a consistent basis.

If the intent of educators of visually handicapped students is to provide services that prepare students for future life endeavors, then one must be willing to develop skills and to create service-delivery models that allow teachers to integrate a more functionally based curriculum. Without a repertoire of socially acceptable behaviors, visually handicapped students are at risk. The development of social skills provides a foundation for independent functioning and for control over one's actions and decisions. The acquisition of social skills is not a natural occurrence for visually handicapped children, but must be trained and nurtured throughout their educational years. At present, there is little empirical evidence to document the long-term strength of social skills training throughout a visually handicapped student's educational experience. The intervention strategies set forth in this chapter, as well as others described, have demonstrated great changes in the students' ability to interact effectively with sighted peers and adults. Further, the introduction of such interventions have given students an enhanced ability to make independent decisions, to take responsibility for his or her own actions, and to feel confident and successful within the sighted environment.

STUDY QUESTIONS

1. Discuss why the social integration of blind and visually impaired students has been particularly difficult to achieve in mainstreamed

Table 5. Social skills activities to promote and facilitate assertive behavior

Assertion Skills: Introductory Unit

Goal: The student will identify feelings by name, recognize self-expressions of emotions, and expressions by others of similar emotions.

Curriculum Item	Instructions to teachers	Pupil behavior/evaluation	Assessment criterion
The class will identify love, hate, anger, joy, jealousy, happiness as emotions or feelings.	Name emotions/feelings in class discussion. Describe causes of named emotions, events that precipitate emotional response.	The students will name at least three feelings on teacher demand. The students will describe a feeling and an event that causes it.	90% class accuracy.
The class will describe their own expressions of emotions.	Name typical expressions of emotions (shouting in anger, laughing when happy, etc.). Name individual responses and behaviors.	The students will be able to describe at least one sign of an emotion/feeling they have experienced.	90% class accuracy.
The class will describe signs of emotion/feeling in others.	The class will review expressions of emotion. The class will name possible feelings in others if they are crying, laughing, shouting, and so forth.	The students will be able to describe one possible feeling from a description of the behavior of another.	90% class accuracy.
The class will discuss the fact that all people have similar emotions and feelings.	Class discussion (teacher led) of the fact that feelings exist in all people. Class discussion of different and similar emotional responses to situations.	The students will agree with teacher's statement that all people have feelings. The students will be able to give two examples of responses to a situation, such as anger shown through crying or shouting as different expressions of the same emotion.	90% class accuracy. 75% class accuracy.

Goal: The student will define communication as the sharing of ideas, feelings, needs, and information. The student will define modes of communication.

Curriculum Item	Instructions to teacher	Pupil behavior/evaluation	Assessment criterion
The student will define communication as the sharing of ideas and feelings.	Review feelings. Share an idea. Define them in telling the feeling or idea to others as communication.	The student will identify the sharing of an idea or feeling as communication.	90% class accuracy.

(continued)

Table 5. (continued)

Curriculum Item (continued)	Instructions to teachers	Pupil behavior/evaluation	Assessment criterion
The student will define communication as the sharing of needs and information.	The student will discuss "need" and "information." The student will define the sharing needs and information as communicating.	The student will define the words "need" and "information," and identify sharing them as a form of communication.	90% class accuracy.
The student will give reasons for communication, and give examples of the positive effects of communications skills.	In class discussion, the students will identify reasons for sharing ideas, feelings, needs, and information. In class discussion, the students will identify the value of communicating ideas, needs, feelings, and information.	The class will name at least three reasons for communication. The class will be able to identify at least three positive effects of communication.	90% class accuracy. 90% class accuracy.
The student will define methods of communication other than verbal.	The class will create a list of alternative communication modes (e.g., tears, laughter, signing, hitting, throwing objects, holding hands, hugging).	The class will be able to name at least three examples of non-verbal communication.	90% class accuracy.

Goal: The student will identify definitions of passive, aggressive, and assertive behaviors, and differentiate among them.

Curriculum item	Instructions to teachers	Pupil behavior/evaluation	Assessment criterion
The student will discuss passive behavior.	Teacher models passive styles of behavior. Class discussion.	The class will either verbally define or demonstrate passive behaviors.	80% class accuracy.
The student will define aggressive behavior.	See above.	See above.	80% class accuracy.
The student will define assertive behavior.	See above.	See above.	80% class accuracy.
The student will identify demonstrated behaviors as passive, aggressive, or assertive.	Teacher models types of behaviors, and assists students in identifying the type.	In a demonstration of different types of behaviors, the class will correctly identify the behavior types.	80% class accuracy.

102

school and community programs. What role must the teacher assume to achieve positive outcomes?

2. Describe some specific strategies parents and teachers can implement with young visually impaired children to maximize social development and integration.

3. Discuss the impact of using nondisabled peers or visually impaired role models to enhance the social competence of blind and visually impaired students.

4. Discuss the impact that limited vision has on developing or interpreting nonverbal social initiations. What are some strategies that can be used to help visually impaired students compensate or adapt?

5. Describe some strategies that can be employed to help students develop assertive behavior. Provide examples that can be implemented in the classroom, in leisure situations, or in the community.

6. What are some specific methods that can be implemented with multihandicapped/visually impaired students to maximize their social competence?

REFERENCES

American Foundation for the Blind. (1954). *The Pinebrook report*. Pinebrook, NY: National Work Session on the Education of the Blind with the Sighted.

Anderson, E.S., Dunlea, A., & Kekelis, L.S. (1984). Blind children's language development: Resolving some differences. *Journal of Child Language, 11*, 645–664.

Apple, M.M. (1972). Kinesthetic training for blind persons: A vital means of communication. *New Outlook for the Blind, 6*, 201–208.

Asher, S.M., & Gottman, J.M. (1981). *The development of children's friendships*. London: Cambridge University Press.

Asher, S.R., Oden, S.L., & Gottman, J.M. (1977). Children's friendships in social settings. In L.G. Katz (Ed.), *Current topics in early childhood* (Vol. 1, pp. 33–61). Norwood, NJ: Able Publishing.

Ball, G. (1974). *Magic circle: An overview of the human development program*. La Mesa, CA: Human Development Training Institute.

Bandura, A. (1977). *Social learning theory*. Englewood Cliffs, NJ: Able Publishing.

Bandura, A. & Walters, R.H. (1963). *Social learning and personality development*. New York: Holt, Rinehart, & Winston.

Bishop, V.E. (1986). Identifying the components of successful mainstreaming. *Journal of Visual Impairment and Blindness, 80*, 939–946.

Centers, L., & Centers, R. (1963). Peer group attitudes toward the amputee child. *Journal of Social Psychology, 61*, 127–132.

Chin-Perez, G., Hartman, D., Sook Park, H., Sacks, S., Wershing, A., & Gaylord-Ross, R.J. (1986). Maximizing social contact for secondary students with severe handicaps. *Journal of The Association for Persons with Severe Handicaps, 11*, 118–124.

Corn, A.L. (1980). *Development and assessment of an inservice training program for teachers of the visually handicapped: Optical aids in the classroom*. Unpublished doctoral dissertation, Teacher's College, Columbia University, New York.

Corsaro, W. A. (1985). *Friendship and peerculture in the early years*. Norwood, NJ: Able Publishing.

Cowen, E.L., Peterson, A., Babigian, H., Izzo, L.D., & Trost, M.A. (1973). Long-term follow-up of early detected vulnerable children. *Journal of Consulting and Clinical Psychology, 41*, 438–445.

Dinkmeyer, D. (1970). *Developing Understanding of Self and Others (DUSO)*. Circle Pines, MN: American Guidance Service.

Dion, K.K. (1972). Physical attractiveness and evaluation of children's transgressions. *Journal of Personality and Social Development, 24*, 207–213.

Eaglestein, S.A. (1975). The social acceptance of blind high school students in an integrated school. *The New Outlook for the Blind, 60*, 447–451.

Fredericks, H.B., Baldwin, V., Groves, D., Moore, W., Riggs, C., & Lyons, B. (1978). Integrating the moderately and severely handicapped child into a normal day care setting. In M.J. Guralnick (Ed.), *Early intervention and the integration of handicapped and nonhandicapped children*. Baltimore: University Park Press.

Gaylord-Ross, R.J., Haring, T.G., Breen, C.G., & Pitts-Conway, V. (1984). The training and generalization of social interaction skills with autistic youth. *Journal of Applied Behavior Analysis, 17*, 229–247.

Gaylord-Ross, R.J., & Pitt-Conway, V. (1984). Social behavior development in integrated secondary autistic programs. In N. Certo, N. Haring, & R. York (Eds.), *Public School integration of severely handicapped students: Rational issues and progressive alternatives* (pp. 197–219). Baltimore: Paul H. Brookes Publishing Co.

Gotlieb, J., & Budoff, M. (1973). Social acceptability of retarded children in nongraded schools differing in architecture. *American Journal of Mental Deficiency, 78*, 15–19.

Gresham, F.M. (1983). Misguided mainstreaming: The case

for social skills training with handicapped children. *Exceptional Children, 48*(5), 321–328.

Harrell, R.L., & Strauss, F.A. (1986). Approaches to increasing assertive behavior and communication skills in blind and visually impaired persons. *Journal of Visual Impairment and Blindness, 80,* 794–798.

Harlow, H.J., & Harlow, M.K. (1962). Social deprivation in monkeys. *Scientific American, 207* (5), 1–10.

Hartup, W.W. (1977). Peer interaction and the process of socialization. In M.J. Guralnick (Ed.), *Early intervention and interaction of handicapped and nonhandicapped children.* Baltimore: University Park Press.

Hatlen, P. (1980). *Mainstreaming: Origin of a concept.* Washington, DC: American Association of Workers for the Blind.

Hendrickson, J.M., Strain, P.S., Trembly, A., & Shores, R.D. (1982). Interactions of behaviorally handicapped children: Fundamental effects of peer interaction. *Behavior Modification, 5,* 345–359.

Hoben, M., & Lindstrom, V. (1979). Evidence of isolation in the mainstream. *Journal of Visual Impairment and Blindness, 74,* 289–296.

Huebner, K.M. (1985). Services for blind and visually impaired. In G.T. Scholl (Ed.), *Quality services for blind and visually handicapped learners* (pp. 8–9). Reston, VA: Council for Exceptional Children.

Jose, R. (1984). *Understanding low vision.* New York: American Foundation for the Blind.

Kekelis, L., & Sacks, S.Z. (1988). Mainstreaming visually impaired children into regular education programs: The effects of visual impairment on children's interactions with peers. In S.Z. Sacks, L. Kekelis, & R.J. Gaylord-Ross (Eds.), *The development of social skills by visually handicapped children* (pp. 1–42). San Francisco: San Francisco State University.

Kleck, R.E. (1968). Physical stigma and non-verbal cues emitted in face to face interactions. *Human Relations, 21,* 19–28.

Mischel, W. (1966). A social learning view of sex differences in behavior. In E. E. Maccoby (Ed.), *The development of sex differences.* Stanford, CA: Stanford University Press.

Naughton, F., & Sacks, S.Z. (1977). *Hey! What's cooking? A kitchen curriculum for parents of visually handicapped children.* Flosmoore, IL: South Metropolitan Association for Low Incidence Handicapped Children.

Piaget, J. (1932). *The moral judgment of the child.* Glenco, IL: Free Press.

Ragland, E.U., Kerr, M.A., & Strain, P.S. (1981). Social play of withdrawn children: A study of the effect of teacher-mediated peer feedback. *Behavior Modification, 5,* 347–359.

Richardson, S.A. (1969). The effects of physical disability on the social development of the child. In D.A. Goslin (Ed.), *Handbook of socialization theory and research.* Chicago: Rand McNally.

Rickelman, B.L., & Blaylock, J.N. (1983). Behaviors of sighted individuals perceived by blind persons as hindrances to self-reliance in blind persons. *Journal of Visual Impairment and Blindness, 77,* 8–11.

Sacks, S.Z. (1987). *Peer-mediated social skills training: Enhancing the social competence of visually handicapped children in a mainstreamed school setting.* Unpublished doctoral dissertation, University of California–Berkeley and San Francisco State University.

Santin, S., & Nesker Simon, J. (1977). Problems in the construction of reality in congenitally blind children. *Journal of Visual Impairment and Blindness, 71,* 425–429.

Scott, R.A. (1969). The effects of blindness on the social development of the child. In D.A. Goslin (Ed.), *Handbook of socialization theory and practice.* Chicago: Rand McNally.

Sisson, L.A., Van Hasselt, V.B., Hersen, M., & Strain, P. (1985). Increasing social behavior in multihandicapped children through peer interaction. *Behavior Modification,*

Strain, P.S. (1977). An experimental analysis of peer social interactions on the behavior of withdrawn preschool children: Some training and generalization effects. *Journal of Abnormal Child Psychology, 5,* 445–455.

Strain, P.S., Cooke T.P., & Apolloni, T. (1976). *Teaching exceptional children: Assessing and modifying social behavior.* New York: Academic Press.

Strain, P.S., Shores, R.E., & Timm, M.A. (1977). Effects of peer social interactions on the behavior of withdrawn preschool children. *Journal of Applied Behavior Analysis, 10,* 289–298.

Turiel, E. (1978). The development of concepts of social structure: Social convention. In J. Glick & K.A. Clarke-Stewart (Eds.), *The development of social understanding.* New York: Gardner Press.

The Ungame Co. (1975). *Tell it like it is with the ungame.* Anaheim, CA: Author.

Van Hasselt, V.B. (1983). Social adaptions in the blind. *Clinical Psychology Review, 3,* 87–102.

Van Hasselt, V.B., Hersen, M., & Kazdin, A.E. (1984). Assessment of social skills in visually handicapped adolescents. *Behavior Research and Therapy.*

Van Hasselt, V.B., Hersen, M., Kazdin, A.E., Simon, J.A., & Mastanuono, A.K. (1983). Social skills training for blind adolescents. *Journal of Visual Impairment and Blindness, 77,* 99–103.

Voeltz, L.M. (1982). Effects of structured interactions with severely handicapped peers on children's attitudes. *American Journal of Mental Deficiency, 86,* 380–390.

CHAPTER 5

INTEGRATING STUDENTS WITH DEAFNESS INTO MAINSTREAM PUBLIC EDUCATION

John W. Reiman and Michael Bullis

The integration of students with deafness into the public education setting is the focus of this chapter. Students with deafness, for the purpose of this chapter, refers primarily to those individuals with severe (65–90 decibel [dB]) and profound (90 dB) prelingual hearing loss who utilize either a visual-manual sign system or sign language in their expressive and/or receptive communication. Although portions of this chapter may be germane to students who communicate orally and possess mild (15–40 dB) and moderate (40–65 dB) hearing loss, space constraints and continuity necessitate a central focus on those using visual-manual communication. The authors intend no disrespect or judgment of value for those exercising an oral-only preference.

Some students with deafness communicate using speech accompanied by an artificial sign system (manually coded English [MCE]) created to exactly follow English word order and syntax. For many of these students, primary identification is with the majority (Hearing) English-speaking culture. Other students with deafness choose not to speak, communicating instead through a natural sign language called American Sign Language (ASL). ASL is a true language with its own syntax and grammar, and bears no resemblance to En-glish. For many of these students, primary identification is with a minority (Deaf) culture. (The reader should note that when "Deaf" and "Hearing" are capitalized, reference is being made to cultural aspects. For example, Deaf students are students with deafness belonging to the Deaf culture. This concept is explained in greater detail in the following section).

For the vast majority of students with deafness in contemporary education, linguistic usage and cultural identification are hybrid in nature—a logical outgrowth of living with hearing loss in a Hearing world. By and large, mainstream instruction of children with deafness emphasizes monolingual (English) proficiency and monocultural (Hearing culture) identification. This exclusive transmission of the values of the Hearing culture and English language may deny some students their inherent personal right to select viable linguistic and Deaf cultural alternatives. Similarly, if the educational environment were to transmit only Deaf culture and ASL, students' learning of Hearing cultural values and English language might be impeded.

To achieve balance and offer students with deafness the benefits of both languages and cultures, a bilingual/bicultural educational model is proposed

The preparation of this chapter was partially supported through Grant #G008630522 awarded by the federal Office of Special Education and Rehabilitative Services. The information presented herein does not necessarily reflect the policy of that agency and no official endorsement should be inferred.

as a long-term goal for the public schools. Research indicates that for bilingual students, bilingual education improves rather than impedes oral language development, reading and writing abilities, mathematics and social studies achievement, cognitive functioning, and self-image (Woodward, 1982). The model must be held as an objective to be reached in the future due to serious attitudinal, economic, personnel, and instructional material limitations at present. It is a goal, however, that can offer clear direction for efforts to responsibly educate children with deafness. Following the presentation of this model, practical strategies and activities are presented that could support the eventual evolution of bilingual/bicultural education. In theory, this model honors and preserves individual differences and personal choice. In practice, the activities and strategies presented seek to create an environment capable of responding to the distinctive needs of an American cultural and linguistic minority, and to foster integration in public education. In order to ground the discussion in a firm context, a brief introduction to the culture of Deaf people and the deaf community is provided first.

DEAF CULTURE AND COMMUNITY

Students with severe and profound hearing loss constitute the largest percentage of students served in deaf education programs in the United States. These students constitute 90% of the residential school population, 80% of the day school population, 70% of the population in special public school classrooms, and 34% of the population in mainstream education (i.e., itinerant programs, resource rooms, interpreted classes, part-time special education classes) (Karchmer, Milone, & Wolk, 1979). Karchmer reports that children with severe or profound hearing loss perform below their less-than-severely impaired age-mates in reading, though closer to them in mathematics. These students depend heavily on manual communication and are unlikely to use their speech,

which tends to be relatively unintelligible. Severe and profound hearing loss are the most prevalent types of hearing loss in the special education population across all age groups.

The educational needs of this group differ significantly from the needs of students with less-than-severe hearing loss. Students' dependence on manual communication requires that the educational environment, whether in special or integrated classes, be transformed by supplementing or replacing aural-oral communication with visual-manual communication. In some cases, this transformation is not simply of communicative mode (i.e., oral to manual), but is accompanied by a shift in sociocultural identification (i.e., Hearing to Deaf).

Deafness is often viewed in a limited context by the dominant (Hearing) society as being an audiological condition with associated educational, social, and psychological problems. What this problem-centered perspective excludes is the reality that many people with deafness aggregate into groups in which members do not experience themselves as deficient and, in fact, have their basic individual needs met. These individuals have their own culture.

> It has been a common practice for authorities concerned in the delivery of education and other services to the deaf, to deny that a deaf society exists . . . These authorities suppose instead, that deaf persons form a handicapped minority that needs a special group of hearing persons to lead it and manage its affairs. (Stokoe, Bernard & Padden, 1976, p. 189)

The term "culture" refers to the set of learned behaviors belonging to a group of people who have their own language, values, rules for behavior, and traditions (Padden, 1980). The Deaf culture constitutes a unique and historically discounted subculture in American society. A culture's values may be represented in positive (what is admired and respected) or negative (what is eschewed) attitudes and behaviors (Padden, 1980). What follows is a brief overview of some identifying values and characteristics of Deaf culture taken largely from Padden.

Language

The language of this group is American Sign Language (ASL). A bona fide language with *no* structural relationship to English, ASL relies on visual rather than auditory encoding and decoding, and has a complex rule-governed phonology, syntax, and morphology (Baker & Padden, 1978). Individuals with deafness born to Deaf parents may have native competence in ASL. Others, with hearing loss, may have the opportunity to become enculturated as Deaf people at later points in life by learning ASL through association with Deaf peers or adults. ASL allows people with deafness to take advantage of their capabilities as normal language-using human beings and serves as a cohesive source of pride and positive identification (Meadow, 1975).

Group Identity

Deaf people are woven together into the fabric of Deaf culture by the thread of American Sign Language. When together, these individuals naturally experience a level of ease in communication rarely experienced in their interactions with the hearing world. Whether in a religious, social, athletic, or educational setting, the company of other people with similar language may provide an environment conducive to free-flowing interaction and expression. Within the group, members are less likely to succumb to the habitually self-critical analysis of communication experienced in and learned through their interaction with the Hearing world. No particular degree of hearing loss is requisite for membership in the Deaf culture. In fact, Padden (1980) notes "there is one name for all members of the cultural group, regardless of the degree of hearing loss: Deaf. The sign 'DEAF' can be used in an ASL sentence to mean 'my friends' which conveys the cultural meaning of Deaf " (p. 100).

Additional supportive evidence for the power of group identity may be drawn from estimates of Deaf people's rate of endogamous marriage (a union with a like person, in this case marriages in which both persons are Deaf), which ranges from 86% to well over 90% (Schein & Delk, 1974). Finally, there exists an elaborate network of organizations to support Deaf people. The National Association of the Deaf; the National Theatre for the Deaf; the National Fraternal Society of the Deaf; local clubs; the Deaf Olympics—local, state, national, and international athletic competitions; and a variety of other groups provide avenues to enhance Deaf group identity.

Speech Communication

Speech, the normative mode for English language interpersonal communication, is not regarded positively by many Deaf people. Traditionally imposed as the requisite vehicle for enculturation into the Hearing-dominant society, speech for some persons has come to represent confinement and denial of a most fundamental need—to communicate deeply and comfortably in one's own language. Although some individuals may opt to use speech in select settings, within the cultural context it is routinely distrusted and deemed inappropriate.

Folklore/Stories/ Literature of the Culture

As with all cultures, there exists a body of information that has as its purpose the perpetuation and support of cultural values and mores. Recorded primarily through visual-manual stories, a legacy reflecting pride and cultural integrity repeatedly emerges. Padden (1980) notes a "typical" example:

> A deaf (non-capitalized "deaf" refers to non-cultural aspects) person grows up in an oral environment, never having met or talked with Deaf people. Later in life, this deaf person meets a Deaf person who brings him to parties, teaches him Sign Language and instructs him in the way of Deaf people's lives. This person becomes more and more involved, and leaves behind his past as he joins other Deaf people. (p. 97)

Conclusion and Summary

The Deaf culture does not exist within a vacuum. Rather, it is located within the multicultural world of people with normal hearing. Between the Hearing world and Deaf culture exists a deaf community. According to Padden (1980), a community is a general social system within which people live together, share common goals, and work collectively toward achieving those goals. More specifically, "a deaf community has not only Deaf members, but also hearing and deaf people who are not culturally Deaf, and who interact on a daily basis with Deaf people and see themselves as working with Deaf people in various common concerns" (Padden, 1980, p. 93). When interacting with non-Deaf individuals in the community, people belonging to the culture of Deaf people, while preferring ASL, may employ varying degrees of written, spoken, and signed English.

To summarize, there exists a unique culture of Deaf people defined by their language, values, and folklore. Many of these individuals will attend public mainstream educational settings. What follows is an educational model that, in theory, responds to the distinctive instructional needs of this population.

EDUCATIONAL MODEL

Children with deafness, the vast majority of whose Hearing parents wish for them to share a Hearing linguistic and cultural heritage, face a serious dilemma. On the one hand, as Erting (1982) observed in a detailed study of interactions among children, their parents, and their teachers, the child experiences a natural and growing allegiance to and identification with Deaf culture. On the other hand, this momentum is placed in dynamic opposition with the child's natural attachment to and dependence on parents with normal hearing.

> The basic contradiction between the deaf individual's social identity, constructed, in part, out of the need for community with others who share fundamentally similar experiences and can communicate them, and the deaf individual's personal identity, resulting, in part, from the physical and emotional bonds between parents and children, very often manifests itself as ambivalence toward both [D]eaf society and [H]ear-

ing society. The challenge to integrate these two identities and resolve the tension these competing and conflicting categories and their symbols generate is perhaps the greatest and most constant challenge faced by the deaf individual. (Erting, 1982, p. 56)

Language is the manifest focal point of this tension. Without sufficient English language skills, the person will find negotiating the everyday Hearing world a pervasive challenge. But without ASL, a sense of belonging to the Deaf culture is at risk. What part has the educational system played in this situation?

In the mid-1800s, Deaf persons had a central role in the education of students with deafness; in fact, in 1863, 40.8% of teachers were themselves Deaf (Gannon, 1981). In 1880, however, at the International Congress on Deafness in Milan, Italy, educators resolved that the use of manual communication inhibited speech and language development (Gannon, 1981). As a result, oralism (communication utilizing speech, speechreading and residual hearing, but no sign communication) prevailed until the mid-1960s when several problems became apparent. First, speechreading depends on prior experience and familiarity with the redundancies and predictability of the language (Moores, 1982). Oralists' contention that language will be learned through speechreading convolutes this fact. Second, reading a written language requires that the reader have linguistic competence in the language of the manuscript's author (Bockmiller, 1981). Oralists' contention that in order to read English, one must have competency in English that will be taught by reading, reflects circular convoluted logic (Barnum, 1984). Third, few persons with prelingual (prior to acquisition of language) deafness—95% of the school-age population—develop speech that can be understood in most social situations (Vernon, 1976).

In the mid-1970s, following a long tradition emphasizing exclusively oral skill development for children with deafness, educational programs initiated a "Total Communication" (TC) approach to the perennial goal of teaching English. Developed to address the right of a child to make use of all forms (speech, speechreading, gestures, sign, body language, etc.) of communication available to develop language competence (Denton, 1972), TC has several inherent difficulties. Cokely (1980) notes first that although the rights of the child received recognition, needed changes in teachers' communicative competence were overlooked. Little emphasis, for example, was placed on having teachers improve either their expressive or receptive American Sign Language skills. The second, and critical, difficulty with TC is that "language competence" is most frequently assumed to mean English language competence (Cokely, 1980). This assumption may deny the child's need to communicate deeply and comfortably, and, as is detailed shortly, may block English literacy skill acquisition. In actual practice, TC may best be described as the use of simultaneous communication: spoken English accompanied by some manual coding of English (Cokely, 1980). Stokoe (1978) cautions that a teacher who learns signs and inserts them into English phrases and sentences will fail to communicate unless the student already understands the sentence- and word-forming systems of English, an assumption that is unlikely. Simply seeing signs that someone *thinks* stand for English words is in no way similar to *learning* the word systems of English. In short, TC has not conclusively proven to be a vehicle either for English language acquisition or for resolution of the tension from competing and conflicting personal identities.

Bilingual/Bicultural Approach

What is called for is a bilingual/bicultural approach that, instead of dichotomously viewing the deaf child as a being to be totally enculturated in Hearing society, honors natural bicultural affiliation and includes the opportunity for development of linguistic and communicative competence in both ASL and English.

Kannapell (1980) suggests the following three ways of classifying students with deafness in terms of bilingualism: 1) ASL-Dominant Bilinguals—more comfortable expressing themselves in ASL than in English (in either printed or signed form); 2) English-Dominant Bilinguals—more comfortable expressing themselves in English and better able to understand English (in printed and signed form) than ASL; 3) Balanced Bilinguals—comfortable expressing themselves in both ASL and English and able to understand ASL and English about equally well.

> Ideally a deaf child should live in the best of two worlds and should be able to freely move from the Deaf community to the [H]earing community and vice versa. He or she should be able to communicate with deaf people in ASL . . . and to participate in their activities, should be able to . . . communicate with hearing people who know signs, and should be able to read and write English fluently. Speech, lipreading, and auditory skills of English should be considered for those who can speak or who have residual hearing. Our goal would be to have as many balanced bilinguals as possible in the Deaf community. (Kannapell, 1980, p. 115)

How can progress toward balanced bilingualism be supported through educational programming? One practical beginning toward this end would be to operationalize the idealized philosophy of Total Communication—the right of children with deafness to use all forms of communication available to develop language competence (Denton, 1972). This would mean that the contemporary monolingual (English) interpretation of TC (i.e., spoken English accompanied by manual coding of English) would need to be extended to include the child's natural visual-manual communication; the inclusion of ASL in a TC program would satisfy this need. If TC is to be what it claims to be (total), it must encompass more than simply coding English in visual symbols (Cokely, 1980). In short, movement toward bilingual education requires that TC's goal of developing "language competence" be clarified and redefined as development of *bilingual* competence in ASL and English.

The use of ASL for instruction is disputed by critics who contend that students with deafness who are deficient in English should be instructed in English (Barnum, 1984). Contemporary research in bilingual education counters this position. Cummins (1979) maintains that "for the minority child, instruction mainly through the native language has been shown to be just as, or more effective in promoting dominant language proficiency as instruction (solely) through the dominant language" (p. 202). Although recent efforts have been made to identify "natural" or "first" language competency in children with deafness entering school (Luetke-Stahlman & Weiner, 1982), it is unlikely that most of these children will have an English language base. Demographic data indicates that 91.7% of children with deafness have parents with normal hearing. Leutke-Stahlman (1982) notes that most of these children do not acquire even rudiments of their parents' language and instead utilize idiosyncratic gestures and isolated words to communicate basic needs (Dalgleish & Mohay, 1979; Greenburg, 1980; Tervoort, 1961). It therefore makes sense not only to build on the isolated words (to build English skills) but also to develop and maximize the child's demonstrated visual-manual potential (to build ASL skills). Complementary pursuit of both skill areas fulfills the real spirit of TC and establishes the opportunity for bicultural affiliation and bilingual development.

Luetke-Stahlman (1982) reports on the work of two researchers with relevance to this issue. The first study suggests that minority-language students obtain English literacy most effectively using their minority language. Monolingual Navajo or Navajo-dominant students who were taught by Navajo teachers and not introduced to English reading until after they read well in Navajo, read two grade levels higher in English by sixth grade than did their peers educated through immersion models (Vorih & Rosier, 1978). The second investigation indicates that English-speaking students instructed mainly through French (i.e., immersion) experienced no negative academic consequences and acquired age-appropriate English literacy skills shortly after introduction of an English language-arts program (Cummins, 1979; Swain, 1978).

These two studies, each representative of a host of similar research, have implications for the inclusion of ASL in bilingual deaf education. Findings suggest that sign (ASL) may be included in the education of students with deafness and cause no negative effects in their learning of either academic language skills or basic interpersonal communication. The intent here is not to promote monolingual instruction with ASL. It is rather to reassert the viability of ASL as a tool for learning English.

Many students with deafness are placed today in single-medium instructional models (Ramirez, 1980), that is, immersion in the dominant language for the entire school day. With these students, English is primarily used by most school staff and is supplemented at times by manually coded English. Attainment of English literacy skills in this model is unlikely (Meadow, 1980; Moores, 1982) since the visual-manual language (ASL) orientation of many students with deafness is not used to acquire proficiency with English.

An instructional program supporting bilingualism and biculturalism might, in theory, eventually assume one of several formats. Luetke-Stahlman (1983) identifies four of these instructional formats with their attendant advantages and disadvantages for deaf students:

1. *Half-day of two languages/systems (L/S).* Instruction is offered in one L/S in the morning and another in the afternoon (e.g., ASL in the morning and MCE in the afternoon). Disadvantages may include excessive early language mixing and potential interference with acquisition of the child's language base, and determination of which subject would be taught in which L/S. A possible advantage, particularly given so few Deaf teachers are presently credentialed, would be that teachers could rotate from the morning to the afternoon, thereby necessitating fewer Deaf teachers.

2. *Bilingual teacher.* The teacher says/signs an

utterance in one L/S, then repeats it in the other L/S. Disadvantages and advantages parallel those of the previous format.

3. *Transition.* The child entering school is instructed in the language and/or system indicated by assessment (Luetke-Stahlman & Weiner, 1982) to be his or her "first" language. In subsequent years, instruction in the dominant language increases as instruction in the "first" language and/or system decreases. Disadvantages center on the difficult, though extremely critical determination through assessment of a child's "first" L/S. Additional concerns may be the grouping of children by language type, not age, and parental reluctance to accept the L/S designated as optimal for the child. The principal advantage would be that children, through proficiency in a first L/S, would have a base on which English literacy skills could be built.

4. *Maintenance.* In an extension of the transition format, instruction in the native language is maintained and never totally eliminated. An advantage may be the continuation of ASL development, which could create heightened potential for bicultural affiliation.

Barriers to the Bilingual/Bicultural Approach

The aforementioned bilingual and bicultural formats, at present, exist mostly in theory only. That these approaches are slow to be practically implemented reflects a dearth of Hearing and Deaf teachers proficient in ASL, an absence of appropriate instructional materials, sociolinguistic problems in implementation, and attitudinal issues (Woodward, 1982). Two problems in particular are that: 1) the push for bilingual education needs to come from within the Deaf community; and 2) attitudes of Hearing and Deaf people need to become positive toward Deaf people, American Sign Language, English, and bilingual education,

before bilingual education can succeed (Woodward, 1982).

Related to the first point, self-advocacy for people with deafness has been difficult historically. Essentially, because of parental and school overprotection and denial of personal decision-making power for young people, the community of adults may be unfamiliar with methods for self-assertion in the public (Hearing) arena (Lane, 1987). Recent events at Gallaudet University reflect an emergent change in this historical passivity. Deaf students at Gallaudet were able to enlist the support of citizens and media nationwide in their assertive and successful effort to secure their institution's first deaf president. The second point, of even greater impact, centers on the widely divergent attitudes between people with deafness and the Hearing people who profess to serve them.

> The hearing establishment serving the deaf and the deaf themselves have two different points of view, two different conceptions of deaf people, and two radically different agendas in America. The hearing leadership of special education believes that the local school offers the least restrictive environment for deaf education; the deaf themselves think it is the most restrictive environment. Hearing authorities view American Sign Language as a crutch, refuse to learn it and discourage its use; the deaf believe it is the equal of English and superior for instructing and communicating with the deaf. The hearing experts are opposed to deaf teachers and blockade their entry into the profession; the deaf organizations think they would be as good or better than hearing teachers and seek their admission. The list goes on and on. The terrible truth is that there is deep rancor between the deaf and those who profess to serve them in America. The fundamental divergence is this: the hearing don't see why the untrained deaf should be consulted, especially as their ideas are so contrary; the deaf don't see why the hearing have the determining say in matters of deafness. (Lane, 1987, pp. 5–6)

Attitudinal barriers coupled with a host of pragmatic issues (e.g., teacher qualifications, economic considerations, material resource availability) present a significant challenge to those presently working toward a bilingual/bicultural approach. Yet in spite of divergent attitudes and related obstacles, respect for individual differences, human dignity, and personal choice require review and modification.

INTEGRATION STRATEGIES

The activities and strategies that follow should be viewed as fundamental and critical steps supporting the evolution of bilingual/bicultural education. Practical guidelines for implementation are included. They seek to maximize visual-manual communication, honor cultural alternatives, utilize technology, assist in the development of appropriate instructional materials, and redress chronic underemployment—all in the service of eventual linguistic and cultural parity in the education of children with deafness.

Visual Communication

In special and integrated classes for students with deafness in public schools, the use of sign *systems,* not ASL, is pervasive. The distinction is that sign *language*—ASL—is an actual language greatly different from English (Stokoe, 1960). Conversely, sign systems follow the grammar of a spoken language (English) and are not regarded as language per se (Bornstein, 1973; Wilbur, 1979). Likely because of their great similarity to spoken language, sign systems are often selected as the proper means of signing in the classroom (D.A. Stewart, 1983). Considerable doubt has been raised regarding the validity of this choice (Battison, 1974; Kluwin, 1981; Stevens, 1976; Woodward, 1973). Concerns center on the feasibility of using a visual mode to represent an aural/oral-based language. The widespread use of sign systems is also perplexing given the fact that ASL is a primary means of communication for signing individuals with deafness (Kannapell, 1982). Nonetheless, philosophic and attitudinal variables combine with generally insufficient teacher preparation in ASL to perpetuate the use of sign systems. Whether sign systems have a place in the education of children with deafness is a point of

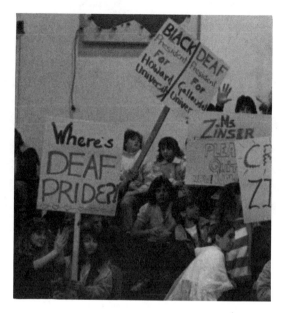

Deaf students at a residential school assert their pride and demands for Deaf leadership.

contention. Whether ASL has a place should easily be resolved in the affirmative for those manually and visually communicating students who naturally and comfortably use ASL in their expressive and receptive communication.

How shall the needs of these students to use ASL be accommodated by mainstream education? Trained and qualified sign language interpreters are vehicles to be used specifically for this purpose. The sign language interpreter takes spoken messages in English and changes them into ASL and vice versa. Interpreting is not simply the matching of equivalent words between languages. It is the re-creation of a message from one language to another in a way that best approximates the spirit and intent of the speaker (or signer) in the source language (Ingram & Ingram, 1975).

The interpreter functions as a member of the educational team and serves to facilitate communication between students with deafness and their teachers (Zawolkow & DeFiore, 1986). The exact nature of the interpreter's role is jointly determined by the teacher and the interpreter who must consider the student's maturity, sign language vocabulary, experience with the use of interpreters, and knowledge of subject matter. The role must be balanced in a manner conducive to maintaining the teacher as ultimately responsible for teaching, the student as ultimately responsible for learning, and the interpreter as ultimately responsible for transmitting messages.

What responsibilities do teachers have in creating an environment conducive to effective interpreting? Practical guidelines for teachers to achieve this goal are listed in Table 1.

It should be noted that the interpreter's re-crea-

tion of the message from one language to another is a necessary, but possibly not sufficient, activity to facilitate student understanding. It may be additionally necessary to develop visual and conceptual resources and strategies to complement interpretation by capitalizing on the student's natural visual-spatial learning style. The delivery of ideas to students with deafness must include two fundamental elements of visual communication (Waldron, 1985). First, the symbols used for communication must be available for review; re-exposure to these symbols is needed before they can be learned. Second, the concepts need to be made

---

Table 1.   Teachers' guidelines for use of an interpreter

Preparation for Class

1. Since the visual environment is critical, there should be sufficient lighting on both the teacher and the interpreter. Ideally, light (nonflickering if fluorescent)should come at a 45° angle from the front. Avoid standing in front of windows or other shiny surfaces capable of generating distracting glare.

2. Arrange seating in a manner that the student(s) using the interpreter can easily switch focus between the interpreter, the teacher, and visual aids. Use of a semicircle is optimal in group discussions.

3. Regularly have available blackboards, charts, overheads, maps, and so forth to visually and conceptually supplement signed interpretations. Have a small low-wattage lamp available to illuminate the interpreter unobtrusively during media use.

4. Be clear on the role of the interpreter. To what extent if any, is the interpreter also in an aide, tutor, or other role?

5. If possible, provide the interpreter with outlines of daily lesson plans to facilitate pre-preparation of difficult signs or concepts and to anticipate necessary classroom seating modifications for discussion, media use, and so forth.

During Class

1. Try to remain in a relatively stationary position and face the students as much as possible. In addition to watching the interpreter, the student may follow the teacher's lip movement, facial expression, and body language.

2. Maintain responsibility for classroom discipline and avoid using the interpreter as a disciplinarian. Allow students to freely sign with one another no more than you would allow students to talk.

3. Maintain responsibility for student understanding. Observation of perplexed expressions and other cues are ultimately the teacher's responsibility.

4. Allow extra time for the interpreter to provide explanations and define terms or concepts, particularly with texts, tests, and handouts written at difficult English reading levels.

5. When demonstrating, be sure the interpreter is close by. Showing (that requires students watch the teacher) and explaining (that requires students watch the interpreter) can split the students' attention.

6. Ask questions directly of students (e.g., "John, what do you think?") and not the interpreter and student (e.g., "Ask John what he thinks.").

7. Control group discussions by insisting that only one person talk at a time. It further helps the interpreter and student if the person talking can either be pointed to or identified by name.

After Class

1. Consult regularly with the interpreter and discuss mutual expectations, student performance, and cooperative strategies. Ongoing communication of this sort ensures stable and positive functioning as a team.

available in graphic pictorial form. For whoever (teacher or interpreter) accepts the responsibility of visually adapting materials, familiarity with both the subject matter and the art of conveying conceptual meaning through signs, graphics, and so forth is imperative (Waldron, 1985). Although all students will not require such adaptations, it remains the responsibility of the teacher to decide when such measures are appropriate.

Waldron (1985) offers three classroom examples of a model for the adaptation of materials. In the first example, a teacher randomly selects mathematics problems from a textbook for oral review. After the problem is identified to the student in sign by the interpreter, the student locates the problem in the book, solves it, and then refocuses on the interpreter either to answer the problem or to see another student's response. To save time and to avoid possible student frustration, the interpreter sitting beside the student may point to the problem as the teacher announces it. Refocusing

from the text to the teacher is thus reduced and the student is freed to synchronize his or her responses with the responses of others. If the interpreter's role is to be strictly that of manual communication, an instructional aide or other student may be used to direct the student's visual attention to specific text passages or problems. In the second instance, a teacher verbally compares the rates of growth of three plants receiving different wattages of lighting, keeping all other variables constant. New vocabulary and concepts may make this material difficult to comprehend for the student receiving it only once from the interpreter. In Waldron's model, the use of a visual representation of the material (See Figure 1) makes the information available for ongoing classroom and home review. A third example centers on the introduction of new vocabulary words. When these words are presented in a transient delivery mode (interpreting) their spelling and/or meaning may not be retained or may be confused if the student pauses

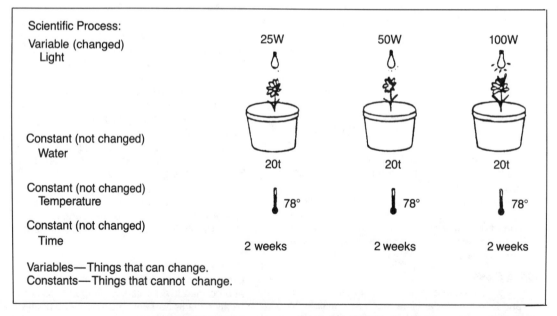

Figure 1.   Set of pictures illustrating experiments using one variable. (From Waldron, M. [1985]. Hearing impaired students in regular classrooms: A cognitive model for educational services. *Exceptional Children, 52;* reprinted with permission.)

to write and then refocuses on the interpreter. If the teacher, interpreter, or aide can write newly introduced words on index cards with a brief explanation of the meaning, a picture, and perhaps a sign, the student is permitted ongoing re-exposure, making learning more likely. In an anecdotal case study (Waldron, 1985) following these models, academic progress, reduced frustration, improved organizational skills, and increased independence were noted.

In the three examples just mentioned and in the previous identification of teacher responsibilities, it becomes apparent that additional visual and conceptual delivery of information clearly supplements interpretation and provides enhanced opportunity for academic integration of students with deafness. Creating opportunities for learning that are commensurate with the students' language and learning style not only offers a chance for fulfillment of personal potential, but also complies with federal law: "No state shall deny educational opportunity to an individual . . . [by] the failure of an educational agency to take appropriate action to overcome linguistic barriers that impede equal participation by its students in its instructional programs" (Title XX of U.S. Code Section 1103 (f) (Lane, 1987).

Reading and Written Materials

Teachers' selection of appropriate reading materials and preparation of written materials play a central role in the instruction of students with deafness, as these students encounter difficulties with idiomatic expressions (Conley, 1976), vocabulary (Trybus & Karchmer, 1977), and English-language grammar and syntax. Thus, it is probable that modifications of existing resources will be necessary and/or new materials will have to be developed.

In selecting printed materials teachers most frequently use informal subjective judgments. At times, however, they may employ one of two more formal procedures (LaSasso, 1980). The first procedure involves determining the student's reading level by using a standardized test (e.g., Stanford Achievement Test–Hearing Impaired) or an informal inventory. A readability formula (Dale & Chall, 1948; Fry, 1968) that assesses grade level is then applied to the material by counting average sentence length, number of syllables, and/or difficult words. The student's reading level is then matched with materials judged to be at an equivalent grade level. The second formal procedure (cloze procedure) involves retyping material from a 250-word sample deemed suitable for a particular student. Every fifth word is then deleted from the sample and replaced by a 15-space underline. Materials are considered appropriate when the student, who is instructed to fill in each blank with a word, can supply 44%–57% of the words correctly. Matching student reading skill level with level of material difficulty is obviously vital to successful academic integration of students with deafness.

Preparation of written materials presents a unique challenge to the deaf educator. The following guidelines (Allen, 1984; Rudner, 1978) may be of value in minimizing the use of problematic linguistic structures:

1. Avoid conditionals (if, suppose, when, etc.).
2. Avoid pronouns with minimal information (someone, it, something, etc.).
3. Avoid comparatives (more than, the most, closer than, etc.).
4. Avoid negatives (without, not, nothing, etc.).
5. Avoid inferentials or qualifications of meaning (because, since, however, etc.).
6. Avoid passive voice.
7. Avoid long sentences.
8. Avoid idiomatic or slang expressions.

Some additional principles for the preparation of written materials may be drawn from Bishop (1979).

1. Reduce complex vocabulary by retaining only necessary technical vocabulary and using simpler words.
2. Reduce concept density by breaking down the lesson into several steps and using supplemental graphic, pictorial, or media resources.

3. Enlist the student's experiential (verbally related in particular) background as a context in which to relate new facts and explore new concepts.
4. Freely use coordinate conjunctions (but, so, for, and, etc.).
5. Keep cause-result and reason-result expressions to a minimum.
6. Analyze difficult vocabulary by identifying meaningful word parts (prefixes or known root words).
7. Hand out a list of guiding questions to help students study new text materials. Questions might address important facts, inferences, vocabulary, and main themes or ideas.
8. Utilize the D.I.G. concept:
   a. *Direct* information to begin.
   b. *Indirect* information next, if needed.
   c. *General* information last.

Most important, view all of the above guidelines as opportunities, not extra burdens. That is, recognize that while some of the suggestions may require additional planning and time, they also result in bright and capable students with a hunger and right to learn.

A review of the research on test development for clients with deafness (Reiman & Bullis, 1987) provides some direction for teachers constructing tests. The results of one study (LaSasso, 1979) indicate that students with deafness find multiple choice items using a *wh* question (e.g., Who wrote the . . .?) significantly less difficult than those using an incomplete statement stem (e.g., _____ wrote the). In another study (McKee & Lang, 1982), data supported the use of multiple-choice tests over true-false tests. Multiple-choice items seemed to be slightly more discriminating, equally reliable, and clearly the preference of students with deafness. A third study (Rogers, 1983) indicated that on a multiple-choice test, use of a separate answer sheet (as opposed to writing responses in a test booklet) did not appear to adversely affect student performance.

Curriculum modification is obviously an essential activity for facilitating the academic integration of minority students. Although by no means

inclusive, the aforementioned guidelines provide direction in the selection of reading materials and in the preparation of written materials. Teachers' efforts in offering comprehensible materials will be appreciated by students with deafness who are not monolingual (English) and who require a sensitive response to their unique linguistic needs.

Social Interactions

The social integration of students into the community is a primary objective of education. A goal of schools is to train children for membership in the school community, and then to extend this sense of membership outward to the state, nation, and world (Cubberley, 1947). Since students with deafness live in a Hearing world, this mainstream socialization process is germane to their economic, social, and vocational future.

Social integration includes four hierarchically arranged interdependent components (Kaufman, Gottlieb, Agard, & Kubic, 1975): 1) physical proximity—students need to be near one another to create social contact; 2) social interactive behavior—verbal and nonverbal communication between students; 3) social assimilation—active inclusion of students into classroom and social activities; and 4) social acceptance—the approval of students by their peers.

In order for social interaction (a building block for assimilation and acceptance) to occur, students with deafness and their peers must have ways to communicate. This communication will likely not happen unless each party makes a sustained and deliberate effort to reach out in the language of the other. Although students with deafness are routinely taught English, sign language training for their hearing peers is not readily available.

Elective sign language classes for students with normal hearing have proven to be exceptionally effective for facilitating social interaction. In one setting (Redding, 1986), the class, taught by a signing teacher and professional interpreter, centered on practicing sign language skills and included guest speakers/signers from the Deaf community, videotapes, games, movies, and panel discussions. As a result of the class, the school's media center was designated as a drop-in area for any students, teachers, or interpreters using sign language. Pre- and posttest questionnaires that followed the sign language class and measured attitudes of students with normal hearing consistently yielded significant changes. Not only did students perceive as friends students with deafness whom they earlier identified only as acquaintances, but they also suggested the possibility of dating students with deafness and asserted the eligibility of those persons to hold school offices. In another school, students with and without hearing were joined to form a singing-signing group that performed songs and poems (Ward, 1985). A questionnaire designed to evaluate the activity showed that both groups enjoyed the contact and hoped that their newly made friendships would continue to grow. A logical outgrowth of these cooperative activities would be the establishment of a "buddy" system. Activities not requiring complex communication might become the focal point for "buddies" who have met in sign classes or performance groups.

Extracurricular activities present an excellent opportunity to maximize this peer interaction and facilitate social integration. A study conducted in a Washington, D.C.–area suburban high school suggests that students with deafness function similarly to their peers with normal hearing in extracurricular activities (Chojnacki & Williams, 1982). Students reportedly enjoyed the particular sport in which they were involved and felt a sense of belonging to a group. Most students reported depending on others for assistance when communication was problematic. It was suggested that written announcements of extracurricular activities be distributed to students with deafness; obviously public address systems are insufficient. Also, interpreters could be utilized for some activities. However, since students with deafness often travel considerable distances to attend public schools, special transportation arrangements may be necessary.

Social interaction and subsequent integration should not be the sole responsibility of students.

Research indicates that physical proximity, while necessary, is in itself not a sufficient condition to create interaction, and that careful planning and evaluation by teachers are essential (Antia, 1982). What specifically might be done to facilitate interaction? Lyon and Oliva (1982) offer the following suggestions:

1. Allow and perhaps insist that students with deafness participate in the planning of orientations to train and sensitize teachers, administrators, and peers.

2. Allow hearing peers to "teach deaf students" about things they normally pick up effortlessly by "over-hearing."

3. Set aside a "deaf awareness" day of the beginning of each school year. Show movies/videotapes without sound and establish groups, using interpreters if necessary, to enable students to share mutual concerns.

4. Create opportunities for older students and adults with deafness to share their experiences with all students and teachers.

5. Involve students with sign language skills in the teaching of other students and teachers.

6. Provide students with deafness with an advocate to serve as a motivator, supporter, and admonisher when necessary.

A useful tool for classroom teachers at any grade level is the structuring of activities to facilitate understanding of the way the "other person sees it." Students who can hear might list or write about how they imagine the experience of deafness and vice versa. Inexpensive foam earplugs can be used by students with otherwise normal hearing for simulation and subsequent processing of the experience with students with deafness.

In addition to providing for interaction and exploration among students, the classroom teacher may also train students in intrapersonal awareness and interpersonal skills. Central to effective social understanding and skills for students with deafness are: 1) the capacity to understand and communicate about social events and emotional responses, 2) the capacity to control one's behavior through internal dialogue, 3) the capacity to take another's point of view, and 4) the capacity to identify with communicatively responsive adults for learning of social rules and norms (Greenberg, Kusché, & Smith, 1982). An excellent social-cognitive training program, Providing Alternative Thinking Strategies (PATHS) (Greenberg, Kusché, Calderon, Gustafson, & Coady, 1983) has been developed for use with children with deafness in the second through sixth grades. Taught by trained classroom teachers for 30 minutes each day for 20–25 weeks, the PATHS program includes the following five topic areas: 1) Affective Understanding (vocabulary and cause-effect attributions); 2) Self-Expression (creative expression through art and drama); 3) Self-Control; 4) Interpersonal Understanding, Role-Taking, and Empathy Training; and 5) Decision-Making and Problem-Solving Skills. This systematic procedure increases student access to a wider variety of activities and may considerably reduce social and academic isolation. Academic achievement may also be improved as an outgrowth of heightened self-control (Greenberg et al., 1982).

Research has been undertaken to investigate the use of classroom aides to arrange opportunities for integrated social interaction (Van den Pol, Crow, Rider, & Offner, 1985). Results suggest that providing data-based feedback to classroom aides regarding the effects of their efforts on children's social performance may be instrumental in their arranging the play environment to enhance social interaction. This is accomplished by encouraging all children to become involved in common activities, and also to prevent them from playing alone by prompting toy play and group participation (Van den Pol et al., 1985).

Finally, the educational community that is intent on fostering social integration must be assistive in the development of a viable home learning environment. Bodner-Johnson (1982) speculates that the following learning environment goals might guide a family intervention program: 1) emphasize to parents the "childness" rather than the "deafness" of their offspring and instill parents with confidence in themselves as competent child-

rearers; 2) restore parental aspirations for their child by providing realistic information on deafness; 3) involve parents as decision makers and restore parental feelings of control and responsibility over their child's schooling; 4) develop parental interest and motivation to communicate with their child; and 5) introduce parents to the Deaf community and reiterate to parents that involvement in this community complements rather than threatens their child's status in the Hearing community.

Ostensibly, when the educational environment can empower parents of children with deafness (90% of whom are Hearing) by providing them with accurate information and active involvement, the parents are more likely to assume functionally helpful roles as agents of socialization. A mutually reinforcing partnership between the educational and home environments creates for students a stable and dependable source of information regarding one's self and one's social interactions in a Hearing world.

Career/Vocational Programs

Educational programs designed to provide career/vocational training to persons with disabilities have expanded greatly in recent years. Such programs have proliferated for students with deafness (Ouellette & Dwyer, 1985). The goal of this section is to provide an introduction to this area. For a more complete discussion the reader is referred to: Bullis, Bull, Sendelbaugh, and Freeburg (1987); Bullis, Freeburg, Bull, and Sendelbaugh (in press); Dwyer (1985); Sacks and Bullis (1987).

The career/vocational movement for students with deafness began in the mid 1960s and roughly paralleled the growth of career/vocational programs for students without disabilities (Marland, 1974) and for students with other disabling conditions (Brolin & Kokaska, 1979). Relatively recent surveys of the status of these programs (Ouellette & Dwyer, 1985; Twyman & Ouellette, 1978) suggest that many have the following general instructional features. The vast majority of residential schools, day school programs, and postsecondary institutions (e.g., community colleges) have active career/vocational preparation classes. Few formal programs, however, exist at the elementary or middle school level. Instead, programs tend to begin in high school and emphasize training in blue-collar trades. Important components of most models include vocational evaluation and varied job placements. Also, career counseling and personal development activities are emphasized.

A major effort in this area is the National Project on Career Education (NPCE), an extensive staff training and systems change endeavor that was initiated in 1978. Although the project is not active now, community-based programs that were established as part of the effort are still operating. More detailed information on NPCE may be found in Cobb and Egbert (1981), Dwyer (1985), Egelston-Dodd (1980), Updegraff and Egelston-Dodd (1982). Originally, 60 schools from around the country were identified to participate in the project. In 1979 and 1980, eight 2-day workshops on career education curricula and program development were conducted with over 120 representatives from these schools. The notion was that these participants would then train others in their respective settings and initiate program development efforts. Overall, the workshops were viewed as extremely helpful by respondents (Egelston-Dodd, Young, Lutz, & Lichty 1983). Follow-up services were provided to all sites on a regular basis and various publications and practical manuals were produced. Currently, the impact of NPCE on selected programs and the students at those respective sites is being conducted (J. Egelston-Dodd, personal communication, May 26, 1987). In sum, NPCE represents an outstanding example of a massive system change effort that led to program and material development.

On an individualized level, several procedural points should be attended to when providing career/vocational education to students with deafness. These concepts include a developmental model of instruction, care in employing career-oriented measures, the inclusion of career decision-making training, active transition planning, and a group-oriented job placement approach.

First, as previously pointed out, it is clear that most existing career/vocational education programs begin in high school. This is unfortunate, as prevailing professional thought embraces a model that begins in the elementary school years and progresses through adulthood. This position has been operationalized in the Comprehensive Career Education Matrix (CCEM) (Galloway, 1978) and is presented in Figure 2. It can be seen that at the elementary grades, career/vocational instruction should focus on awareness and basic work-related behaviors (e.g., punctuality) and extend to vocational exploration and preparation in the later years. Adherence to the CCEM is encouraged, though there are few materials for teachers to use at the elementary level. Clark (1979) provides examples of curricula packages that could be adapted for these students.

Second, the career/vocational assessment of students plays a major role in instructional programs, as such information is invaluable in structuring optimal training and placements. In recent years several manuscripts have been published that provide in-depth information on work aptitude and interest measures (e.g., Stewart, 1986a) and work sample systems (Shiels, 1986; Sligar, 1983) for individuals with deafness. However, most instruments have been neither designed expressly for nor standardized on members of this population. Thus, the psychometric properties of many of these measures are suspect (Bullis et al., in press; Holm, 1987; Watson, 1979). In essence, then, one is unsure of whether the tests are measuring true vocational abilities or merely the individual's competence in communication. Further, studies conducted on the criterion validity of career/maturity measures (White & Slusher, 1978) and work samples (Bullis & Marut, 1986) with persons with deafness are not encouraging. Therefore, one must be extremely cautious in interpreting the results of career/vocational testing (Stewart, 1986a). Accordingly, it makes sense to include trial job placements and situational/obser-

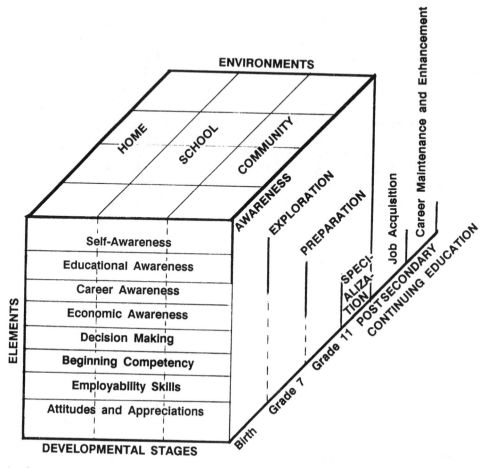

Figure 2. Comprehensive Career Education Matrix. (Developed by the Ohio State University; From Galloway, V. *Overview of a career development model* (p. 22). Washington, DC: Gallaudet College Press; reprinted with permission.)

vational assessments to gain a notion of the individual's behavior and skill in job placements, and to expose the student to a variety of different vocations.

Third, a content area in which persons with deafness appear to need intensive instruction is in career/vocational decision-making (critical thinking) skills (Bullis, 1985; DiFrancesca, 1980; Greenberg & Kusché, in press; Lang & Stinson, 1982). Several promising curricula packages have been developed to address this issue (DiFrancesca, 1978; G. Long, 1986; N. Long, 1986).

Basically the materials provide a format by which students are taught the process of critical thinking through the identification of a goal, the development of a plan to reach that goal, implementation of the plan, evaluation of the results of the action, and—if needed—a reinstituting of the process. The response of teachers to these programs has been positive (Boone, Long, & Long, 1987; Bullis, 1988; Di Francesca, 1978), but the impact on students has not been demonstrated empirically at this point.

Fourth, a concept that has become widely used

in recent years relates to the transition of students with disabilities from the school to the community (Will, 1984). This movement has become part of the field of deafness and two projects have been funded recently to investigate this process for persons with hearing impairments (Bullis, 1986; Watson, 1986). It should be noted that discrepancies exist between representatives of vocational rehabilitation and special education agencies over the specific responsibilities in this process, and it appears that many students are not afforded cooperative transition planning from both agencies (Sendelbaugh & Bullis, 1988). Furthermore, as many students with deafness go on to some type of postsecondary or community-based training after leaving high school (Ouellette, 1986; Schrodel, 1986; Stewart, 1986b), it is imperative that teachers be aware of local (e.g., community colleges and rehabilitation facilities) and national (e.g., colleges and universities) postsecondary training opportunities, and vocational rehabilitation services.

Finally, the teacher must be aware of the importance of training students in job-seeking skills. Unemployment rates among persons with deafness run as high as 50% (Bullis et al., 1987; Passmore, 1983); a fact that may be due, at least in part, to weaknesses in job-seeking skills (Anderson, 1986). A technique that can be utilized to promote job placement is the "Job Club" (Azrin & Besalel, 1980). The Job Club is a structured teaching model in which small groups of participants ($n = 8-12$) are instructed in how to find jobs on their own. Excellent programs using this approach exist for persons with deafness (e.g., Long & Davis, 1986; Torretti & Hendrick, 1986) and at least one curriculum designed specifically for persons with deafness is available (Justl, McMahon, & Lewis, 1983). A brief overview of one such package is provided here.

The Florida Deaf Services Project (FDSP) adapted the original Job Club for a clientele of persons with deafness. Participants are taught to identify job leads, contact job leads, prepare résumés, interview effectively, and learn appropri-ate rules of work behavior. The particulars of these aspects of the job-search process are taught in the morning, and participants are required to go out into the community to practice these skills in the afternoon (i.e., actual job leads are located, contacts are made, and interviews are conducted). Components of the program include the use of interpreters in the job-search process, and adaptations that the worker and/or employer may need to make regarding the worker's hearing loss. The FDSP program runs for 2 full weeks and offers a supportive, reinforcing environment in which participants are encouraged to seek work.

Technology

Major technological advances have been achieved in the past decade. An area with immense practical application for educators across the instructional continuum is the use of computers and sophisticated media equipment as teaching resources and tools. In this part of the chapter, technological advances and their application in fostering the integration of students with deafness are discussed. Specifically, three broad areas are addressed: library services, computer-assisted instruction, and visual media.

Library Services   A major part of any school setting is the library. The library serves as a depository for journals and books, and provides an area where students can meet and study. Given the visual-manual communication orientation of many students with deafness (i.e., ASL or a manually coded system) it may be difficult to access these services and resources. It follows that students' independent learning, by accessing and reading specific books and/or magazines, can be limited. For example, in a survey conducted in Maryland in 1982 (cited by Dalton, 1985) it was found that many persons with deafness did not use the library because of the "foreign" nature of the facility.

Thus, steps must be taken to ensure the availability of the general school library to this population. A logical place to start in this endeavor is with the staff (Dalton, 1985; Macon, 1982). Unless the library is operated in a residential school or the staff have knowledge of the unique characteristics of these students, it is probable that some type of inservice program will be necessary (Wright, 1979). This type of program would include information on deafness, the proper way to talk to a person with hearing loss (e.g., looking at the person and speaking slowly), and the correct way to use an interpreter in an interaction.

Other methods to make a library a more interesting and friendly place for students with deafness are discussed in detail by Dalton (1985), and Junor and Taylor (1984). These include the establishment of a special periodical section devoted to articles, magazines, and books on persons with deafness. A special day might be developed to celebrate the achievements of persons with deafness, and both students with deafness and other community members with deafness could serve on an advisory board to ensure that the library is accessible. Of course, by involving these students in such activities and by recognizing them as an important segment of society, far more than the increased use of the library will be accomplished (i.e., it is probable that these persons will be viewed in a more positive fashion by their peers).

Specific to the improvement of reading, Ernst (1982) provides an excellent description of a program implemented in a library. Study guides providing simple-to-complex overviews of specific stories and/or books were developed. By "layering" the difficulty of the guides in advancing levels, one is better able to match materials with a student's unique reading skills. In this way a student with minimal reading ability could understand parts of *Romeo and Juliet,* for example, through a relatively simple study level. It is hoped that this understanding would lead to greater awareness and advancement in learning and reading.

Increased access to educational materials will not, in and of itself, help a person with deafness to acquire knowledge. Steps must be taken to encourage and structure instruction. Techniques that

use computer-assisted methods toward this end are discussed next.

Computer-Assisted Instruction (CAI) The explosion of instructional software has been one of the most significant educational developments of recent years. Only a few studies, though, document the effects of many of these programs for persons with disabilities (Arcanin & Zawolkow, 1980; Galbraith, 1978; Geoffrion & Goldenberg, 1981; Irwin, 1982; Pollard & Shaw, 1982; Prinz, Nelson, & Stedt, 1982; Stepp, 1982). Still, CAI systems proliferate and it is logical to believe that they do affect learning in a positive manner to some degree. Further, configurations of computer equipment and software (e.g., games) can be used to promote interactions between students with deafness and their hearing peers. Two representative programs are described briefly below. Descriptions of other such programs may be found in Arcanin and Zawolkow (1980) and Cronin, MacKall, and Richardson (1979).

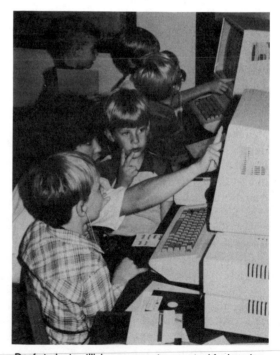

Deaf students utilizing a computer as a tool for learning.

Garvey (1982) describes a program designed for secondary-level students in both resource rooms and self-contained classes. In this model, use is made of "canned," commercially available programs for instruction in language, reading, math, home economics, sciences, and career exploration. It is Garvey's position that programs developed by school staff to address particular local curriculum issues are most beneficial, as they accurately reflect the content covered in class and the specific needs of the student. Most important, the linking of words with visual concepts (e.g., the word "apple" with a picture of an apple) appears to enhance the learning situation. Of special interest is the fact that many students in this program seek out the computer as a way to spend free time; consequently, computer access has become a primary reinforcer for appropriate behavior and academic achievement.

Brady and Dickson (1983) describe a computerized game designed to foster the acquisition of oral communication skills. The program is designed to be used by pairs of students who sit side by side in front of the keyboard. A picture is isolated to the "sender" who describes the image for the "receiver" through the keyboard. If the image is not understood initially, the receiver types questions regarding the image, prompting an exchange between the pair. Eventually, the receiver guesses what the picture is and the computer signals "RIGHT." Another image is then offered and the procedure repeated. A pilot study of the program with 10 students with deafness who were paired with hearing peers indicated that the verbal abilities of the former group improved. All students stated that they enjoyed the game. The hearing peers indicated that the game was one of the few times they had had the opportunity to interact with persons with deafness and that they learned a lot from the experience. Also, the teacher response to the program was very favorable.

To conclude, CAI for students with deafness is a new, but growing, instructional technique that has great potential application. In addition to im-proving the learning and social interaction of this group, technology of this type can also be used to tailor instruction to specific students and to monitor individual progress.

Visual Media Since visual presentation of information may be most appropriate for many students with deafness, the school's media center can be a valuable resource. Staff of such centers may need an inservice on the characteristics of this particular group. Petrie (1982) makes specific suggestions for adapting visual media to persons with deafness. These include the appropriate use of captioning, collecting special materials specific to persons with deafness, and film/filmstrip selection. It should be noted that many captioned films can be secured through state residential schools, state departments of education, and vocational rehabilitation offices.

Instructional approaches that embody a visual presentation can have significant applications for use with students with deafness. Sheie (1983) describes an interesting project that involved secondary-level students in a mainstreamed setting using photography and word-processing equipment. Specifically, students were involved in the production of a photo-journalism model to create a photo exhibition and a class newspaper. The project fostered interaction among these students and many of the skills (e.g., word processing) were utilized in other classes. The success of the project seemed to provide students with deafness with a great deal of status in the eyes of their hearing peers.

Technological application with broad-reaching utility and importance is described by Stuckless (1983). Real-time graphic display (RTGD) is a system for transcribing the spoken word into visual display. It was developed at the National Technical Institute for the Deaf to aid in the integration of students with deafness into mainstreamed classes. Essentially, a stenographer translates speech verbatim, the message is displayed immediately on a screen, and the receiver reads the message. It is possible to produce a hard copy of the content that is covered within minutes of completion of the class or lecture. Extensive work has been conducted to reduce the error rate of the transliteration (Stuckless & Matter, 1982a, 1982b) and to improve the visual presentation of the material (Stuckless, 1982). Although the actual effect of this system is not known (Stuckless, 1983), it would seem that its potential to foster accurate exchanges for persons with severe hearing loss is high. As such competence forms a foundation for learning and interaction, it is possible that this technological advance will lead to greater opportunities for the social integration of persons with deafness. Of course, given the problems in English competence manifested by many persons with deafness, this exact translation of material may be of questionable benefit.

SUMMARY

Many students with deafness may identify with the Deaf culture, which is characterized by distinctive language (ASL), values, rules for behavior, and traditions (Padden, 1980). For this group and for other students with severe and profound hearing loss, mainstream public education is responsible for providing appropriate and effective instruction. Single-medium (immersion) instruction that emphasizes English throughout the school day (Ramirez, 1980) ignores these students' natural visual/manual communication and need for bicultural affiliation, and also reduces the likelihood of English literacy skill attainment (Meadow, 1980).

Bilingual/bicultural instruction, instead of dichotomously viewing the child as either Hearing or Deaf, honors bicultural affiliation and offers the opportunity for the development of linguistic and communicative competence in both ASL and English. In a fully developed bilingual/bicultural model, a significant portion of instruction would be provided in ASL. However, due to an absence of teachers skilled in ASL, a dearth of appropriate instructional materials, attitudinal issues, and so-

ciolinguistic problems in implementation, this is not possible.

Therefore, it is necessary to implement strategies and undertake practical activities that will provide a foundation for, and support the eventual evolution of bilingual/bicultural education for students with deafness. To this end, the educational environment must be optimized through the use of sign language interpreters and graphic-pictorial presentations of concepts. Selection of reading materials and preparation of written materials must follow guidelines that minimize problematic linguistic structures and maximize access for students not claiming English as their first language. Social interaction must be promoted through special classes, extracurricular activities, teacher support, and training in intrapersonal awareness and interpersonal skills. Use of technology must be developed to assist in instruction and promote interactions between students with deafness and their hearing peers. Career and vocational programs must be tailored to provide appropriate assessment, decision-making skills, job-search techniques, and work behavior.

A great deal more research must be undertaken and countless legislative, practical, and financial issues need to be addressed before bilingual/bicultural education for individuals with deafness can become widespread (Johnson, 1987). Hearing parents, educators, and politicians need to be shown the wisdom of encouraging schools to promote people's linguistic and cultural identification and heritage (Johnson, 1987). For now, however, the activities and strategies described in this chapter may be implemented as deliberate steps leading to responsible and effective instruction for a neglected linguistic and cultural minority.

STUDY QUESTIONS

1. Describe the ASL/English controversy from the viewpoints of: the child with deafness, the parent who is hearing, and the educational system.

2. List the four instructional formats for bilingual/bicultural education and describe the pros and cons of each.

3. How can written material be linguistically, conceptually, and presentationally modified to meet the reading level of the student with deafness?

4. What factors determine social integration and how can they be incorporated into mainstream education for students with deafness?

5. Outline the components of career/vocational education across the age spectrum.

6. How can technology and media be used to enhance education for students with hearing impairments?

REFERENCES

Allen, T.E. (1984). Test response variations between hearing-impaired and hearing students. *The Journal of Special Education, 18,* 119–129.

Anderson, G. (1986). Employability enhancement skills training for deaf rehabilitation clients. In D. Watson, G. Anderson, & M. Taff-Watson (Eds.), *Integrating human resources, technology, and systems in deafness* (pp. 306–312). Silver Spring, MD: American Deafness and Rehabilitation Association.

Antia, S. (1982). Social interaction of partially mainstreamed hearing-impaired children. *American Annals of the Deaf, 127,* 18–25.

Arcanin, J., & Zawolkow, G. (1980). Microcomputers in the service of students and teachers—Computer assisted instruction at the California School for the Deaf: An update. *American Annals of the Deaf, 125,* 807–813.

Azrin, N., & Besalel, V. (1980). *Job club counselor's manual: A behavioral approach to vocational counseling.* Baltimore: University Park Press.

Baker, C., & Padden, C. (1978). *American Sign Language: A look at its history, structure and community.* Silver Spring, MD: T. J. Publishers.

Barnum, M. (1984). In support of bilingual/bicultural education for deaf children. *American Annals of the Deaf, 129,* 404–408.

Battison, R. (1974). Phonological deletion in American Sign Language. *Sign Language Studies, 5,* 1–19.

Bishop, M. (1979). *Mainstreaming: Practical ideas for educating hearing impaired students.* Washington, DC: Alexander Graham Bell Association for the Deaf.

Bockmiller, P.R. (1981). Hearing-impaired children learning to read a second language. *American Annals of the Deaf, 126,* 810–813.

Bodner-Johnson, B. (1982). The interaction of family and school in the academic achievement of the deaf child. In B. Culhane & C. Williams (Eds.), *Social aspects of deafness: Vol. 2. Social aspects of educating deaf persons* (pp. 199–215). Washington, DC: Gallaudet College Press.

Boone, S., Long, G., & Long, N. (1987). Adapting and evaluating social skills curricula for use with deaf adolescents. In G. Anderson & D. Watson (Eds.), *Innovations in the habilitation and rehabilitation of deaf adolescents* (pp. 235–249). Little Rock, AR: Rehabilitation Research and Training Center on Deafness and Hearing Impairment.

Bornstein, H. (1973). A description of some current sign systems designed to represent English. *American Annals of the Deaf, 118,* 454–463.

Brady, M., & Dickson, P. (1983). A microcomputer communication game for hearing impaired students. *American Annals of the Deaf, 128,* 835–861.

Brolin, D., & Kokaska, C. (1979). *Career education for handicapped children and youth.* Columbus, OH: Charles E. Merrill.

Bullis, M. (1985). Vocational decision making: A career education approach. In M. Bullis & D. Watson (Eds.), *Career education for hearing-impaired students: A review.* (pp. 77–95). Little Rock, AR: Rehabilitation Research and Training Center on Deafness and Hearing Impairment.

Bullis, M. (1986). *Transition study of persons who are hard of hearing, deaf, or hearing impaired with secondary handicapping conditions.* Washington, DC: National Institute on Disability and Rehabilitation Research.

Bullis, M. (1988). Career education. In S. Boone & G. Long (Eds.), *Enhancing the employability of deaf persons: Model interventions* (pp. 21–30). Springfield, IL: Charles C Thomas.

Bullis, M., Bull, B., Sendelbaugh, J., & Freeburg, J. (1987). *Review of research on the school to community transition of adolescents and young adults with hearing impairments.* Washington, DC: The Catholic University, National Rehabilitation Information Center.

Bullis, M., Freeburg, J., Bull, B., & Sendelbaugh, J. (in press). Adolescents and young adults with hearing impairments. In R. Gaylord-Ross (Ed.), *Issues and research in special education (Vol. 1).* New York: Teacher's College Press.

Bullis, M., & Marut, P. (1986). Vocational evaluation recommendations and rehabilitation outcomes. In L. Stewart (Ed.), *Clinical rehabilitation assessment and hearing impairment: A guide to quality assurance* (pp. 111–118). Washington, DC: National Association of the Deaf.

Chojnacki, M.R., & Williams, C.M. (1982). The extracurricular participation of deaf adolescents integrated into an academic program. In B. Culhane & C. Williams (Eds.), *Social aspects of deafness: Vol. 2. Social aspects of educating deaf persons* (pp. 243–258). Washington, DC: Gallaudet College Press.

Clark, G. (1979). *Career education for the handicapped child in the elementary classroom.* Denver: Love Publishing.

Cobb, S., & Egbert, M. (1981). *A career education bibliogra-*

phy: Annotations of studies and programs for handicapped Americans. Washington, DC: Gallaudet College Press.

Cokely, D. (1980). Sign Language: Teaching, interpreting, and educational policy. In C. Baker & R. Battison (Eds.), *Sign language in the deaf community: Essays in honor of William C. Stokoe* (pp. 137–156). Silver Spring, MD: National Association of the Deaf.

Conley, J. (1976). The role of idiomatic expressions in the reading of deaf children. *American Annals of the Deaf, 12,* 381–385.

Cronin, J., MacKall, P., & Richardson, J. (1979, August). *Computer based education for the hearing impaired: A look to the future.* Paper presented at the Third National Computer Symposium on Instructional Technology, Vancouver, WA.

Cubberley, E.P. (1947). *Public education in the United States.* Boston: Houghton Mifflin.

Cummins, J. (1979). Cognitive/academic language proficiency, linguistic interdependence, the optimum age question and some other matters. *Working Papers in Bilingualism, 19,* 197–205.

Dale, E., & Chall, J. (1948). A formula for predicting readability. *Educational Research Bulletin, 27,* 11–20.

Dalgleish, B., & Mohay, H. (1979). Early holophrastic communication without a mature language model: Gesture types at 20 to 26 months. *Sign Language Studies, 23,* 161–166.

Dalton, P. (1985). *Library services to the deaf and hearing impaired.* Phoenix, AZ: Oryx Press.

Denton, D. (1972). A rationale for total communication: The state of the art. *American Annals of the Deaf, 124,* 53–61.

DiFrancesca, S. (1978). *The step method: Learning and practicing thinking skills.* New York: Psychological Corporation.

Dwyer, C. (1985). Career education: A literature review. In M. Bullis & D. Watson (Eds.), *Career education of hearing impaired students: A review* (pp. 3–25). Little Rock, AR: Rehabilitation Research and Training Center on Deafness and Hearing Impairment.

Egelston-Dodd, J. (Ed.). (1980). *Trainer's manual for career education/planning skills.* Rochester, NY: National Technical Institute for the Deaf.

Egelston-Dodd, J., Young, M., Lutz, J., & Lichty, D. (1983). Inservice training in career education and planning skills. In G.D. Tyler (Ed.), *Critical issues in rehabilitation and human services* (Vol. 6, pp. 61–88). Silver Spring, MD: American Deafness and Rehabilitation Association.

Ernst, M. (1982). Tapping literature's language growth potentials for the secondary school hearing-impaired students— The study guide. *Volta Review, 84,* 109–120.

Erting, C.J. (1982). *Deafness, communication and social identity: An anthropological analysis of interaction among parents, teachers, and deaf children in a preschool.* Unpublished doctoral dissertation, American University, Washington, DC. (University Microfilms No. 83-06-972).

Fry, E. (1968). A readability formula that saves time. *Journal of Reading, 11,* 513–516, 575–578.

Galbraith, G. (1978). An interactive computer system for teaching language skills to deaf children. *American Annals of the Deaf, 123,* 706–711.

Galloway, V. (1978). *Overview of a career development model.* Washington, DC: Gallaudet College Press.

Gannon, J.R. (1981). *Deaf heritage: A narrative history of deaf America.* Silver Spring, MD: National Association of the Deaf.

Garvey, M. (1982). CAI as a supplement in a mainstreamed hearing-impaired program. *American Annals of the Deaf, 127,* 613–616.

Geoffrion, L., & Goldenberg, E. (1981). Computer-based exploratory learning systems for communication-handicapped children. *Journal of Special Education, 15,* 325–332.

Greenburg, M. (1980). Mode use in deaf children: The effects of communication method and communication competence. *Applied Psycholinguists, 1,* 65–79.

Greenberg, M., & Kusché, C. (in press). Intellectual, emotional & social growth of deaf children. In M. Wang, H. Walberg, & M. Reynolds (Eds.), *The handbook of special education: Research and practice (Vols. 1–3).* Oxford, England: Pergamon Press.

Greenberg, M.T, Kusché, C.A., Calderon, R., Gustafson, R.N., & Coady, B.A. (1983). *The PATHS curriculum (2nd ed.).* Seattle: University of Washington, Department of Psychology.

Greenberg, M.T., Kusché, C.A. & Smith, M. (1982). A social-cognitive model of psychosocial difficulties and their prevention in deaf children. In B. Culhane & C. Williams (Eds.), *Social aspects of educating deaf persons* (pp. 221–242). Washington, DC: Gallaudet College Press.

Holm, C. (1987). Testing for values with the deaf: The language/cultural effect. *Journal of Rehabilitation of the Deaf, 20* (4), 7–19.

Ingram, R.M., & Ingram, B.L. (Eds.). (1975). *Hands across the sea: Proceedings of the first international conference on interpreting.* Washington, DC: Registry of Interpreters for the Deaf.

Irwin, M. (1982). CAI at CSDF: Organization strategies. *American Annals of the Deaf, 127,* 487–492.

Johnson, R.C. (1987). Research reports: Bilingual, bicultural education for deaf students: A deaf researcher's perspective. *Perspectives for Teachers of the Hearing Impaired, 5* (5) 6–9.

Junor, L., & Taylor, C. (1984). The integration of hearing-impaired students into regular education programs: Some ramifications for library-resource personnel. *Australian Library Journal, 33* (4) 29–35.

Justl, J., McMahon, B., & Lewis, F. (1983). *Curriculum for the employability skills training of deaf/hearing impaired persons.* Tallahassee, FL: Office of Vocational Rehabilitation.

Kannapell, B. (1980). Personal awareness and advocacy in the Deaf community. In C. Baker & R. Battison (Eds.), *Sign Language in the Deaf community: Essays in honor of William C. Stokoe* (pp. 105–116). Silver Spring, MD: National Association of the Deaf.

Kannapell, B. (1982). Inside the Deaf community. *Deaf American, 34,* 23–26.

Karchmer, M., Milone, M., & Wolk. S. (1979). Educational significance of hearing loss at three levels of severity. *American Annals of the Deaf, 124,* 97–109.

Kaufman, M.J., Gottlieb, J., Agard, J.A., & Kubic, A. (1975). Mainstreaming: Toward an explication of the construct. *Focus on Exceptional Children, 7,* 1–13.

Kluwin, T.N. (1981). The grammaticality of manual representations of English in classroom settings. *American Annals of the Deaf, 124,* 417–421.

Lane, H. (1987, July). *Is there a 'psychology of the Deaf'?* An address presented to the U.S. Department of Education, Office of Special Education Programs Conference of Research Project Directors, Washington, DC.

Lang, H., & Stinson, M. (1982). Career education and the occupational status of deaf persons: Concepts, research, and implications. In J. Christiansen & J. Egelston-Dodd (Eds.), *Social aspects of deafness: Vol. 4. Socioeconomic status of the deaf population* (pp. 95–121). Washington, DC: Gallaudet College Press.

LaSasso, C. (1979). The effect of WH question format versus incomplete statement format on deaf students' demonstration of comprehension of text-explicit information. *American Annals of the Deaf, 124*, 833–837.

LaSasso, C. (1980). The validity and reliability of the cloze procedure as a measure of readability for prelingually, profoundly deaf students. *American Annals of the Deaf, 125*, 359–363.

Long, G. (1986). *Goal setting skills training.* Little Rock, AR: Rehabilitation Research and Training Center on Deafness and Hearing Impairment.

Long, N. (1986). *The effects of assertiveness training on assertiveness, social adjustment, and impulsivity of deaf adults.* Unpublished doctoral dissertation, Northern Illinois University, DeKalb.

Long, N., & Davis. G. (1986). Self-directed job seeking skills training: Utilization in a projects with industry program. In D. Watson, G. Anderson, & M. Taff-Watson (Eds.), *Integrating human resources, technology, and systems in deafness* (pp. 313–324). Silver Spring, MD: American Deafness and Rehabilitation Association.

Luetke-Stahlman, B. (1982). A philosophy for assessing the language proficiency of hearing-impaired students to promote English literacy. *American Annals of the Deaf, 127*, 845–851.

Luetke-Stahlman, B. (1983). Using bilingual instructional models in teaching hearing-impaired students. *American Annals of the Deaf, 128*, 873–877.

Luetke-Stahlman, B., & Weiner, F. (1982). Assessing language and/or system preferences of Spanish-deaf preschoolers. *American Annals of the Deaf, 127*, 789–796.

Lyon, S.M., & Oliva, G.A. (1982). The role of classmates and peers in the socialization process of mainstreamed hearing-impaired students. In B. Culhane & C. Williams (Eds.), *Social aspects of deafness: Vol. 2. Social aspects of educating deaf persons* (pp. 221–242). Washington, DC: Gallaudet College Press.

Macon, M. (1982). *School library services to the handicapped.* Westport, CT: Greenwood Press.

Marland, S. (1974). *Career education: A proposal for reform.* New York: McGraw-Hill.

McKee, B.G., & Lang, H.G. (1982). A comparison of deaf students' performance on true-false and multiple-choice items. *American Annals of the Deaf, 127*, 49–54.

Meadow, K. (1975). The Deaf subculture. *Hearing and Speech Action, 43*, 16–18.

Meadow, K. (1980). *Deafness and child development.* Berkeley, CA: University Press.

Moores, D.F. (1982). *Educating the deaf: Psychology principles and practices.* Boston: Houghton Mifflin.

Ouellette, S. (1986). Preliminary results of a descriptive analysis of 46 postsecondary education programs for hearing im

paired students in the United States. In D. Watson, G. Anderson, & M. Taff-Watson (Eds.), *Integrating human resources, technology, and systems in deafness* (pp. 420–428). Silver Spring, MD: American Deafness and Rehabilitation Association.

Ouellette, S., & Dwyer, C. (1985). A current profile of career education programs. In M. Bullis & D. Watson (Eds.), *Career education of hearing impaired students: A review* (pp. 27–56). Little Rock, AR: Rehabilitation Research and Training Center on Deafness and Hearing Impairment.

Padden, C. (1980). The Deaf community and the culture of Deaf people. In C. Baker & R. Battison (Eds.), *Sign Language in the Deaf community: Essays in honor of William C. Stokoe* (pp. 89–103). Silver Spring, MD: National Association of the Deaf.

Passmore, D. (1983). Employment of deaf people. In D. Watson, G. Anderson, W. Ford, P. Marut, & S. Ouellette (Eds.), *Job placement of hearing impaired persons: Research and practice* (pp. 5–16). Little Rock, AR: Rehabilitation Research and Training Center on Deafness and Hearing Impairment.

Petrie, J. (1982). *Mainstreaming in the media center.* Phoenix, AZ: Oryx Press.

Pollard, G., & Shaw, C. (1982). Microcomputer reading comprehension improvement program for the deaf. *American Annals of the Deaf, 127*, 483–486.

Prinz, P., Nelson, K., & Stedt, J. (1982). Early reading in young deaf children using microcomputer technology. *American Annals of the Deaf, 127*, 529–535.

Ramirez, A. (1980). Language in bicultural classrooms. *National Association for Bilingual Education Journal, 4*, 61–80.

Redding, J. (1986). Three cheers for sign language class. *Perspectives for Teachers of the Hearing Impaired, 4* (4), 21–23.

Reiman, J.W., & Bullis, M. (1987). *Research on measurement procedures for persons with hearing impairments: An annotated bibliography.* Monmouth: Teaching Research Division, Oregon State System of Higher Education.

Rogers, W.T. (1983). Use of separate answer sheets with hearing-impaired and deaf school-age students. *British Columbia Journal of Special Education, (7)*, 63–72.

Rudner, L.M. (1978). Using standard tests with the hearing-impaired: The problem of item bias. *The Volta Review, 80* (1), 31–40.

Sacks, S., & Bullis, M. (1987). The training and employment of persons with sensory handicaps. In R. Gaylord-Ross (Ed.), *Vocational education for persons with special needs* (pp. 417–444). Palo Alto, CA: Mayfield.

Schein, J.D., & Delk, M. (1974). *The Deaf population of the United States.* Washington, DC: Gallaudet College Press.

Schrodel, J. (1986). A national study of the class of 1984 in postsecondary education with implications for rehabilitation. In D. Watson, G. Anderson, M. Taff-Watson (Eds.), *Integrating human resources, technology, and systems in deafness* (pp. 267–286). Silver Spring, MD: American Deafness and Rehabilitation Association.

Sendelbaugh, J., & Bullis, M. (1988). Special education and rehabilitation policies for the school to community transition of students with hearing impairments. *Journal of the American Deafness and Rehabilitation Association, 21*(4), 15–20.

Sheie, T. (1983). Photo journalism: Microcomputer text editing and photography—Synthesis and divergence. *American Annals of the Deaf, 128,* 653–661.

Shiels, J. (1986). Vocational assessment. In L. Stewart (Ed.), *Clinical rehabilitation assessment and hearing impairment: A guide to quality assurance* (pp. 95–110). Washington, DC: National Association of the Deaf.

Sligar, S. (1983). Commercial vocational evaluation systems and deaf persons. In D. Watson, G. Anderson, P. Marut, S. Ouellette, & N. Ford (Eds.), *Vocational evaluation of hearing impaired persons: Research and practice* (pp. 35–56). Little Rock, AR: Rehabilitation Research and Training Center on Deafness and Hearing Impairment.

Stepp, R. (1982). Microcomputers: Macro-learning for the hearing-impaired. *American Annals of the Deaf, 127,* 472–475.

Stevens, R.D. (1976). Children's language should be learned and not taught. *Sign Language Studies, 11,* 97–108.

Stewart, D.A. (1983). The use of sign by Deaf children: The opinions of a Deaf community. *American Annals of the Deaf, 128,* 878–883.

Stewart, L. (Ed.). (1986a). *Clinical rehabilitation assessment and hearing impairment: A guide to quality assurance.* Washington, DC: National Association of the Deaf.

Stewart, L. (1986b). State VR agencies policies for sponsoring deaf students in postsecondary education and training. In D. Watson, G. Anderson, & M. Taff-Watson (Eds.), *Integrating human resources, technology, and systems in deafness* (pp. 287–297). Silver Spring, MD: American Deafness and Rehabilitation Association.

Stokoe, W.C. (1960). *Sign language structure: An outline of the visual communication system of the American Deaf.* Buffalo, NY: University of Buffalo.

Stokoe, W.C. (1976). The use of sign language in teaching English. *American Sign Language, 120,* 417–421.

Stokoe, W.C. (1978). Sign language and the verbal/non-verbal distinction. In Sebeok (Ed.), *Sight, sound, and sense* (pp. 157–172). Bloomington: Indiana University Press.

Stokoe, W., Bernard, H., & Padden, C. (1976). An elite group in deaf society. *Sign Language Studies, 12,* 189–210.

Stuckless, R. (1982). *Deaf and hearing undergraduate students' ability to detect and correct word errors in the real-time graphic display of spoken lectures.* Rochester, NY: National Technical Institute for the Deaf.

Stuckless, R. (1983). Real-time transliteration of speech into print for hearing-impaired students in regular classes. *American Annals of the Deaf, 128,* 619–624.

Stuckless, R., & Matter, J. (1982a). *Word accuracy and error in steno/computer transliteration of spoken lectures into real-time graphic display.* Rochester, NY: National Technical Institute for the Deaf.

Stuckless, R., & Matter, J. (1982b). *Word accuracy in translation of spoken lectures into real-time graphic display for deaf students: First year.* Rochester, NY: National Technical Institute for the Deaf.

Swain, M. (1978). French immersion: Early, late, or partial. *The Canadian Modern Language Review, 34,* 577–586.

Tervoort, B. (1961). Esoteric symbolism in the communicative behavior of young deaf children. *American Annals of the Deaf, 106,* 436–480.

Torretti, W., & Hendrick, P. (1986). A job club approach with severely disabled deaf clients. In D. Watson, G. Anderson, & M. Taff-Watson (Eds.), *Integrating human resources, technology, and systems in deafness* (pp. 325–339). Silver Spring, MD: American Deafness and Rehabilitation Association.

Trybus, R., & Karchmer, M. (1977). School achievement scores of hearing impaired children: National data on achievement status and growth patterns. *American Annals of the Deaf, 122,* 62–69.

Twyman, L., & Ouellette, S. (1978). Career development programs in residential schools for the deaf: A survey. *American Annals of the Deaf, 123,* 10–12.

Updegraff, D., & Egelston-Dodd, J. (1982). The national project on career education: Past, present, and future. *Directions, 2*(4), 15–23.

Van den Pol, R.A., Crow, R.E., Rider, D.P., & Offner, R.B. (1985). Social interaction in an integrated preschool: Implications and applications. *Topics in Early Childhood Special Education, 4*(4), 59–76.

Vernon, M. (1976). Deafness and mental health: Some theoretical views. In *Gallaudet today: Special issue on mental health and deafness.* Washington, DC: Gallaudet College, Department of Publications.

Vorih, L., & Rosier, P. (1978). Rock Point community school: An example of a Navajo-English bilingual elementary school program. *TESOL Quarterly, 12,* 263–269.

Waldron, M. (1985). Hearing impaired students in regular classrooms: A cognitive model for educational services. *Exceptional Children, 52,* 39–43.

Ward, G.B. (1985). Bale's talking hands. *Perspectives for Teachers of the Hearing Impaired, 3*(3), 17–18.

Watson, D. (1979). Guidelines for the psychological and vocational assessment of deaf rehabilitation clients. *Journal of Rehabilitation of the Deaf, 13,* 27–57.

Watson, D. (1986). *Application for the funding of a research and demonstration project for a national study of transition from school to work for deaf youth.* Washington, DC: National Institute on Disability and Rehabilitation.

White, K., & Slusher, N. (1978). *Measuring career development among post-secondary deaf adults* (Paper No. 25). Rochester, NY: National Technical Institute for the Deaf.

Wilbur, R.B. (1979). *American Sign Language and sign systems.* Baltimore: University Park Press.

Will, M. (1984). *OSERS program for the transition of youth with disabilities: Bridges from school to working life.* Washington, DC: Office of Special Education and Rehabilitative Services.

Woodward, J. (1982). *How ya gonna get to heaven if ya can't talk to Jesus: On depathologizing deafness.* Silver Spring, MD: T.J. Publishers.

Woodward, J.C. (1973). A program to prepare sign language specialists to work with the deaf. *Sign Language Studies, 2,* 81–83.

Wright, K. (1979). *Library and information services for handicapped individuals.* Littleton, CO: Libraries Unlimited.

Zawolkow, E.G., & DeFiore, S. (1986). Educational interpreting for elementary- and secondary-level hearing-impaired students. *American Annals of the Deaf, 131,* 26–28.

CHAPTER 6

INTEGRATING STUDENTS WITH CHALLENGING BEHAVIORS

Joy Casey-Black and Peter Knoblock

Achieving integrated educational opportunities for students exhibiting a diverse range of needs may be a complex and, at times, difficult task for teachers. This is often particularly true when students demonstrate extremely challenging behaviors. Such behaviors may act to distance the student from others, inhibit communication, interfere with activity performance, and contribute to a negative self-image. The characteristics of students who present difficult behaviors within school settings certainly vary, but such behaviors may be particularly evident in populations of students labeled as "emotionally handicapped," "autistic," or "severely emotionally disturbed." This chapter proceeds from a problem-solving perspective, regarding the occurrence of extremely challenging behaviors, examining their functions and the contexts surrounding them, and discussing the implications of teachers in planning for and implementing integrated activities. Descriptions of three different operating models of educational programs serving students who exhibit challenging behaviors follow. Within these models, the classrooms described are structured (with respect to physical environment, classroom groupings, scheduling, etc.) for the purpose of achieving an intensive educational environment through integration. A series of specific integrated activities, developed within the contexts of these educational models, is presented, covering an age span from preschool to middle school students.

A CASE STUDY

The discussion of the educational processes the authors' use in developing an individualized schedule of integrated activities for a student with difficult behaviors begins with an observation of Danny, a 13-year-old middle school student labeled as "autistic." This observation illustrates key questions teachers should raise regarding the impact of challenging behaviors on planning for and implementing integrated activities.

On a cold and snowy December afternoon, Danny was standing on a busy downtown street corner with two of his classmates and his teacher, waiting for the city bus to arrive. The group had just completed a fitness routine at the YMCA, and was returning to school just prior to the end of the school day. The teacher commented that the bus would arrive in approximately 5 minutes. Danny began shifting from foot to foot, tugging on the teacher's arm and saying, "Bus now! Bus now!" Although the teacher referred Danny to his digital wrist watch to check the remaining time, Danny continued to tug at his teacher, shouting, "Now! Now!" When the bus approached, the teacher reminded the group about waiting in line to enter the bus, and stood directly behind Danny as the group joined others waiting to board. As one elderly woman came down the bus stairs,

Danny started to lunge forward, but stopped as his teacher took hold of his coat and reminded him to wait. Once having entered the bus and been guided to a seat in the rear, Danny began to slap and grab at his teacher who was seated next to him, and tried to turn the teacher's face toward his. The teacher ignored these actions, talking instead to the other students across the bus aisle. When Danny quieted, the teacher turned to him and calmly asked about his visit to the YMCA.

In many instances, the behaviors described above would be viewed as sufficient evidence for disallowing students with intense behavioral needs from participating in integrated environments, whether in school or in the community. However, the expectation demonstrated in this middle school program, that all students have the right of access to the full range of environments enjoyed by their peers, is intertwined with processes for enhancing student competencies and for problem solving around difficult behaviors.

What are the contexts of the challenging behaviors?

Danny's teacher operated from an ecological perspective in designing and carrying out an integrated educational plan for his student. Rather than viewing the source of Danny's difficult behaviors as residing solely within him, the teacher examined the interaction between Danny and the larger ecosystem in which he functioned. Ecological theory (Apter & Conoley, 1984) focuses on the interaction of an individual with the social and physical environments in which she or he operates, with a view to how well the individual matches the expectations of the environment. When the various aspects of a person's ecosystem are working together, the system is regarded as "balanced" and the person seen as normal. When this level of congruence does not exist, the person's behaviors are likely to be seen as deviant or incompetent. Those points at which the person's behaviors fail to match the expectations of the sys-

tem are called "points of discordance." The resulting conflict has been described as: "a mismatch between a child's abilities and the demands of his or her environment. Consequently, either an increase in a child's skills or a decrease in environmental pressures can prevent the occurrence of school situations that produce or exacerbate disturbance" (Apter & Conoley, 1984, p. 83). From this perspective, Danny's teacher approached the issue of designing integrated activities for his student not from a readiness viewpoint (Was or was not Danny "ready" to be integrated?), but from a viewpoint of skills training and environmental support strategies. Given this perspective, the implications for the teacher's role becomes clear. Teacher tasks then focus on determining critical skill areas for targeting, assessing present skill levels, and deciding on best instructional practices as well as levels and kinds of environmental support.

What functions do the behaviors serve?

In an article entitled "Analyzing the Communicative Functions of Aberrant Behavior," Donnellan, Mirenda, Mesaros, and Fassbender (1984) assert that all behavior "has functional message value" (p. 202). All behavior is considered to be communicative, whether clearly articulated through spoken language or an alternative system of communication, or inferred from a functional analysis of behavior. This perspective on the communicative functions of language is known as "pragmatics." Pragmatics is the study of language within its social context, focusing on both verbal and nonverbal means of message delivery. Employing a functional analysis of behavior seeks to discover the underlying messages of behaviors, or their communicative intent. If one reexamines Danny's behaviors before and during his bus ride, one can probably make some sound interpretations as to the messages he was sending: "I'm anxious, I want to go now!" (Shifting from foot to foot, saying "Bus now!"); and "Pay attention to me!" (slapping, grabbing, and turning the teacher's face toward his). This level of interpretation around student behaviors suggests a much different means of intervening around teaching more appropriate means of communicating the message, rather than simply decreasing the behavior.

How do behaviors relate to skill level?

Learning theorists would describe the occurrence of maladaptive or challenging behaviors as deriving from a lack of skills necessary to perform the behaviors appropriate to the situation. From this perspective, the prescription of choice would be systematic instruction in areas of skill deficiency. Goldstein, Sprafkin, Gershaw, and Klein (1980), in their book *Skill-streaming the Adolescent,* comment that what have traditionally been viewed as disruptive behaviors within school settings may more appropriately be seen as a lack of or weakness in "the necessary skills and behaviors that all people need to lead effective and satisfying personal and interpersonal lives" (p. 1). Whether the observed behaviors are aggressive, withdrawn, or immature and inadequate in nature, if their source is a deficit of skills, a systematic approach to skill instruction is indicated. The authors advocate the use of "Structured Learning . . . a psychoedu-

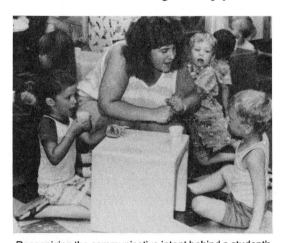

Recognizing the communicative intent behind a student's behavior enables teachers to provide spoken and sign language models for the intended message. (Photo by Susan Gelling.)

cational intervention designed specifically to enhance the prosocial, interpersonal, stress management, and planning skills" (p. 11) of students experiencing maladaptive behavior patterns (Goldstein et al., 1980).

How do behaviors relate to students' self-concept?

Far too often, educators examine the occurrence of challenging behaviors solely from an outside perspective (e.g., "How are these behaviors perceived by others in the environment?" or "How can I keep the behaviors from interfering with my instruction?") rather than seeking to understand the behaviors from the student's viewpoint. One would do well to ask instead how the behaviors relate to issues of respect and autonomy, to the student's ability and opportunity to make choices around participation in activities, and the perceptions of the student regarding the success, functionality, and reward value of the behaviors. In the example about Danny, when he began to slap, grab at, and attempt to turn his teacher's face toward himself after having been guided toward his seat, was he only saying, "Pay attention to me!" or could the message have been, "I want to pick my own seat" or, "I want to sit alone"? Whatever the case, did Danny perceive his behaviors to be successful and rewarded (the teacher ignored Danny until he quieted, then began to converse with him); or would he have felt more successful if the teacher had given Danny a more appropriate alternative means of expressing himself (e.g., "If you want my attention, touch my shoulder") and responded to (rewarded) Danny for that behavior?

How do teachers respond to the challenge of integrating students with difficult behaviors?

The questions outlined above provide a framework for problem solving around the major issues that may arise when designing an integrated educational experience for students with challenging behaviors. As is evident in the illustration about

Danny, the issues these questions address do not typically arise in isolation; that is, the issues are often interrelated and the solutions, of necessity, are complex. In addition, the interventions chosen are not "the right way," irrespective of time and situation. Teachers must continuously reassess the success of integration plans for students, and adapt the plans prescriptively as the situation warrants. With this in mind, the chapter first discusses particular integrated educational models, and then, specific integrated activities developed within those models. (The reader should note the variety of ways in which integration is achieved, and perhaps explore the possibilities for adapting the activity examples given for particular student needs.)

INTEGRATED EDUCATIONAL MODELS

The specific integrated educational models presented in this section are currently in operation in Syracuse, New York. These programs represent a continuum of integrated services from preschool to middle school, and with the exception of Jowonio, the preschool program, operate in the Syracuse City School District's regular public schools. The driving force behind the creation of the continuum was parents and educators who, having witnessed the possibilities and opportunities available to students within existing integrated educational settings, advocated strongly for the extension of an integrated program from preschool to elementary to middle school, as students transitioned into these settings.

Jowonio School

Background

Jowonio was created in 1969 as a private alternative learning environment for school-age students who, for a variety of reasons, had begun to react negatively to public school. Beginning with 10 students and one teacher, Jowonio focused on the creation of a "learning community" where stu-

dents were seen as active learners, growing through their interactions with the people in their environment (both peers and adults), as well as through exploration of materials. In 1975, Jowonio responded to the requests of parents of three preschool-aged children with special needs to provide educational programming in the absence of home school district programs. With the addition of three graduate students in special education from Syracuse University, Jowonio extended its educational program to include these children with special needs. What began as a parallel educational program (located in a separate classroom, with different teachers and activities) soon became much more interactional (with labeled and nonlabeled children sharing space, materials, and teachers). The basic premise of children learning through interaction with the people in their environment was then realized to apply not only to "typical" children, but to their peers with special needs as well. Although the parents and staff at Jowonio did not begin with the conception of the school as an integrated learning environment, they soon discovered the benefits as well as challenges this option presented.

Class Groupings

Jowonio currently serves children with special needs from 1 to 4 years of age. The 1- and 2-year-old classrooms are composed of eight children, four of whom are labeled as having special needs. In the two 3–4-year-old classrooms as well as the kindergartens, the groupings are larger, with 6 labeled children in each class of 16. Classroom placement of individual children is decided based upon various factors, including: age, intensity of need/severity of disability, as well as the existence of, or best matches for, the development of peer relationships. Every attempt is made to create a classroom grouping that is heterogeneous along such student variables as presence of challenging behaviors, intensity of communication needs, and cognitive and social skills. For the most part, students remain within their primary classroom group for whole group and independent activities.

Children with special needs may receive additional services, either within or outside the classroom, from various resource staff, either individually or partnered with a "typical" classmate.

Curriculum

The focus of curriculum at Jowonio spans a range of developmental areas including behavior, communication, socialization, cognition, and motor skills. An individualized education program (IEP) is developed for each of the children with special needs, identifying learning objectives in each of these areas, using *Developmental Therapy* (Wood, 1975) as a guide. The individual learning objectives identified in the IEP are then translated into specific classroom activities in a weekly planning session for all classroom staff. Inclusion of specific materials or adaptation of existing materials/procedures within group activities is discussed at this time to ensure that there are avenues of participation available to students who are presenting a range of behavioral needs and operating at varying skill levels.

Staffing/Administrative Support

Each classroom team is made up of a number of adults, varying with the size/age level of the classroom (as described above). Every class has a lead teacher and an assistant teacher who have trained and worked in various special education, early childhood, and elementary education settings. In addition, graduate and undergraduate university interns, volunteers, and parents complete the classroom teams to provide for a consistent group of full-time adults in each class (minimum of three for the 1- and 2-year-old rooms, and four for the other classrooms). Additional itinerant members of the classroom teams include a speech-language therapist, a physical therapist, an occupational therapist, and a resource teacher. This level of adult resources allows for sufficient individual in-class support for students exhibiting very challenging behaviors, as well as the opportunity for many contributions to problem-solving discussions.

Administrative support systems include a designated support person from among the administrative staff for each classroom. Support people meet with each of their classroom teams at least weekly to facilitate problem-solving discussions around classroom issues. Clinical team meetings occur on a rotating basis around issues relating to specific children, incorporating input from additional administrative, resource, and other classroom staff. Weekly inservice seminars are held for all school staff to provide ongoing support around issues of integration.

Edward Smith School

Background

The integrated program at Edward Smith School, a regular public elementary school, became the "feeder" program for students leaving Jowonio to enter the public schools. This continuum of integrated classrooms became a reality due to efforts by Jowonio staff and parents. Significantly, parents of nondisabled students were equally active in requesting integrated classrooms for their children; and in some instances where friendships had developed, these parents asked to have their children placed in the same classrooms with their friends. This transition process took 1½ years and, in 1980, a combination third-fourth grade was created for the three students with autism who, at 8 years old, were leaving Jowonio School. The ability and willingness of teachers, parents, and administrators to plan ahead for the next environment was a crucial element in the change process (Vincent et al., 1980).

During this protracted planning process, local school officials were informed by parents and Jowonio staff of the names, ages, and projected needs of the students who would be transitioning into the public schools. The reality of having to plan a program for specific students coupled with parent involvement expedited the planning process. In addition, because the children had begun their school lives in integrated classrooms and had grown socially and cognitively, these parents could look forward to groupings that maintained such diversity.

Class Groupings

The practice of placing older and younger children together in one classroom, referred to as cross-age grouping, was used at Jowonio School when it began integrating students with autism, and it was continued in the third-fourth grade combination classroom at Edward Smith School. This model, staffed by regular education teachers and a special education teacher, was maintained for the next several years as those 8-year-olds moved up the grade ladder toward middle school. Class sizes were maintained at 25 to 30 students, with no more than 5 or 6 students with special needs assigned to each team. The students with special needs were grouped in a heterogeneous fashion with respect to the intensity/severity of the needs they presented. Thus, the two teachers had the flexibility of grouping students a variety of ways: small integrated reading lessons were taught by one teacher while the other did a large group lesson; one teacher functioned as a support teacher to special needs students taking part in large or small group instruction, some students took part in community-based activities with one teacher while the other remained in school, and so forth.

As one might expect, any one classroom grouping model has advantages and disadvantages. For some teachers, sharing skills and learning from one another was viewed as an opportunity; for others, collaborating with other staff was not considered to be an advantage. In this latter group, two teachers were assigned to one group, but they actually divided the students between them and did not engage in joint planning. Other teachers preferred to work alone with two or three special needs students placed into their classroom with a slightly reduced number of nondisabled students. Rather than discourage this proliferation of models, the teachers, administrators, and parents at Edward Smith School encouraged the creation of grouping options.

Today, kindergarten through grade six have integrated classrooms, and the models differ, as Table 1 indicates. For example, the first and third grades have maintained the team-teaching model developed in 1980; but the second and fourth grades have adopted radically different grouping models. Three of the second-grade classes have each reduced their total number of students to 17, with 2 special needs students in each classroom. There is a teacher and a teaching assistant in each classroom and the staff of the two rooms plan collaborative activities and engage in joint planning when appropriate. Also, there are less severely involved special needs students integrated into each of the other second-grade classrooms.

The fourth-grade team decided to assign the students with special needs to each of the five fourth-grade classrooms. By placing one student in each fourth-grade classroom, that team, composed of four regular teachers and one special education teacher, has moved closer to the concept of natural proportions by avoiding the clustering of special needs students in one classroom. Of course, if one is to approximate natural proportions, or the placing of students into classrooms or schools according to the proportion found in that community, then the large numbers of students with severe disabilities could not be placed into one school as has been done at Edward Smith School. It was originally felt that the clustering of students to maximize available resources justified such grouping arrangements. That logic may sound familiar when one remembers that proponents of special class groupings designs used that argument to justify clustering students in one classroom. Gradually, the Edward Smith program appears to be moving toward more of a dispersal strategy, and the fourth-grade grouping model is an example of that effort. As one fourth-grade teacher said, "I'm a teacher, and if I'm any good I can teach any student."

Curriculum

Teachers in this program, and in all public school programs, are under increasing pressure to "guar-

Table 1.   Integrated program at Edward Smith Elementary School, Syracuse, New York

Grade level	Number of teachers		Number of children		
	Special education	Regular education	Special needs students	Nonhandicapped students	Number of Classes
Kindergarten	1	1	6	21 (split sessions)	1
First Grade	1	1	6	25	1
Second Grade	1	2	2 per class	15 per class	3
Third Grade	1	1	6	25	1
Fourth Grade	1	4	1 per class	22 per class	5
Fifth Grade	1	1	6	23	1
Sixth Grade	1		5	17	1

antee" skills acquisition by students. This issue is further complicated by the need to individualize instruction for students with special needs included in regular classrooms with their nondisabled peers. For students with challenging behaviors, a sound curriculum should include activities and materials that facilitate social interaction as well as addressing cognitive and communication needs. The teaching staff at Edward Smith School, at each grade level, strives to continue the efforts made by teachers at the previous grade level. This provides continuity of instruction as the teaching staff emphasizes the teaching of functional skills, independent functioning, choice making, and preparation for and participation in community-based instruction. These priorities are accomplished by skillful arranging of schedules, groupings, and teacher collaboration. Fenwick (1987), a lead teacher in the Edward Smith program, summarizes this curriculum approach when she writes:

> In addition to presenting academic instruction in all curriculum areas—including reading, language, art, spelling, writing, mathematics, social studies, science, and health—teachers in integrated classes also include in their daily schedules meeting [whole group discussion of classroom issues] and choice times [loosely structured period, with choice of games and other socially oriented activities]. While integrated classes emphasize skill development, mastery, and independence and enjoyment in application, as other typical classes do, and while they

participate in all activities that classes at the same grade level participate in, teachers set aside approximately 30 minutes a day for a class meeting time and another 30 minutes each day for an individual choice-making time. (p. 271)

Staffing/Administrative Support

The integrated classes at Edward Smith School coexist with segregated classrooms for students labeled mentally retarded and with regular classrooms with students identified as mildly disabled or with no identified special needs students. This situation calls for unique administrative and staff support.

Administratively, the principal has provided a degree of leadership that allowed the integration to occur initially and to sustain its evolution from one team-teaching model at the third-grade level to integrated classes at all grades in the school. At the same time, it has been necessary for her to continually interpret the integrated program's purpose to the rest of the staff and encourage the efforts of the other teachers in the school. The principal's leadership role was recently apparent when she responded to a fourth-grade teacher's suggestion to involve each of the other fourth-grade teachers. Together, the teacher and the principal first obtained the support of the other teachers on that grade level, and then arranged for a presentation to the board of education by parents and teachers describing the new model.

One of the unique features of this integrated program is the degree of support that teachers provide to one another. For the past several years they have met as a group to provide catharsis and technical assistance to each other. Representatives of this group have met with the principal on an ongoing basis to make suggestions for improving the program. These included the assigning of a person to function as a program supervisor and support person; the development of schedules to maximize the effectiveness of school support staff members (e.g., language therapists, physical therapists, and occupational therapists); and the hiring of sufficient numbers of teacher aides to assist the lead teacher and assistant teachers placed in each classroom.

Levy Middle School

Background

This program for students with special needs ages 12 to 16 was initiated to maintain students from Edward Smith School and other programs in integrated educational programs. The teacher who created this program, in consultation with school administrators and Syracuse University consultants, faced unique organizational and content issues.

At the middle school level, programs for students with special needs face a very different challenge than that posed for teachers of preschool and elementary-age children. The structure of the school changes; academics become departmentalized according to their subject areas; students move through six different classroom environments, each with different teachers, different peers, and different expectations; and students are expected to exercise increasing levels of responsibility and independence with regard to their school functioning. The focus of the adolescent's life, which has been shifting progressively toward greater association with his or her peer group, becomes almost institutionalized in the school, where there is no longer one primary adult with which to identify, but many. Additionally, the dwindling number of remaining school years prompts teachers to give even greater focus to the types of skills students will need to successfully negotiate the vast array of nonschool environments within which they will operate.

Class Groupings

The Levy Middle School program is cognizant of the above issues and attempts to respond to each. It currently serves eight students, ranging in age from 12 to 16. It is located in a public school building, and is designated as semi–self-contained (integrated for parts of the school day). The classroom serves as an integrated homeroom, in which the special needs students and their nondisabled peers spend the first 20 minutes of the school day together. Then, each of the special needs students attends classes responsive to each of their particular needs. For example, two students attend reading class in a regular classroom; three students attend shop; two students attend adaptive physical education class; and another learns functional reading in the reading lab. The first-period grouping plan is followed in the second and third periods by students attending regular education social studies and mathematics classes, and being involved in functional domestic skills instruction such as generating a picture-symbol grocery shopping list or learning to cook in the homeroom. After the third and final period of the morning, each student has a plan to function in the community in a recreational and job-site opportunity. Thus, the program is intensive, individualized and both school and community based.

Curriculum

With regard to curriculum, an excerpt from the class's program description states:

> The ideal middle school curriculum for Autistic students had yet to be formulated. We hope to make a significant contribution to this effort. As a starting point, our programmatic goals are to promote optimum student functioning, possibility of choice, and participation of Autistic students in a wide range of school, non-school, and post-school environments . . . The extent of departure from developmental ac-

ademic curriculum will be based on: student interests and age, parental input, and a longitudinal analysis of the skills necessary for students to function in current and future school, vocational, domestic, and community environments. (Black, 1983, p. 1)

School-based instruction breaks down into three major categories: classroom-based instruction that is primarily self-contained, activities employing reverse integration strategies, and participation in mainstream regular education classes (with varying levels of support). In-room instruction centers on functional academics—reading and math as they relate to functional life activities (e.g., reading and measuring ingredients for a recipe, or compiling a shopping list and estimating the price of items to determine if one has adequate money for purchases). Such instruction is performed either individually or in small groups. Activities employing reverse integration include a daily first-period homeroom, a once-weekly teacher advisement group (designed to give students a "home base"), and a sign-up system for use of classroom equipment and materials. A word about the physical environment is warranted here. The class is quite unlike a typical middle school room. In addition to the work tables, desks, chalkboards, and shelves piled with books and materials, the classroom holds: a complete fitness center with weights, two exercycles, a rowing machine, and a punching bag; a potters wheel; a complete kitchen; and a personal computer with software ranging from "Pac Man" to video basketball. Talk about materials that engage! This room looks like an adolescent's dream. One would guess that such creative environmental design would go a long way toward drawing interest and involvement of the larger school population, and in fact, it has. The final component of the school-based curriculum is participation in mainstream classes. All eight of the program's students are integrated in regular education classes for part of their school day, with times ranging from 4 hours per week to 12 hours per week (excluding integrated lunch periods).

How was integration achieved for all students, some of whom have abilities and needs quite different from their typical peers? The teacher reported that, when his program first opened, before students even entered the building, he did an in-service presentation to all school staff on the nature of his program and the needs of his students. He ended by stating that he would probably be approaching departmental teams and individual teachers about integrating his students in some of their classes. He then followed up his presentation by initiating contact with eight teachers of subjects most suited to the needs of his students. Classes targeted included those focusing on reading skills (e.g., reading, English, and social studies) as well as the so-called "specials": shop, art, home economics, and physical education. All those approached agreed, most with enthusiasm. The teacher made a teaching assistant available to the regular education teachers to be utilized in whatever manner they found most beneficial—supporting the integrated student, running a small group, or assisting with paperwork. Before long, many of the regular education teachers politely said that the students were doing quite nicely, and they no longer needed the support of the teaching assistant. Not all integrated situations went quite as smoothly, however. One student was withdrawn from an industrial arts class because he consistently turned the power on to many of the big machines, creating a safety concern. Similar difficulties should be met with a "back to the drawing board" approach to select a better fit between the student and the environment and expectations of the class.

The other major aspect of this unique program is its emphasis on community-based instruction. Roughly one-half of each student's school program takes place outside the school walls. Sample nonschool environments include: a domestic training apartment donated for daytime use by a local citizen; various neighborhood stores and nearby shopping malls; several on-site or nearby vocational training placements ranging from custodial to clerical to grocery clerking; community restaurants; and a range of leisure/recreation environments including parks, riding stables, bowling alleys, video arcades, public libraries, and the local YMCA.

Staffing/Administrative Support

The Levy Middle School program is staffed by a special education teacher, two teaching assistants, and one Syracuse University graduate student intern. The lead teacher works very hard to establish working relationships with other teachers in the school and considers it an essential part of his job to keep the principal very well informed. Also, the teacher and his staff spend a considerable amount of time developing job sites in the community and soliciting the support of community persons in recreational and work settings.

INTEGRATED ACTIVITIES

The specific integrated activities included in this section were envisioned within the integrated educational models described in the previous section. As described, these integrated models span a wide range of ages (from preschool to middle school); they also reflect diverse strategies for achieving integration of students with challenging behaviors. The activities are outlined with a fairly high level of specificity with regard to such variables as student groupings, materials, and manner of implementation. This has been done to create a clear picture of the integrated activity, enabling the reader to carry out the activity as designed. However, the reader is encouraged to use the activities outlined as a springboard—adapting instructional variables as necessary to tailor activities to his or her own students' needs, as well as the structure of the integrated environment within which instruction occurs.

Activities described are grouped into five instructional domains targeted as significant areas of instruction for students exhibiting challenging behaviors, and are derived from an examination of students' IEPs. The majority of the domains selected represent a focus on the development of

positive social interaction skills, so critical to successful functioning in a range of integrated environments. Instructional domains include: social skills, play/leisure skills, self-concept, and communication. In addition, a cognitive/academic domain is included to address the significant question of how best to integrate students with challenging behaviors into academic instruction, ensuring that instruction is relevant to the learning goals of the special needs student, as well as being intensive enough for typical learners. Here, the skills are learned in context of the ultimate, or minimally adapted, environments in which they will be practiced. Each instructional domain includes two specific activities at differing age/grade levels. Again, the reader is invited to explore the possibilities for expanding and adapting the activity ideas presented to particular student needs and learning environments.

SOCIAL SKILLS

Special Friends Program—Middle School Level

Rationale

The Special Friends Program was developed in Hawaii as an attempt to foster a smooth transition to public school services for students experiencing severe disabilities. The program focuses on cultivating a school environment that is receptive to the integration of students with challenging needs, as well as structuring systematic opportunities for "positive and mutually rewarding interactions" (Voeltz, 1984, p. 175) between regular education students and their classmates with special needs. In the context of these interactions, social skill building is facilitated within a normalized, integrated environment.

Participants

As the name implies, one of the major goals of this activity is the development of a friendship between a student with challenging behaviors and a typical age/grade-peer. This goal dictates that group size for any given activity be no larger than two: one student with challenging behaviors and one typical classmate. Since the Special Friends Program was not designed to be a tutoring situation, the requirement that participants be similar age/grade-peers maximizes the equality of the interaction and also ensures the utilization of age-appropriate and stimulating materials.

Setting

The setting for the partnered interaction should be within the school building, with the exact location dependent upon the preferences and scheduling flexibility of the students involved. Possibilities include the school cafeteria (eating lunch); the library (listening to music at listening centers); the computer lab (playing computer games); the gym (jogging or lifting weights); and the integrated homeroom (enriched with such engaging materials as a fitness center and a mini-workshop). Scheduling options may be as limited as shared lunch times, or as flexible as within the context of a regularly scheduled class (e.g., computer lab) or substituting for a study hall.

Materials

Determination of specific materials is linked to the selection of the location for the partners' activity. The guiding idea should be the opportunity for interactive as opposed to parallel participation (e.g., turn taking in the use of computer games or negotiating about the particular tape to choose at the listening center, as opposed to each independently looking at books). Again, assessing student preferences prior to selecting specific materials will maximize sustained interest and successful participation.

Intervention

Student participants are matched according to their expressed preferences for similar types of activities. Individual schedules are checked to ascertain possible times for the "special friends" to get together on a consistent basis (e.g., daily lunch in the cafeteria, or Tuesday and Thursday afternoons for weightlifting in the gym). Finally, the type and degree of needed individual support for the student with special needs must be determined and planned for (e.g., adapting the complexity of the task in selecting a computer game by limiting the choice to two; designing strategies for waiting in a turn-taking activity with the exercycle; or assigning an individual support teacher to facilitate the interaction).

Structured Learning— Elementary School Level

Rationale

According to its authors, Structured Learning is "a psychoeducational, behavioral approach for providing instruction in prosocial skills" (McGinnis, Goldstein, Sprafkin, & Gershaw, 1984, p. 9) that focuses primarily on instruction within public school settings. The skills targeted in Structured Learning deal with issues arising around group membership, with skill deficiency presumed to be a major factor in contributing to interpersonal conflict. The use of Structured Learning in integrated environments offers a direct approach to addressing classroom issues in a manner that acknowledges the contributions and impact of challenging behaviors with regard to the total classroom environment.

Participants

Structured Learning sessions may be conducted with the entire classroom group, to maximize the likelihood of consistent ongoing models of the targeted skill in the natural setting. Reinforcement sessions may be planned as necessary with particular students within the larger classroom group to give additional practice within a structured setting.

Setting

A once-weekly inclusion of Structured Learning concepts in the classroom's daily "meeting time" allows for a concentrated focus on building particular social interaction skills, with opportunities to practice in a supportive and reinforcing environment throughout the remainder of the week. Small group reinforcement sessions would most appropriately be scheduled at alternative times (e.g., as part of language arts or social studies) when the class breaks up into small groups for more individualized content work. The physical setting should be arranged so that participants are seated comfortably around a "stage" area, where the role-playing aspect of Structured Learning can unfold.

Materials

A chart or chalkboard is needed to display the individual steps that lead to the overall skill (derived from a task analysis of the skill). Steps may be listed in pictorial and/or written form, depending on the skill levels of the participants. Materials in the "stage" area should be selected to resemble, as much as possible, those in the setting where participants will be required to display the targeted skill.

Intervention

The selection of a specific skill is made based on a combination of teacher and student input, with student input gathered via a simple questionnaire. Once the skill is selected, a sequence of behavioral steps is constructed. The teacher and support staff (or a skilled student volunteer) model the initial demonstration of what the skill looks like, in a clear and nonambiguous way. For example, in teaching the skill "Responding to Teasing," the "actors" are each given a specific role to play, either as the person who is doing the teasing, or as the one who is being teased. The student who is responding to the teasing models the following steps, in sequence: 1) Stop and count to five; 2) Think about your choices (e.g., ignore, state how you feel, ask the person to stop); 3) Act out your best choice (McGinnis et al., 1984, p. 147). Then, students are selected to role-play the situation, attempting to match their performance to the model. Members of the "audience" share perfor-

mance feedback with the actors, specifying how well they played their roles. Social reinforcement for following the behavioral steps outlined occurs in this segment of Structured Learning. Finally, homework assignments are given that relate to practice of the targeted skill in the settings of concern to enhance practice and mastery of the skill. The subsequent Structured Learning session begins with a review of the previous week's homework, then proceeds through the additional steps as described above.

PLAY/LEISURE SKILLS

Turn-Taking Games—Preschool Level

Rationale

When focusing on social interaction during the preschool years, issues of sharing and turn taking are paramount. During loosely structured play times, many opportunities arise for teachers to model a problem-solving approach to conflicts around sharing, helping the children to generate solutions to the problem and arrive at a mutually agreed-upon strategy for sharing (e.g., "Michael's turn for two more minutes, then my turn!"). For some youngsters, however, reliance on naturally occurring episodes of conflict about sharing as a strategy for teaching turn-taking skills targets instruction at a time when they are least likely to be receptive to learning. Conflicts around sharing can be highly arousing, producing a great deal of anger and frustration within the child, thus inhibiting his or her ability to remain open to a problem-solving approach. For this reason, teachers often structure planned and controlled episodes of turn taking through enjoyable games, as a means of skill building in a more neutral context.

Participants

For the purposes of instruction, group size should be limited to two children initially, to minimize the amount of time that each child needs to wait for his or her turn. When the specified criterion is achieved for successful turn taking in a group of two (e.g., participating in a turn-taking activity with one other child for 5 minutes), group size may be expanded systematically to include other children, up to the number that would normally participate in classroom games.

Setting

Because the content of the turn-taking activity is planned to be motivating to the participants, it is likely that it would attract the interest of many other children in the classroom. Since the success of the activity is dependent upon a controlled group size, the teacher may either plan to have enough of the materials available to run several groups of two simultaneously (with additional adult support), or choose to use a more private part of the room, where the activity would attract less attention.

Materials

Individual student preferences will guide the selection of specific materials, as will other IEP goals that relate to play (e.g., expanding the use of simple cause-and-effect toys, or engaging in pretend-play activities). Initially, materials chosen should be those that promote brief, easily observable turns (e.g., a top, a toy radio). As the participants learn that their waiting will always be rewarded by another turn and have some way to predict when that will occur, the complexity of the turn-taking activity can increase with respect to duration, number of participants, and amount of time each child must wait for his or her turn.

Intervention

The teacher labels the activity and the materials to be used, and demonstrates the desired action, such as activating the toy. She or he then outlines the sequence and duration of turns, so there is a predictable routine for the activity. Once the action is begun, the teacher gives support, as needed, to each child as he or she waits for a turn. Individual strategies for waiting may be employed, such as countdowns or waiting songs, while directing the waiting child's attention to the action of the other participant.

Video Arcade—Middle School Level

Rationale

A survey of the out-of-school recreational activities practiced by typical middle-school students shows a fair amount of time spent in video arcades. Integrated instruction in such game-playing skills not only achieves high interest and motivation for participation on the part of students, but also builds skills and, sometimes, friendships that carry over to afterschool activities.

Participants

A small group of about four students made up of two sets of partners (one special needs student and a typical peer) allows for intensive instruction and supervision as well as a level of independence.

Setting

The first choice for the setting would be an actual video arcade, outside of school in the nearby community. An approximation of this setting would be a community restaurant that had a few video machines located on the premises. In some communities, such establishments are located no more than a 5-minute walk from the school. If these opportunities are unavailable, an in-school approximation using computers and video games software is an alternative. A word is warranted here about different types of integration. While it may be impractical to plan activities that include regular education students that would necessitate their being absent from school for a prolonged period of time (e.g., 2 hours), this is not sufficient reason for discarding longer community activities from the schedule of a student with special needs. A teacher may simply need to think about integrated activities on two different levels: in school, with peers, as in the computer video game example; and integrated into the community, as in the video arcade.

Materials

Materials include either video arcade games and cash (from student accounts or from home), or a computer with video game software.

Intervention

Depending on the student, instruction may begin in the community at an actual video arcade, or in an adapted setting such as with computers in school. The student should be instructed in the use of a variety of video arcade machines. The teacher should assess the necessity for specific instruction or individual adaptations in the requisite skills, such as turn taking or use of money. If instruction is undertaken in school, a plan should be in effect for how carry over to the real-life environment of the video arcade will be implemented.

SELF-CONCEPT

Child of the Week—Preschool Level

Rationale

The main objective behind Child of the Week is to give each student an opportunity to share special interests, talents, and skills with his or her classmates. In addition, the role of Child of the Week carries with it particular privileges involving classroom jobs and choices. These elements of individual positive focus, and choice/control of certain features of classroom life are designed to yield an increase in positive feelings about the child's self-worth and status within the class.

Participants

The group setting most appropriate to featuring Child of the Week is the entire class group. At the preschool level, most activities are conducted ei-

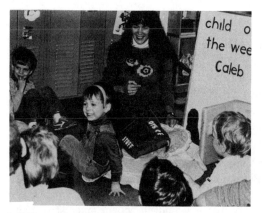

Activities such as this "Child of the Week Show" highlight the individual characteristics and interests of each child, enhancing his or her positive self-concept. (Photo by Susan Gelling.)

ther as loosely structured "choice" times, or in small structured groups. Therefore, the appropriate whole group time for Child-of-the-Week activities is the daily "circle time."

Setting

The physical setting should be the same as where the daily "circle time" routine is conducted. Space may be designated for the Child of the Week at the head of the circle, next to the leader, to convey the specialness of this role.

Materials

One day during the week is designated as Child-of-the-Week show day, where the child takes a special chair at the head of the circle, wears a crown, and shares with the class some photographs for the Child-of-the-Week bulletin board, as well as a few favorite toys brought from home. In addition, the teacher may want to feature the child's favorite food as a classroom cooking activity (necessitating the gathering of specific ingredients), or may stock the language area with favorite books and music.

Intervention

In addition to the Child-of-the-Week show described above, preferred classroom tasks can be assigned to the Child of the Week, either individually, or partnered with a classmate of his or her choice. Such jobs may include: preparing the classroom snack, taking the attendance to the office, calling the other children to the table for snack and lunch, or choosing a friend to be the line leader for times when the group leaves the classroom.

Project Adventure— Middle School Level

Rationale

Project Adventure is an adaptation of Outward Bound, a program of increasingly difficult physical challenges undertaken in a supportive group atmosphere. Project Adventure was an attempt to translate the goals and outcomes of Outward Bound into the curriculum of public schools. The program focuses on individual personal growth, on building a sense of group identity, and on building skills for positive interaction within the group. The author of *Cowstails and Cobras* (Rohnke, 1977) specifies that the stated aim of the activities is "to allow the students to view themselves as increasingly capable and competent" (p. 7). Within such an atmosphere, the student may begin to build true self-esteem.

Participants

Project Adventure has been used successfully in schools both within the context of the regular physical education curriculum and in specialized programs for adolescents with challenging behaviors. The natural extension of these successes is to combine the two populations into an integrated group format. Optimal group size would be 10–12 students, about half of whom are labeled as having special needs, and the rest nondisabled classmates.

Setting

Adventure activities can be carried out in the school gymnasium or outdoors on the athletic field.

A ropes course, consisting of high and low elements (with respect to distance from the ground) can be constructed either inside or out.

Materials

Materials are needed only for the ropes course. Ropes course designs are somewhat standardized, and many materials are available through Project Adventure, or in local lumber stores. Specifics for construction are supplied by Rohnke (1977).

Intervention

Instruction proceeds in a predictable sequence from meeting to meeting. Project LEAP (Levy Education through Adventure Program), a Project Adventure–style program for 12 students in the Syracuse City School District, Syracuse, New York, was designed to run for 12 weeks. During those 12 weeks, a group of 12 disabled and nondisabled students met twice weekly for 1½ hours per session. The sessions were structured to include warm-up exercises, stretching, group initiative problems (where group members must work together to solve a logistical problem such as getting the entire group over a 14-foot wall without any material aids), and selected ropes course elements. Each session ended with a group discussion designed to focus on the "feelings, experiences, conflicts, failures, and successes" (Black, 1984) of the Project LEAP participants. Such a model for integrated social interaction skill development and increased self-esteem has a great deal to recommend it, provided that it is administered by a knowledgeable and conscientious teacher.

COMMUNICATION

Partnered Snack—Preschool Level

Rationale

At times the complex environment of the integrated classroom must be broken down into smaller structured subgroups to focus specifically on particular goals and objectives. One of the domains to which this type of structuring applies is the area of communication. Communicative exchange between two people involves many discrete steps, from gaining the listener's attention, to shifting to a new topic, to bringing closure to the communicative exchange. Reducing the complexity of the social environment in a way that requires the child to focus only on one other peer often facilitates progress toward successful communication with peers.

Participants

Students are grouped in pairs, with each child with a special need having a typical peer as a partner. Pairs are created with individual student characteristics in mind, in a manner that complements students' strengths and needs (e.g., a student whose verbal responses are often negative and teasing might be paired with a student who does not seem to pay much attention to the teasing and the tone).

Setting

Partners are grouped "picnic" style, on blankets for two around the classroom. One of the partners is given the role of "keeper of the snack" to promote opportunities for communication (e.g., requesting, responding to a peer's request).

Materials

Materials needed include food, a small pitcher of juice, cups, and a blanket for each set of partners.

Intervention

At the transition to snack time, the names of the partners are called, and they are directed to particular "picnic" spots around the classroom. Support teachers are assigned as necessary to pairs of students to model the appropriate communication behavior, and to give the children strategies for successful communication (e.g., calling the partner's name if she or he is not listening).

Other partnered activities might include: art

projects where partners share one large piece of paper and set of paints, necessitating their talking together about what colors to use; a cooking activity where one partner is in charge of the bread and the other has the peanut butter, requiring the pair to communicate and share to make their sandwiches; or a "grocery store" play situation where one partner operates the cash register, and the other is the customer, necessitating communication about what the customer wants to buy and how much money he or she must pay to the cashier.

Following Directions Game—Elementary School Level

Rationale

There is, perhaps, no more powerful tool for teaching the impact of positive communication than a lesson that allows students control over the actions of their peers. The Following Directions Game achieves just that, by enabling students to take turns being the leader who directs the activity of classmates.

Participants

Since this is an action-oriented game, it is most successfully done in small groups. Small groups facilitate organized participation, as well as allow for more frequent turns as leader for each of the participants.

Setting

The activity level of the game requires that the game either be conducted in an area of the classroom that can be sectioned off so as not to disturb other students working on more quiet projects, or be held outside of the room (e.g., in the gym or an empty classroom).

Materials

Teacher-made cards with simple action-oriented directions printed on them, with the complexity of directions dependent upon the abilities of the students (e.g., one-step directions for younger students, three-step directions for older elementary-age students) are needed. For students who are not yet reading, directions may be expressed in picture forms.

Intervention

The teacher designates the sequence of turns in some logical fashion (e.g., going from left to right). Students take turns picking a card from the top of the pile, and then read it aloud to communicate the specified action to peers. The group then follows the directions read (e.g., "Jump on your left foot and pat your head"). Leadership rotates through the group.

COGNITIVE /ACADEMIC SKILLS

Grocery Store Math— Elementary School Level

Rationale

Grocery Store Math not only makes math instruction fun, but allows for targeting widely varying skill levels within an integrated academic group. Math instruction could range from teaching one-to-one correspondence (e.g., handing out one shopping bag or one coupon to each shopper), to multiplication (e.g., constructing a list that calls for three cans of fruit for $.89 each).

Participants

Small, heterogeneous skill groups allow opportunity for a higher level of individualization. In addition, mixed skill groups allow for greater teacher flexibility in direct instruction, yielding opportunities for a greater proportion of independent work for students who may succeed at that, as well as more direct contact with students who need extra help.

Materials

Materials needed include a cash register, money (either pretend or real), different types of empty food containers marked with prices, pencils and paper to add/multiply prices to arrive at a total, shopping bags, and possibly a calculator.

Intervention

Food containers are marked with prices that correspond to the numbers targeted for students to recognize, add, or multiply. Each student should have an individual list of items to buy, as well as a prescribed amount of money. The student gathers items on his or her list, adds together or multiplies, and determines when there is enough or not enough money to complete the purchases. Students then move to the cash register to buy their grocery items, counting out the correct money to the cashier.

Mainstream Class— Middle School Level

Rationale

At the middle school level, when academic instruction in regular education becomes departmentalized, the issue of integration for students with special needs takes a somewhat different focus. This is the point in the student's school career when the focus shifts toward a higher level of community integration. Choices must be made on an individual basis as to the balance of in-school academic instruction (depending upon the student's present and perceived potential for success in particular subject areas), and community-based experiential learning (e.g., utilizing restaurants, public transportation, leisure environments, and vocational settings).

Participants

When it is decided that a student would be well placed in a mainstream academic classroom, she or he becomes a member of a large classroom group. The special education teacher who is referring the student for mainstream class placement must consider several factors when selecting a successful mainstream situation. These factors include such things as the interests of the student (e.g., is she or he more interested in science or woodworking?); the student's skill level in the subject area; possible accommodations that might be made to compensate for skill deficits (e.g., tape recording class lectures if the student has difficulty taking notes); the openness of the mainstream class teacher to the student's presence in the class; and the available supports to help facilitate the placement (e.g., an assistant teacher who could accompany the student to class if necessary, or opportunities for repeated practice of important skills within the special education classroom).

Once the student has been placed within the mainstream class, he or she will participate in the normal grouping for activities that occur within the classroom, including large group demonstrations and lectures, small group projects, and independent work. However, the student with challenging behaviors may require additional task structuring or teacher support when the demands for focused attention and/or independent work are high. Such support may take the form of outlining the steps/requirements of the task, seating the student in close proximity to the teacher, or giving intermittent words of encouragement or direction to help the student remain on task.

Setting

The student will attend the mainstream class, with additional practice and reinforcement of learning supplied by special education staff. Reinforcement of learning might include such activities as assistance in using the school library to gather information for a homework assignment; planning some in-class cooking activities that follow the same format as those in the mainstream home economics class, for practice in following a recipe; reviewing class notes, checking for student understanding; or helping the student to learn organizational skills (e.g., writing down homework assignments, assembling materials needed for class).

Materials

Materials and assignments may require adaptation to match the student's academic levels and ability to deal with complex information (e.g., selecting materials that cover similar content, but are written on a lower reading level). Reinforcement exercises that target the same content in new ways to avoid boredom will encourage repeated practice to mastery. In addition, tests may need to be adapted to assess knowledge of content without penalizing the student for areas of skill weakness (e.g., individual, oral administration of a test for a student who has difficulty reading and following written test directions).

Intervention

The nature of the mainstream activity may be as varied as the types of classes offered in the particular middle school. As noted earlier, the decision about the specific type of mainstream class selected for an individual student is made based on student interests and skills, as well as the potential for adapting instructional content and techniques to meet the student's skill level. Possibly the most critical factor in the success of a mainstream placement is the level of communication between the regular class teacher and the special education teacher. Knowledge should be shared around what kinds of skills the student brings to the class, the particular successes and difficulties the student experiences, and the manner of adaptations and individualized support necessary to maximize success.

SUMMARY AND CONCLUSION

This chapter has illustrated a problem-solving approach to the issue of integrating students with challenging behaviors. An ecological perspective on behavior was described and demonstrated via an examination of the types of variables that teachers must consider when facing challenging behaviors. Significant variables to consider include the contexts and hypothesized functions of the behavior; the manner in which the behavior relates to the student's skill levels; the impact of the behavior on the student's self-concept; and the implications for the teacher in planning for and implementing integrated educational activities.

Descriptions followed of three different operating models of educational programs serving students who exhibit challenging behaviors. All three programs operate in Syracuse, New York. Together they offer a continuum of integrated services for students from preschool to middle school level. Programs were examined on fundamental aspects of operation such as background, class groupings, curriculum, and staffing/administrative support.

Finally, a series of ten integrated activities were outlined, spanning a wide range of ages (from preschool to middle school) and reflecting diverse strategies for achieving the integration of students with challenging behaviors. The integrated activities described were grouped into five instructional domains derived from an examination of students' individualized education programs (IEPs), and representing significant areas of instruction for the development of positive social interaction skills. Instructional domains included: social skills, play/leisure skills, self-concept, communication, and cognitive/academic skills.

The reader is encouraged to explore the possibilities for expanding and adapting the activity ideas presented to specific student needs and the particular structure of the integrated educational environment in which she or he teaches. In an integrated classroom, it is the teacher's responsibility to design programs, activities, and interventions to facilitate positive social and instructional interactions for students—by focusing on the strengths of each student, and structuring the environment to promote a successful match between the student and the demands of the class.

STUDY QUESTIONS

1. When problem solving around a challenging behavior that a student may exhibit, teachers address the following issues: the context and functions of the behavior, its relationship to the student's skill level, and the impact of the behavior on his or her self-concept. How do each of these variables affect behavior?

2. Describe three models of integrated educational programs for students with challenging behaviors.

3. Discuss the different challenges around integration that occur at the middle school level (e.g., departmentalized curriculum, community-based integration).

4. What factors should educators consider in the creation of groupings for integration in the formation of classrooms, and within the classroom for activities?

5. Give examples from the chapter of appropriate curricular domains to target for students with challenging behaviors at various age levels. What guidelines should educators use in making decisions about curriculum areas to target?

6. Using the format given in the chapter, design integrated activity plans in two of the following areas: social skills, play/leisure skills, self-concept, communication, and cognitive/academic skills.

REFERENCES

Apter, S.J., & Conoley, J.C. (1984). *Childhood behavior disorders and emotional disturbance*. Englewood Cliffs, NJ: Prentice-Hall.

Black, J. (1983). *Program description: Levy middle school program students with autism*. Unpublished manuscript.

Black, J. (1984). *Mini-grant proposal: Project LEAP (Levy Education through Adventure Program)*. Unpublished manuscript.

Donnellan, A.M., Mirenda, P.L., Mesaros, R.A., & Fassbender, L.L. (1984). Analyzing the communicative functions of aberrant behavior. *Journal of The Association for the
Severely Handicapped, 9*(3), 201–212.

Fenwick, V. (1987). The Edward Smith school program: An
integrated public school continuum for autistic children. In
M.S. Berres & P. Knoblock (Eds.), *Program models for
mainstreaming: Integrating students with moderate to severe disabilities* (pp. 261–286). Rockville, MD: Aspen
Systems.

Goldstein, A.P., Sprafkin, R.P., Gershaw, N.J., & Klein, P.
(1980). *Skill-streaming the adolescent: A structured learning approach to teaching prosocial skills.* Champaign, IL:
Research Press.

McGinnis, E., Goldstein, A.P., Sprafkin, R.P., & Gershaw,
N.J. (1984). *Skillstreaming the elementary school child: A
guide for teaching prosocial skills.* Champaign, IL: Research Press.

Rohnke, K. (1977). *Cowstails and cobras: A guide to ropes
course, initiative games, and other adventure activities.*
MA: Project Adventure.

Vincent, L.J., Salisbury, C., Walter, G., Brown, P., Gruenewald, L.J., & Powers, M. (1980). Program evaluation and
curriculum development in early childhood/special education: Criteria of the next environment. In W. Sailor, B. Wilcox, & L. Brown (Eds.), *Methods of instruction for severely
handicapped students* (pp. 303–328). Baltimore: Paul H.
Brookes Publishing Co.

Voeltz, L.M. (1984). Program and curriculum innovations to
prepare children for integration. In N. Certo, N. Haring, &
R. York (Eds.), *Public school integration of severely handicapped students* (pp. 155–183). Baltimore: Paul H. Brookes
Publishing Co.

Wood, M. (1975). *Developmental therapy.* Baltimore: University Park Press.

CHAPTER 7

STUDENTS WITH HANDICAPS WHO HAVE CULTURAL AND LANGUAGE DIFFERENCES

Maximino Plata and Philip C. Chinn

WHAT IS CULTURE?

Every child in every classroom has culture. It is culture that determines the way each individual thinks, feels, and ultimately behaves in society. Culture can be considered a blueprint for perceiving, believing, evaluating, and behaving (Gollnick & Chinn, 1986). While culture includes an individual's ethnicity, it involves much more than ethnic background or national origin. Most individuals in this country share at least a part of the macroculture or core culture, but in addition all also belong to numerous sub- or microcultures.

Culture is manifested in many ways. What one eats, when one eats, and how often one eats are all determined by culture. The clothing one wears and one's hair style is determined by culture. Politics and religious beliefs are determined by culture. Student's behaviors, speech, and music preferences are all a function of their culture. A child's feelings about being touched or hugged by a teacher may be culturally influenced, as some cultures are contact cultures while others are not. The learning style of a student may also be related to his or her cultural background.

The Macroculture

The social and political institutions in the United States are deeply rooted in Western European traditions. Thus the schools and the value systems to which children are exposed are Western European in origin. Throughout this country's infancy and formative years of development, the dominant force was white, Anglo Saxon, and Protestant (WASP). From this group evolved the basic values that influence government, schools, and citizenry. While the composition of the dominant group has changed, WASP values remain and have been adopted by the new dominant group, the middle class. While whites continue to dominate the middle class in numbers, the group comprises individuals from all ethnic and religious groups (Gollnick & Chinn, 1986). The macroculture in the United States is the universal or national culture that is shared by most of the nation's citizenry. The group most identified with the macroculture is the middle class.

There is a core of universal cultural traits shared by most individuals. Traits that characterize the macroculture are industriousness, ambition, competitiveness, individualism, independence, and

149

the belief that humans are separate from and superior to nature (Gollnick & Chinn, 1986). The overpowering value, however, is self-reliance—the belief that every individual is his or her own master, with control of his or her own destiny. While these traits and values are not shared to the same degree by each member of the macroculture, they are shared to some extent by nearly all.

Microcultures

In addition to the macroculture, there are a number of microcultures or subsocieties in every country. These groups share certain traits and values that are not common to all members of the macroculture. While sharing some cultural patterns with the macroculture, they have their own distinctive cultural patterns. The most common microcultures in the United States are based in ethnicity or national origin, religion, gender, age, socioeconomic status, language group, geographical region, and exceptionality.

The way one thinks, perceives, and behaves is very much a function of the microcultural group to which one belongs or in which one was raised. As a group, the poor tend to have values and behaviors different from the middle class and, to a greater extent, from the upper class. Individuals who come from devout Roman Catholic families often have different perceptions as well as behaviors from those who have Protestant or Jewish backgrounds. Typically, boys are socialized with values and behaviors different from girls. The deaf and blind communities often develop some traits, values, and behaviors that differ from the seeing/hearing world.

Cultural Differences in the Classroom

Educators, especially those in special education, need to be acutely aware of the implications of culture on the behavior of their students. Many special education students come from lower socioeconomic backgrounds. As such, many of their values are not congruent with those of their middle-class teachers. Special education classes in general, and some exceptionalities in particular, have disproportionately large groups of children from ethnic minority backgrounds (Office of Civil Rights, 1986).

For example, in some special education classes, disproportionately large numbers of children may be from Hispanic homes. Since Hispanics are more likely to fall into the poverty levels because of their lower earning power and income than whites (U.S. Bureau of Labor Statistics, 1984), it is likely that many Hispanic students in special education classes are also poor. In addition, they are also likely to be Catholic. Thus the white special education teacher with Hispanic students in the classroom may be faced with cultural values incongruent with his or her own. Even the middle-class Hispanic teacher may have many values quite different from lower-class Hispanic students.

Between 1978 and 1984, the percentage of ethnic minority children in U.S. schools increased from one fourth to over one third (Office of Civil Rights, 1986). In several states there are large black and/or Hispanic communities, so that ethnic minority groups actually form the numerical majorities. In addition, the nation is experiencing large waves of immigration, particularly of Hispanic and Asian groups. In the last decade over 750,000 Southeast Asians have entered the United States (Chinn & Plata, 1986). To compound the situation, some immigrants arriving in this country are entering school for the first time in their lives.

At a time when ethnic minority students are increasing in numbers, there is a disproportionately low number of ethnic minorities entering the teaching profession. Competency testing and state preservice testing, coupled with enhanced opportunities for minorities in other disciplines, are rapidly decreasing their numbers in the education ranks. Many states are moving perilously close to having all-white teacher cadres (Chinn, 1987).

The overrepresentation of ethnic minority students in special education has been a pressing and volatile issue for educators in the past 2 decades (Heller, Holtzman, & Messick, 1982). More ethnic minorities are served in some classes for handicapped students than would be expected from their numbers in the general population. In addition there are disproportionately low numbers of American Indians, blacks, and Hispanics in classes for gifted and talented students. These disproportionate representations are not a new phenomenon. What is new are the changing patterns of minority representation in the various categories of exceptionality (Chinn & Hughes, 1987).

Attention was first brought to focus on overrepresentation by Dunn (1968) in his seminal article "Special Education for the Mentally Retarded—Is Much of it Justifiable?" In the article Dunn pointed out that in 1968 one third of the special education teachers nationally were teachers of students with mental retardation. Dunn further reported that 60%–80% of these students were ethnic minority students from low socioeconomic backgrounds.

Mercer (1973) reported that in Riverside, California, in public school special education classes, blacks and Mexican-American children were grossly overrepresented in classes for educable mentally retarded (EMR) students. Mexican-Americans constituted 11% of the general school population, but 45.3% of the EMR population. The placement of blacks in EMR classes was three times greater than their numbers in the general school population, while placement of whites was disproportionately low.

Surveys of Student Placement

Since 1968, the Office of Civil Rights (OCR) has surveyed schools and school districts regarding student enrollment and placement. The OCR report is issued every 2 years and is released approximately 2 years after the data are gathered. The data provided are extensive. However, the data of particular interest to special educators are the numbers of students reported in the following categories of exceptionality: gifted and talented (G/T), educable mentally retarded (EMR), train-

able mentally retarded (TMR), speech impaired (SI), seriously emotionally disturbed (SED), and specific learning disabilities (SLD). Data on the following racial/ethnic groups are also reported: American Indian, Asian, Hispanic, black and white.

Chinn and Hughes (1987) made an analysis of the four most recent OCR surveys (1978, 1980, 1982, 1984) to determine if there were any changes in the nature of the representation of minorities in special education between 1978 and 1984. The data analyzed by Chinn and Hughes are national data only, which obscures data of individual states that may differ substantially from national statistics. The analysis of the data suggests that as a group, blacks are disproportionately represented in EMR, TMR, and SED classes. The disproportion of blacks in EMR classes is the largest disproportionate representation in classes for handicapped students. In 1978, the percentage of blacks in EMR classes was 38.01% as compared to 15.72% in the total school enrollment. In 1984, the percentage of blacks in EMR classes had increased to 48.30% as compared to 24.52% in the total school enrollment. While the ratios have decreased between 1978 and 1984, the disproportion of blacks in EMR classes still remains high.

Hispanic representation in EMR, SI, SED, and G/T classes is disproportionately low. However, the national data obscure some data in states with large Hispanic populations. For example, in 1984, Arizona and New Mexico reported disproportionately large representations in EMR, TMR, SI, and SLD classes. Colorado reported disproportionately large percentages in EMR and TMR classes.

There is a disproportionately high representation of American Indian children in SLD classes for all 4 reporting years, in EMR classes in all but the last reporting year, and in TMR classes in 1984. There is underrepresentation in G/T classes for all 4 years. Asian and Pacific Islanders are underrepresented in all categories except G/T, where there is overrepresentation.

In contrast to ethnic minority groups, whites are underrepresented in EMR and TMR classes in all 4 reporting years and overrepresented in G/T classes in the last 3 reporting years. They are proportionately represented in all other areas.

Since the advent of PL 94-142 (Education for All Handicapped Children Act) and the increased awareness of the problems of overrepresentation, some special education enrollment patterns have apparently shifted. For example, between 1975 and 1987, the national statistics on the overrepresentation of minorities in EMR classes changed, considerably so for Hispanics. Even in those states where overrepresentation existed, it was not at the 1973 levels that Mercer found in Riverside. Disproportions among blacks in EMR classes was still a serious problem in 1987, but there was an indication that the disproportions were becoming slightly smaller. Ortiz and Yates (1983) conceded that the overrepresentation of Hispanics in EMR classes has lessened, but point out the concurrent increase of Hispanics receiving SLD services. While there is no conclusive evidence that a shift from EMR to SLD is taking place, the latter could be considered by some a "safer" category, in which less challenges and lawsuits over improper placements are likely to occur. Chinn and Hughes (1987) state:

> The evidence appears to be overwhelming that many children in the past, and in all likelihood today, are part of the overrepresentation due to faulty identification procedures. What is not known with certainty is if overrepresentation exists in part due to children who have been appropriately referred, diagnosed and placed . . . Some ethnic minority children may be appropriately placed in special education classes and receiving intervention appropriate to their needs. In such situations, whatever benefits accrue should be recognized as such and continued as long as it is in the best interest of the child. However, the problem of disproportionate identification for special education placement due to faulty procedures must continually be attacked as long as it exists. (p. 45)

Judicial Decisions

In the last 2 decades, a number of major court decisions have had a profound impact on the education and services provided to culturally and linguistically different children. Among the promi-nent court cases are *Diana v. State Board of Education* (1970), *Larry P. v. Riles* (1974), *Lau v. Nichols* (1974), and *Lora v. Board of Education of the City of New York* (1978).

Diana v. State Board of Education (1970) and *Larry P. v. Riles* (1974) were major cases that challenged the testing procedures used for the placement of minority children in special education classes. *Diana,* involving Mexican children, resulted in an agreement that required school districts to test in the children's primary language, to use nonverbal tests, and to collect and utilize extensive supporting data. *Larry P.* involved black students whose parents maintained they were inappropriately identified and placed in classes for mentally retarded students. The case resulted in a ban against the use of standardized IQ tests, setting a precedent around the country in which some school districts have either restricted or abolished IQ testing.

Lau v. Nichols (1974) was a class action suit on behalf of 1,800 Chinese students in the San Francisco unified school district. The plaintiffs charged that the children were not receiving appropriate educational opportunities when the instruction was not in their native language. The court agreed, stating that "there is no equality of treatment merely by providing students with the same text books, teachers, and curriculum; for students who do not understand English are effectively foreclosed from any meaningful education" (*Lau v. Nichols,* 1974, p. 566). Although no specific remedy was prescribed by the court, the decision became the basis for many bilingual and English as a Second Language (ESL) programs in the United States.

Lora v. Board of Education of the City of New York (1978) was initiated in 1975 on behalf of black and Hispanic children assigned to schools for emotionally handicapped students. In July, 1979, a U.S. District Court ruled that the students had not been properly placed. The school board was ordered to improve identification, referral, evaluation, and placement procedures, and to reevaluate placement policy guidelines for emotionally handicapped students.

The above court decisions, coupled with the provisions of PL 94-142, have provided the impetus needed to better address the needs of culturally diverse exceptional children. Today school districts are making greater efforts to ensure that procedures are in place to guarantee due process and appropriate programming for their culturally diverse exceptional children. Some teacher education programs are beginning to recognize that a large number of the children who will be served by special education are from cultural backgrounds different from those of the teachers they are preparing. If teachers are to be effective, they must be able to recognize the cultural differences that may exist between them and their students, a major step toward providing all students with the free and appropriate education promised them in PL 94-142.

EDUCATING STUDENTS WITH CULTURAL AND LANGUAGE DIFFERENCES

Schools, as extensions of the community, should embrace and impart values and skills that will serve *all* students well. Educational strategies utilized should inculcate values and teach skills that will prepare students to get along with culturally different individuals and to become productive members of society. The educational concept that addresses cultural diversity and the provision of equal educational opportunity in schools is *multicultural education*. This concept is based on the following fundamental beliefs and assumptions:

1. The U.S. culture has been fashioned by the contributions of many diverse cultural groups into an interrelated whole.
2. Cultural diversity and the interaction among different groups strengthen the fiber of U.S. society.
3. Social justice and equal opportunity for all people are inalienable rights of all citizens.
4. The distribution of power should be distributed equitably among members of all ethnic groups.
5. The education system provides the critical func-

tion of modeling attitudes and values necessary for continuation of a democratic society.
6. Teachers and other professional educators must assume a leadership role in creating an environment that is supportive of multiculturalism. (Gollnick & Chinn, 1986, p. 27)

As classroom teachers impart information about different values, life-styles, religions, and ethnic backgrounds, these differences must not be described as inferior to the educators' own. Taking into account the students' ethnic background recognizes cultural differences as reflected in learning, human relations, motivational incentives, and communication styles. Indeed, students should be helped to develop openness, flexibility, and receptivity to cultural diversity and alternative life-styles (Gay, 1977a). Teachers must be as open to sharing, discussing, and changing their own culturally and ethnically based perceptions as they expect their students to be (Piper, 1986).

Gollnick and Chinn (1986) believe that the competencies to function comfortably in multicultural settings should lead to: 1) increased self-awareness and self-respect, 2) a greater respect for cultural groups that differ from the student's own, 3) the extension of cultural pluralism and equity in the United States, and 4) fewer intergroup conflicts caused by ignorance and misunderstanding.

Because of the complex problems these students bring to school, educating culturally and linguistically different handicapped students is no easy task. Furthermore, there are no easy solutions to these students' academic, social, and language problems. The difficulty teachers face in teaching these students may be due, in part, to the complex interaction effects among the social, educational, psychological, and linguistic factors these students encounter in their daily lives, which have yet to be specified through research.

It appears, however, that children's cognitive and academic development is a direct function of their interaction with adults both in the home and school and whatever can be done to strengthen this process of cultural transmission is likely to contribute to the children's overall personal and intellectual growth. (Cummins, 1984, p. 127)

There is little literature validating differences or similarities in learning style, achievement, values, and so forth between students with cultural and language differences who are handicapped (A. Ortiz, 1983). As a consequence, most researchers superimpose existing knowledge about nonhandicapped bilingual students into their arguments for treatment of bilingual handicapped students.

There is a danger in this approach. Teaching and learning principles may differ for these students. But until research efforts result in the development of such principles, one must continue to use strategies and methods that have been found successful with bilingual students. One caution is in order, however. If existing bilingual methodology is to be used with bilingual handicapped students, it is suggested that special education and bilingual education personnel be made part of a team effort, regardless of the discipline from which such efforts originate. This coordination and cooperation between disciplines will ensure that the commitment to bilingual handicapped students is shared by various disciplines, and that basic principles and methods that are successful in special and bilingual education are integrated into the discipline's approaches in educating bilingual handicapped students.

Three factors are addressed in the following section: 1) student characteristics, 2) teacher competencies and skills, and 3) curriculum and instructional materials. Several points are discussed as they relate to the education of handicapped students with cultural and language differences. Finally, suggestions and/or guidelines for working with bilingual handicapped students are offered, including suggestions for the teacher and suggestions for curriculum development.

Student Characteristics

To be successful in teaching culturally and linguistically different handicapped students, one needs to become aware of these students' characteristics and needs (see Table 1).

Value Orientation

Because bilingual handicapped children come from a social class and/or culture different from their mainstreamed peers, their value system will also differ (Vasquez, 1979). The conflict between these students' values and those of the mainstream society has resulted in an array of problems. For example, in special education it is an accepted fact that learning is enhanced through reinforcement. However, this principle, if traditionally applied, may be in jeopardy with bilingual handicapped students, especially if the student is a Hispanic male. Many of these Hispanic students come from families where instruction and discipline are the duty of the father, never that of the mother or other females. Therefore, female classroom teachers should take advantage of this information and orient their reinforcement with consideration of the family. For example, instead of the female teacher saying to a Hispanic male student "Roberto, you did a good job on your paper; *I'm* proud of you," the teacher should say "Roberto, you did a good job on your paper; *Your father* will be proud of it."

Locus of Control

Some students perceive that they are responsible for their grades and similar outcomes; some students perceive outsiders or outside forces to be in control of their achievements. Those who believe they are in control of their achievements are said to be "internally" controlled (Norwick & Strickland, 1973; Vasquez, 1978).

Research has demonstrated that students who perceive themselves to be in control of their academic achievements are usually white and middle class. Some ethnic minorities tend to think that outside factors such as luck, chance, "powerful others," and task difficulty are instrumental in determining grades (Norwick & Strickland, 1973). This characteristic may have considerable implication for teaching some bilingual handicapped students. As yet, there is no evidence to suggest that bilingual handicapped students would react differently than their normal bilingual peers.

Table 1.   Culturally/linguistically different pupils: What to look for

1.   Achievement—slow, confused; inability to respond to academic demands. Overly cautious on class-work. Full attention is given to the task being done, forgetting about the time constraints applied to task completion.

2.   Behavior—shyness, especially in novel situations or with strangers. May be submissive or withdrawn under certain conditions. Shows fear of failure, nontrusting attitudes, or ambivalence toward authority figures. Could be assertive/aggressive to indicate frustration, lack of success within the system. Loses hope for success within the system.

3.   Does not complain about anything. Does not ask for assistance regarding personal problems or academic problems because of shame it brings to themselves and/or the family. Trait may be more prevalent in Asians, American Indians, Hispanics.

4.   Totally obedient and courteous behavior, followed by an overzealousness for pleasing the teacher or other authority figures. May be more prevalent in young, culturally different exceptional students, including Asians, American Indians, and Hispanics. Also seen in students of parents who recently immigrated to U.S.

5.   Poor self-esteem due to lack of acceptance by peers, teachers, and significant others. May also be due to lack of success and achievement.

6.   Delinquency—extremely aggressive behavior, especially when forced into role that conflicts with culture's value system or when they have little hope for success within the system. May be the results of disorganization in the home. Accumulation of failures in school and at home. Turned to delinquency due to the immediate results of such activity.

7.   Confused during diagnosis or problem-solving situations.

8.   May try to use memorization of materials as a coverup or overcompensation for disabilities.

9.   Poverty background, resulting in disheveled appearance, worn clothes, poor nutrition, and health problems.

10.   Language differences and/or underdeveloped language system. Limited-English speaking and limited-English proficient. May also be limited in native language proficiency.

11.   High sensitivity to others' feelings and problems.

12.   Withdrawal when situations seem insoluble, when reprimanded, or when challenged with tasks perceived to be beyond their potential.

13.   Usually are followers—not leaders under normal circumstances, especially in an ethnically integrated situation.

Adapted from Chinn and Kamp (1982, pp. 371–390).

(Table 2 presents information related to the effects of internality and externality on school performance.) Because these students may fail to perceive their own efforts as important causes of success or failure, this could influence a teacher's perceptions and expectations that maintain a cycle of failure, reinforcing the students' learned helplessness (Henderson, 1980).

Cognitive Style

Cognitive style is the way one mentally organizes and approaches problem solving. Many of these skills are gained through the socialization process in early childhood. For bilingual handicapped children, there are numerous factors that mold their cognitive style. At the very base of the cognitive style development process are cultural values (Ramirez & Castaneda, 1974). Cultural values affect socialization practices, which in turn affect learning styles, incentive-motivational styles, human relational styles, and communication styles. The cumulative effect of these styles constitutes the essence of one's cognitive style.

Culturally and linguistically handicapped pupils' cognitive styles, no doubt, have been formu-

Table 2. Effects of internality and externality on students' school performance

	Internal	External
Self-reliance	Work independently. Curriculum and classroom activities and expectations are structured for independent learners.	Dependent on others for task completion. Have difficulty approaching task assignments demanded by curriculum.
Level of aspiration	Able to plan and implement strategies that yield desired outcomes.	Fail to see the relationship between actions and outcomes. Therefore, have tendency to ignore planning or learning strategies.
Expectations of success	Attribute success to own behavior, abilities, skills, and efforts. Able to change behaviors or level of effort to ensure success.	Do not use analytical skills to determine relationship between behaviors and outcomes. Therefore, do not appear to profit from experiences, even with feedback or ordinary reporting procedures.
Achievement	Show visibly that they want to achieve. More likely to meet the aspirations/expectations of teachers.	Judged to lack motivation and/or desire for achievement. Apparent lack of interest to learn produces frustration/irritation for teachers who are likely to be internal themselves.
Intensity of work	Challenge conventional, imposed structure. React to success/failure experiences as products of self-determination.	Conform to or willing to accept imposed structures. Ego strength not involved, unlikely to reflect upon experiences as either successful or unsuccessful. Desire to please others, especially individuals who are perceived as authority figures.
Performance under skill conditions	Challenged by situations that require a display of skills (e.g., in test taking, analyze difficulty of test items and complete easier items first).	Do not use analytical skills (e.g., in test taking, may recognize difference in difficulty of test items but begin with the first test item and work in sequence until frustrated or time is exhausted).

Adapted from A. Ortiz (1983, pp. 7–8).

lated through this process. However, what is yet to be discovered through research is how the handicapping condition affects the final cognitive style of students. It is suggested, then, that known information on the cognitive styles of nonhandicapped bilingual students be used with those who are bilingual and handicapped. Documentation of similarities and differences in cognitive style between nonhandicapped and handicapped bilingual students would contribute greatly to the knowledge base on how best to educate these students. For example, field-sensitive or field-dependent individuals depend on external factors in gauging their behavior; field-independent individuals do not rely on these external cues. (An extended discussion on these traits is given later in this chapter.) Table 3 presents additional information on the effects of field-sensitivity (field-dependence) and field-independence on observable student behavior.

Teacher Competencies and Skills

A multicultural curriculum is essential in teaching all students, including the bilingual student who is handicapped. However, equally as important is the teacher's attitude toward individual differences. Saville-Troike (1978, p. 44) captures the essence of the importance of attitude in the teacher-learner process when she states that "teacher attitudes and behavior may be much more significant than curriculum content." In addition, she believes that "teachers are models; what they value and respect is often valued and respected by their students as well" (Saville-Troike, 1978, p. 44).

To offset prevailing attitudes that ethnic minority students' low academic achievement is student based, it is imperative that teachers: 1) gain knowledge of these students' cultures; 2) gather information about the relationship between culture and values, and their implications on learning/schooling; and 3) integrate into the curriculum those activities that will teach pluralistic values according to the students' learning style.

A creative, sensitive teacher with knowledge of teaching strategies and a working philosophy of cultural pluralism can "multiculturalize" physical education, mathematics, science, art, music, language arts, reading, and even vocational arts. The key question the teacher must answer is, "How do I include all students who have a rightful place in this lesson?" The teacher is the key to the students' academic success as well as to their gaining an understanding of a pluralistic society. The degree of success in each depends on the teacher's understanding of different ethnic cultures, and upon his or her ability to develop teaching strategies appropriate for cognitive growth and attuned to the philosophy of cultural pluralism (Baptiste & Baptiste, 1977).

The teacher faces a double-edge responsibility when choosing, adapting, or developing materials (Baptiste & Baptiste, 1977). Materials must pro-

Table 3. Effects of field-sensitivity or field-dependence and field-independence on observable student behavior

Field-sensitive or Field-dependent	Field-independent
Peer relationships	
1. Likes to work with others	1. Prefers to work independently
2. Likes to help others	2. Likes competition, recognition
3. Sensitive to feelings/opinions of others	3. Task oriented; inattentive to social environment when working
Teacher relationships (personal)	
1. Expresses positive feelings for teacher	1. Avoids contact with teacher
2. Sees teacher as role model; seeks to emulate teacher's tastes and personal experiences	2. Interaction with teacher is task oriented.
Teacher relationships (instructional)	
1. Seeks guidance and demonstrations from teacher	1. Likes to try tasks without teacher's help
2. Seeks to please teacher, leading to stronger bond with teacher	2. Impatient to begin tasks; likes to finish first
3. Highly motivated when teacher helps individually; seeks teacher reward	3. Seeks nonsocial reward; internal reward system
Thinking style	
1. Responds to detailed explanations and modeling of lessons	1. Focuses on detail and parts of things
2. Learns concepts when presented in humanized and story format	2. Excels in math and science concepts
3. Learns well when curriculum content is relevant to experiences/interests	3. Likes discovery or trial-and-error learning

Adapted from Cox and Ramirez (1981, p. 67).

mote both academic and cognitive growth and a sense of unity within cultural diversity, as well as include humanizing teaching strategies. Castañeda (1976) provides suggestions to help educators who are concerned with providing appropriate education to Mexican-American students. These suggestions may also be helpful in working with handicapped students from other than a Hispanic background. Castañeda's suggestions are:

1. Be sensitive to the child's feelings, remembering that a child-centered rather than a task-centered approach is more effective with traditional Mexican-American children.
2. Use personalized rewards that make your relationship with the child closer.
3. Use as much Spanish as possible in the classroom.
4. Implement English as a second language (ESL) training.
5. Introduce materials with a Mexican, Mexican-American, and Spanish heritage into the curriculum.
6. Have staff who can converse and interact with Spanish-speaking parents. Adequate parent-school communication is an essential element of a successful school program.
7. Involve parents actively in the educational process.
8. Make bilingualism and cultural experiences available not only to Mexican-American children but all children.

Curriculum and Instructional Materials

A. Ortiz (1983) indicates that there is little evidence to suggest that factors impinging upon the achievement of Hispanic handicapped students are similar to those that hinder nonhandicapped Hispanic learners. Little attention has been given to the curricula, instructional methods, and content and processes of educational planning for students who are bilingual and handicapped. Educators are thus at a loss as to how to develop programs for bilingual handicapped students consistent with PL 94-142's "appropriate education" criteria. They

are unsure of the instructional guidelines to apply, not only in terms of handicapping conditions, but also in terms of linguistic, cultural, and other student background variables that may affect the learning process.

Materials used to teach bilingual handicapped students must be relevant to their needs and learning styles (Chinn, 1979; Chinn & Kamp, 1982; Vasquez, 1979). A lack of relevance will either cause frustration in the students' initial efforts to learn and accomplish tasks and assignments given them, or heighten students' existing frustration that may have been brought about by the cumulative effects of the handicapping condition. As a consequence, interest in school wanes, resulting in a *cumulative deficit* phenomenon (Deutch, 1965).

It is unrealistic to expect the non-English speaking handicapped students to read and understand materials with which they come in contact, especially if the materials are saturated with figurative language (Adkins, 1970). For example, sentences such as, "*Like a flash* he ran through the woods," "A little old woman *popped out of* the room in the back," and "Nathan was having trouble *speaking his mind*" would be troublesome for non-English speaking or limited-English speaking students. Words or phrases similar to those italicized in the sample sentences that are abstract, subtle, supernatural, or are not used in their usual or exact sense would contribute to the non-English speaking handicapped students' inability to understand reading material. While it is true that learning activities must be structured toward the goal of mastery, the process must be gradual, starting with language encounters with which students can achieve a measure of success. Thus, linguistic "puzzles" in the form of figurative speech, which are common in reading texts, must somehow be surmounted by the classroom teacher.

Based on their studies of second language acquisition, Dulay, Burt, and Kreshen (1982) provide guidelines for teaching ESL. These guidelines are also appropriate for educators to follow in instructing bilingual handicapped students.

1. Maximize the student's exposure to natural communication.
2. Focus on the message being conveyed, not the linguistic form of the message.
3. Incorporate a silent period at the beginning of the instructional program so that students will be able to listen to the second language without being pressured to speak it.
4. Encourage and create situations in which students can interact with native speakers of the language.
5. Use concrete referents to make the new language understandable to beginning students.
6. Devise specific techniques to relax students and to protect their egos.
7. Learn the motivations of students and incorporate these into lessons.
8. Create an atmosphere in which students are not embarassed by their errors.
9. Do not refer to, or revert to, the student's native language when teaching the second language. To do so may create a situation in which the student, instead of focusing attention on the second language, simply waits for the teacher to repeat utterances in the native language.

Finally, learning activities must be created to serve all children in all grades, regardless of their ethnic identity. In developing and/or adapting classroom materials for bilingual handicapped students, recommendations by Grant and Grant (1977) are useful.

1. Reflect the pluralistic nature of society as a positive feature of the nation's heritage by not presenting cultural, racial, and individual differences in isolation from each other.
2. Include a wide representation of all cultures and races in all curriculum materials from kindergarten to 12th grade.
3. Help students recognize and appreciate the racial and cultural contributions of different people to science, education, business, commerce, and fine arts.
4. Teach the cultural, racial, and individual differences of people in society by using words

and phrases that are complimentary and honest, connoting positive attitudes and acceptance of others.
5. Do not restrict the explanation of different cultures to special occasions (e.g., the study of American Indians during Thanksgiving, blacks during Black History Week, Mexican-Americans on Texas Independence Day). Instead, examine real problems and real people, not just heroes and highlights. Portray culturally and racially different people as displaying various human emotions, toiling and achieving in many aspects of life.
6. Examine the social, economic, and political forces and conditions that optimize or minimize opportunities for individuals on the basis of their race, culture, sex, age, or physical difference.

INSTRUCTIONAL AND SOCIAL INTEGRATION ACTIVITIES

Language Development

Rationale

Educators should not perceive the bilingual handicapped child as being deficient in language. These students *do* have a language base but are hindered in academic achievement due to factors such as limited knowledge of the English language, locus of control, learning styles, cognitive styles, and the handicapping condition itself. Therefore, it is appropriate to help these students gain language concepts necessary to succeed in school. These concepts can best be developed using the students' experience and his or her native language (Cummins, 1980; Kreshen, 1982; Saville-Troike, 1984). However, if the teacher is unable to instruct in the students' native language, he or she should follow suggestions given by Castāneda (1976); Gallegos, Gallegos, and Rodriguez (1983); A. Ortiz (1984); and Rodriguez (1979). By using the students' experiences and native language background, the teacher is providing a foundation that bilingual handicapped students can use to understand concepts being addressed or to add new knowledge to their repertoire.

The type of language development activities chosen is critical. Cummins (1980) has made a distinction between the language competency necessary to survive socially and the language competency necessary to survive academically. He believes that basic interpersonal communication skills (BICS) are those skills used in social interaction and that BICS are a superficial language competency that does not help bilingual students in accomplishing cognitively demanding academic feats. BICS are learned in rather personal and meaningful contexts with fairly immediate goals. Therefore, BICS are not good indicators of academic success because proficiency in BICS is superficial and focuses on pronunciation, vocabulary, and grammar aspects of the language process and not on knowledge, comprehension, and application of the cognitive process. Academic-oriented pursuits demand thinking and language that move beyond the BICS context and make entirely different demands on the student. For academic-oriented activities it becomes necessary for the student to focus on the semantic and functional meaning of the language process and on the cognitive processes of analysis, synthesis, and evaluation. These cognitive-oriented skills have been termed cognitive academic language proficiency (CALP) and are skills that are formally and informally assessed in academic pursuits. Because many bilingual handicapped students do not have the wealth of experiences from which CALP skills develop, they tend to do poorly in many academically demanding tasks.

Participants and Setting

Manuel is a learning disabled Hispanic student in a rural elementary school. He is 7 years old and has only attended school in Mexico. His family has been in the United States for about 6 months. His father, Domingo Alverez, works for Mr. Tarpon, a rancher in the community. Mr. Tarpon is also a member of the school board for the Mope Independent School District.

When Mr. Tarpon heard about Manuel's learn-

ing problems, he insisted that Mr. Alvarez take advantage of the Mope School District's reputation for helping children with learning difficulties. Mr. Tarpon initiated a meeting between Mr. Alvarez and Mrs. De Leon, the first-grade teacher at Mope Elementary School. Mr. Tarpon knew that Mrs. De Leon would be the link in providing successful school experiences for Manuel.

Intervention

Mrs. De Leon is a highly motivated teacher. Using her personal experiences of being a non-English speaking student, Mrs. De Leon developed a program consistent with the many guidelines she had learned in her teacher training program, especially those developed by Williams and De Gaetano (1985). These guidelines seemed appropriate even though they were written for those teaching English as a second language. The guidelines are:

1. Work on those concepts children already know in their first language.
2. Introduce a limited amount of new vocabulary at one time.
3. Embed new vocabulary in a natural context.
4. Use action activities.
5. Use objects familiar to the children.
6. Allow children to manipulate and explore the objects.
7. Provide opportunities for natural repetition. Do *not* drill.
8. Use songs and games as frequently as possible.

Mrs. De Leon developed activities that were familiar to the students (i.e., consistent with their cultural background). Mrs. De Leon selected art, music, and language development activities about animals, insects, and vegetation typically found on the farm or ranch. For example, Mrs. De Leon selected "Old MacDonald Had a Farm" as the type of song for her students to sing. For art, she asked the students to draw their perception of Old MacDonald's farm. For language development activities each student was given the opportunity to talk about their drawing of Old MacDonald's farm. She allowed her students to talk about anything related to their own farm experiences, including activities in which they or their family members were involved. For the more reluctant speakers, Mrs. De Leon would ask *wh* questions (Saville-Troike, 1984).

In essence, Mrs. De Leon was interested in the students' concept development. She applied the principle that each student learns the language of a concept as they learn the concept (Galvan & Brodie, 1977; Gonzales, 1981; Saville-Troike, 1984). Because Manuel was a non-English speaker, she was providing the opportunity to listen and interact with native speakers of the language (Dulay et al., 1982). This practice is consistent with research results that demonstrate the acquisition of a second language in about 2 years and that listening to the second language (in this case, English) is a characteristic of the initial stage of learning the language (Cummins, 1984; Dulay et al., 1982; Saville-Troike, 1984).

Mrs. De Leon initially permitted Manuel to listen to the other students as they talked about their drawings. As the students described their drawings, Mrs. De Leon wrote on the blackboard as many as five vocabulary words the students had used in their discourse. This made the students feel good because Mrs. De Leon had used "one of their words."

Using these vocabulary words, Mrs. De Leon made duplicate language master cards with each word on two cards. Then, she taught her students how to play "Concentration" with the cards. Two students were allowed to play the game. On a rotation basis, each student was allowed to turn over any two cards of his or her choice. If the two cards matched, the student was required to say the words on the card. The student would verify the correct pronunciation of the word by running the card through the language master, a machine that provided Mrs. De Leon's prerecorded message on the card. If the student was correct, he or she could keep the card pair. If the student was incorrect, the cards were taken out of the game set to be

used later in practicing the correct pronunciation of the word.

The game promoted the visual match of like words; it provided a safe competitive atmosphere, allowing the student to detect a relationship between successful outcome (number of card pairs) and memory skills; and it provided audio verification of the students' pronunciation of the word.

Mrs. De Leon also asked her students to count the number of animals on each of their drawings. As the students counted the number of animals, Mrs. De Leon wrote the numeral on the board. Manuel was allowed to listen to the pronunciation of the number concepts. The use of their drawings to count the number of animals provided the students with visual imagery of number concepts that were *meaningful*—a guideline that is extremely useful in teaching initial concepts (Williams & De Gaetano, 1985). Students were then given worksheets that provided practice in matching "concrete" symbols with numerals.

Later in the school year, Mrs. De Leon used words from the students' discourses as sight vocabulary.

Summary

Language development activities may prove invaluable as motivators, especially for non-English or limited-English speaking students. Using concepts with which students are familiar allows students to use expressive language skills in discussing concepts.

The success of language development activities may be found in the level of communication of students. Affective indicators expressed by bilingual handicapped students, such as initiative, achievement motivation, interest, and enthusiasm, are just as important in the initial stages of acquiring the English language as in acquiring the academic skills themselves.

Academic Skill Development

Rationale

Some ethnic minority children are characterized as low achievers. In his comparison of achievement scores of Spanish-speaking children in the early 1930s with achievement scores in 1959, Manuel (1965) found that in both time periods there was a tendency for achievement scores for Spanish-speaking children to be lower than for English-speaking children. In addition he found lower scores in reading than in arithmetic for Spanish-speaking children. Similar achievement patterns for Hispanics in comparison to their peers are reported in the literature (Coleman et al., 1966; Development Associates, 1980; National Assessment of Educational Progress, 1977, 1981; U.S. Commission of Civil Rights, 1975).

Many professionals believe that much of these students' difficulties are caused by an irrelevant curriculum—one that does not take into consideration the students' background (Garcia, 1978), values (Vasquez, 1978), or cognitive and learning styles (Cox & Ramirez, 1981). Saville-Troike (1981) places part of the blame on the school for non-English speaking students' delays in and out of school. But, she suggests that schools *can* succeed in teaching these students if they follow accepted principles.

> Where schools hired members of the students' ethnic group as regular teachers and administrators, and have developed strong academic programs which respect, utilize and build upon the students' native language and culture, achievement has exceeded national norms in English, reading, and mathematics. Where the school has hired staff from the minority group only in subordinate positions, or not at all, and has given only lip service to the more superficial aspects of the group's culture—food, dress, holidays—the reality of social inequities beyond the school has been telegraphed to minority students, whose achievement has been depressed accordingly. (Saville-Troike, 1981, p. 80)

Participants and Setting

Cecelia Lightfoot is a 12-year-old Navajo Indian girl. Cecelia lives in Tupu, a city of about 360,000 inhabitants. She lives with her mother, Mrs. Alma Lightfoot, her brother Eric, age 14, and her baby sister Gloria, age 18 months. They live in a two-bedroom frame home on the south side of the city.

The neighborhood is a mixture of blacks, American Indians, and Hispanics.

At school Cecilia and Eric are extremely quiet, both in and out of the classroom. They seem apprehensive and reluctant to interact with their Hispanic and black peers. Cecilia has been teased by some Hispanic girls about her surname, Lightfoot. They called her *pata pesada* (heavy foot). This was humiliating to Cecilia but she did not fight back—rather, she was intimidated. Cecilia tries to learn her subjects but she cannot understand how to do some of her assignments.

Intervention

In her attempts to help her students, Mrs. Farber requested certain information from the students. She asked them: 1) the number of people in their family, their ages and how many children of each gender there were; 2) where their parent(s) worked, how far they had to travel to work; 3) whether their family owned an automobile; 4) where the family did its shopping; and 5) to describe their favorite meal, place to study, place to relax, place for recreation, and hobby. Mrs. Farber asked the students to make two copies of their answers, one for her and one to keep in a manila folder.

Mrs. Farber believed that the teaching of mathematics, especially at the elementary-school level, takes place in a cultural context. Accordingly, Lovett (1980) states that "good mathematics teachers, sensitive to the real world experiences of their pupils, have always searched for the mathematics existing within these experiences as well as for ways to exploit these experiences by superimposing mathematical tasks on them" (p. 16). Using the information from her students, Mrs. Farber developed mathematical tasks. She used the students' names in math problems that included the following skills adapted from Wallace and Larsen (1979, p. 438):

1. Expressing fractions in lowest terms
2. Expressing fractions as decimals
3. Adding and subtracting like fractions

4. Adding and subtracting with decimals
5. Applying addition and subtraction skills to whole numbers
6. Applying multiplication skills to problems involving numbers with at least four digits
7. Applying division skills to problems with division with up to two digits
8. Determining time and time periods
9. Solving word problems involving time and requiring a combination of operations

In addition, Mrs. Farber found that Plata (1986) has provided a lesson plan model helpful in developing a bilingual approach to classroom instruction with limited-English speaking handicapped students (see Figure 1). The lesson plan model gives the classroom teacher the opportunity to delineate several components that comply with the essential elements of effective teaching (Galloway, 1976; Mann, 1971; Walker, 1981). The components of the lesson plan include:

1. *Objectives* obtained from the IEP and/or skills hierarchies resulting from task analysis
2. *Procedures (steps)* to carry out objectives, in English and the students' native language
3. *Safety precautions,* especially those in laboratory settings such as biology and vocational shops, in English and the students' native language
4. *Rules of conduct and instruction,* especially those that enhance the students' level of proficiency in meeting teacher expectations, in English and the students' native language
5. *Core vocabulary,* especially that which is predicted to enhance the students' effectiveness in achieving the lesson's objectives (may be obtained from other components of the lesson plan model and should be translated into the students' native language)
6. *Materials/tools/equipment* necessary to accomplish objectives, in English and the students' native language
7. *Suggested activities for skill acquisition* that would enhance individualization
8. *Prerequisite skills* necessary to accomplish

the lesson's objectives, especially in the quantitative, language, cognitive, perceptual, psychomotor, and social areas

Furthermore, the model complies with practices used to teach bilingual and handicapped students, including the use of ESL techniques and techniques for individualizing instruction. Finally, the instructional management plan meets the specific criteria of a lesson as stated by Besvinick (1960, p. 431), namely, "(a) the teacher should be able to teach from it; (b) someone else who is qualified in that subject area should be able to teach from it, and (c) it should be useful as a basis for planning the lesson if it is taught again sometime in the future."

In developing math problems for her students, Mrs. Farber made sure to integrate the food items, clothing items, and so forth mentioned in the students' personal information sheets. These efforts personalized mathematical tasks for the students. After developing mathematics problems (both computational and word problems), Mrs. Farber used components of Plata's (1986) lesson plan model to teach her class. First, she made a list of mathematical terms needed to solve mathematical tasks. In addition, Mrs. Farber developed a list of words that she used in the word problems. Second, she made sure that her students understood the meaning of each of the terms and/or concepts on her lists. For example, in a mathematics problem involving common fractions, Mrs. Farber reviewed the meaning of "common fraction," "numerator," and "denominator." She used the chalkboard to explain each of the terms, identifying and labeling the numerals in sample math problems.

Mrs. Farber made sure that the introduction of a new mathematics skill was followed by several (up to 10) practice problems. Providing opportunity for practice on one concept at a time and providing immediate feedback are practices that attempt to apply basic learning principles with handicapped students (Kirk & Gallagher, 1983). (For additional suggestions on how to individualize the math

Dates	Procedures (Steps) (English)	Student Progress			Dates	Procedures (Steps) (Nat. Lang.)	Student Progress		

Student: _____ Year: _____ Subject Area: _____
Objective: _____

Safety precautions (English)

Safety precautions (Nat. Lang.)

Rules of Conduct (English)

Rules of Conduct (Native Lang.)

Vocabulary (English)

Vocabulary (Native Language)

Initiation date / completion date — Introduced / Developed / Competent — Initiation date / Completion date — Introduced / Developed / Competent

Materials/Tools/Equipment (English)

Materials/Tools/Equipment (Nat. Lang.)

Suggested Activities for Skill Acquisitions:

Prerequisite Skills

A. Cognitive and Academic Skills

B. Perceptual/psychomotor/social

Figure 1. Instructional management model for bilingual handicapped students. (From Plata, M. [1986]. Instructional planning for limited English proficient students. *Journal of Instructional Psychology, 13* [1], 34; reprinted by permission.)

lessons see Plata and Cavin [1984] and Plata and Tolliver [1978].)

To offset the possible negative effects of individualized instruction on bilingual and limited-English proficient students, Mrs. Farber instituted a language development discussion group. This group allowed students to discuss their work, their problems in understanding specific assignments, and lack of knowledge of procedures used for resolving mathematical tasks. She assured students that they would not be teased for making errors in pronouncing words in English or in formulating verbal descriptions, or for errors in academic work.

Since instructional activities differ for field-independent and field-dependent (or field-sensitive) learners, at every possible opportunity, Mrs. Farber attempted to incorporate ESL, bilingual education, and direct teaching strategies to ensure that both types of learners could develop their cognitive-academic learning potential (Cummins, 1980). As noted earlier in this chapter (refer to Table 3, for example), students who are field-independent believe that they are in control of or are accountable for their behavior and its subsequent outcomes. Thus, they do not require the motivational strategies needed by students who are field-dependent. Field-independent students are self-starters, good organizers and problem solvers. Conversely, students who are field-dependent or field-sensitive believe that their behavior and its subsequent outcomes are controlled by environmental variables, authority figures, or luck. Thus, these students require a great deal of prodding, structure, guidance, feedback, and rewarding. In essence, their success depends, to a large extent, on the teacher's planning, organization, flexibility, direct teaching skills, and other hands-on involvement in the teaching-learning process.

Mrs. Farber was also cognizant that each learner, whether field-independent or field-dependent, should learn to approach learning situations using the opposite preferred cognitive learning style. Lovett (1980) suggests that each student should learn: 1) how to attack nonroutine, open-ended problem situations as well as highly structured problems; 2) material with social content as well as impersonal material requiring analytical skills; and 3) to work independently as well as with others. Having the facility to switch back and forth between approaches or strategies characterizing field-independent and field-dependent styles (bicognitive skill) (Ramirez & Castãneda, 1974) may provide students with advantages not otherwise afforded. By applying bicognitive strategies such as those outlined by Lovett (1980), students with cultural and language differences may be better able to meet challenging and urgent educational tasks.

Summary

Classroom teachers are in a dilemma when it comes to dealing with bilingual handicapped students. However, in their attempts to teach academic skills to bilingual handicapped students, classroom teachers must be sensitive to—and understand—the dilemma of the bilingual handicapped student. These students are battling barriers that, to them, seem insurmountable. They do not need the added burden of being preoccupied with the overtones resulting from the teacher's negative attitude. Curriculum objectives *must* include academic skill development: This is the role of the school. But academic skills should not be developed at the expense of the bilingual handicapped students' language, cultural background, or values. Used wisely, these cultural variables can become growth enhancers instead of growth detractors.

Teaching Reading through Writing

Rationale

Critics believe that teacher expectation, perception of student behavior, and assumptions about the student's English proficiency affect the quality of instruction. A number of studies have shown that teachers tend to use positive interaction more often with students whom they perceive as high achievers than with students perceived as low achievers (Good & Brophy, 1971; Kerman, Kimball, & Martin, 1980; McDermott, 1977; Rist, 1970). Furthermore, Roberts, Hutton, and Plata (1985) found teachers to rate similar behaviors significantly differently when they were exhibited by black and Hispanic students than when exhibited by white students.

The traditional approach to teaching reading and writing as separate components of the curriculum may also contribute to the bilingual students' problems. Many teachers who teach reading use the *bottom-up approach,* one that requires the analysis of visual units, such as letters and words, before meaning is realized (Chall, 1967; Gough, 1972).

The narrow view of the bottom-up approach to teaching reading contradicts what is known about the acquisition of language. Theorists concerned with the acquisition of reading and writing skills also advocate the application of principles compatible with language acquisition theories. These principles have been incorporated in the reciprocal interaction model (K. Goodman & Goodman, 1977; Y. Goodman & Burke, 1980; Graves, 1983; Holdaway, 1979, 1984; Smith, 1978, 1982). Essentially, these theorists argue that in order to develop effective literacy skills, children need to be *actively* involved both in generating meaning from texts and in expressing their thoughts and feelings in writing.

Participants and Setting

Young Sook Kim is a 13-year-old Asian-American female who has been mainstreamed into an English class from a special education resource room. The particular English class into which she was placed was developed for students who had been referred for placement into special education classes but had not met the eligibility criteria. The make-up of the group is rather typical of special populations who experience difficulty in school—there is an overrepresentation of male ethnic-minority students. The group members have poor academic track records, especially in subjects requiring reading and writing skills. Further, negative attitudes toward school and school personnel have been internalized.

Mr. Washington, the teacher for the special English class, was assigned to the class upon personal request. He had been teaching remedial reading for 3 years since his graduation from the local university with a major in English, and an interdisciplinary minor in remedial reading and special education.

Intervention

Using the reciprocal interaction model, Mr. Washington focused on writing as the vehicle to advance cognitive growth in his students. He knew that the chosen instructional activities had to be interesting and relevant, yet must challenge the cognitive potential of the student. With the writing activity Mr. Washington wanted to dispel the myth that these students were passive, dependent, and lacked motivation to learn.

On the first day of class Mr. Washington told the students that a class writing project—a newsletter—would dominate the class activities. He initiated class discussion and requested and encouraged students to interject comments, discuss ideas at length, and suggest their own ideas. Most students participated in the discussion, while some students listened, and some remained skeptical about the whole idea of a newsletter. Young Sook listened intently and observed her peers' behaviors—both those who were serious about school and those who seemed to dismiss school.

After a reasonable amount of discussion, Mr. Washington expressed his appreciation to the class for having participated in the discussion about the group's writing project. He then asked the class to list the advantages of writing a newsletter. While the students made comments, Mr. Washington wrote the major points on the chalkboard. The following advantages were produced:

1. All class members can participate.
2. It is an ongoing activity.
3. Several areas of interest in and out of school could be covered.

4. It gives students opportunities to interact with various groups of people.
5. Class members will be viewed positively by their peers.
6. It allows class members to work in small and large groups.
7. Students will learn to use the computer to produce the newsletter.
8. Class members will learn to be responsible.

Mr. Washington suggested that the students copy the eight points from the board so they could discuss them with their parents, other family members, and/or their friends. Finally, Mr. Washington also requested the students to think about the components of the newsletter over the weekend.

Mr. Washington contacted Mr. Fitzhugh, the editor of the local newspaper, to see if the newspaper staff could help the class with ideas on how to get started. Mr. Washington invited Mr. Fitzhugh to visit the school and provide the class with suggestions about writing a newsletter. Following is a list of topics discussed by Mr. Fitzhugh with the class:

1. Designs or formats for newsletters
2. Tips/suggestions/guidelines that would be helpful in developing the newsletter
3. Tips/suggestions/guidelines for gathering information for newsletter entries
4. Samples of writing that would be appropriate for different topics or issues for newsletters

The next step for the students was to practice writing on topics with which they were familiar. Some students seemed timid and were reluctant to write because they could not spell some of the words and they could not think of anything to write. Mr. Washington assured the class that he was not concerned, at this time, with misspelled words or how well they wrote. He was only interested in the class members writing down their ideas. He also assured the class that all errors would be corrected later. This procedure follows findings by Elley (1981, p. 12) that "pupils who had no formal grammar lessons for three years

were writing just as clearly, fluently, and correctly as those who had studied much grammar." The only apparent difference between the groups was that the pupils who had not studied grammar enjoyed English more. Furthermore, Chomsky (1972, p. 120) suggests that students "ought to be directing their activities and make decisions, not you [the teacher]. They ought to pick the words and write them, with your guidance. Or, if you suggest the words, as you will sometimes do, they ought to know that it is up to them to come up with their own spellings."

After several days of practice writing, Mr. Washington assigned predetermined topics to groups of three students. As each student group received a topic, Mr. Washington recorded the topic, the students' names responsible, and the deadline date for the feature story each group was to write.

Mr. Washington made arrangements with Ms. Wilkerson, the computer lab manager, for the students to use the computers. She offered to assist students who did not know how to use the computer for the development of their newsletter.

As the year progressed, the students in the special English class and Mr. Washington were the "talk of the school," indeed the talk of the town. They were featured in the local newspaper, thanks to Mr. Fitzhugh. The students selected topics, and wrote articles and poems and drew cartoons about: politics; education; children's school, home, and summer activities; people in the community; employment problems; health-related issues; drugs; people in the school; entertainment; and themselves.

At the end of the year Mr. Washington, in his evaluation of the special English class, wrote:

Indeed, this class was *special*. But they did not become *special* without a lot of hard work on their part. They have learned a great deal, and so have I. Following are just some of the things I believe these *special* students have learned:

1. To believe in themselves; that they can do things of which they were fearful initially.
2. To plan ahead and to work cooperatively and to become responsible for their own behaviors.

3. To believe that someone does care about them, their education and their ideas.
4. To interact with different business people in the community, with different school personnel and with each other, regardless of ethnicity, cultural background, gender, or socio-economic background.
5. About what went on in their school; who does what, when, where, and how; that it takes cooperation from everyone to make school a good place to be.
6. A different perspective of education. That they have to become involved in what they learn and that, they, not *the other guy* are responsible for what they learn.
7. More than just how to read and write (the ultimate goal for the class) they became informed about sociological-economical-political-educational issues with which people are confronted.

. . . In a nut-shell, these students have become literate. (Washington, personal communication, February 16, 1987)

Summary

The ability to read is treasured, especially among students. But writing may be the one skill that ascertains the academic prowess of an individual more quickly than even reading or analytical skills. Without the written word, reading would no longer be required.

It is not surprising, then, that linguists are advocating the importance of writing as a vehicle for learning. Saville-Troike (1984) believes that the language skill most likely to produce academic success in limited-English proficient students is writing. However, Saville-Troike (1984), among others, also advocates using the richness of the students' culture in developing learning activities, be they in the affective or the cognitive domains. By doing so, these students will be motivated to learn because learning is relevant.

Teaching reading through writing is an approach worthy of initiating. The advantage of this approach is that it can be used successfully with all students, nonhandicapped and handicapped, limited-English proficient, bilingual, and monolingual English speakers.

Teaching Multicultural Concepts

Rationale

The United States is a multicultural nation of persons of different ethnic backgrounds, religions, socioeconomic levels, and native languages. In addition there are natural differences such as skin color, gender, age, and physical and mental abilities (Gollnick & Chinn, 1986). Every day one is reminded of and exposed to these differences in many ways, including: news on radio and television and in newspapers; and families and neighbors' attitudes. Not only are students made aware of such information through these methods, but they are also confronted with it at school—through teachers' attitudes, peer attitudes, and the curriculum. Often, this information about persons' "differences" is distorted or ethnocentric. Therefore, all students need to learn appropriate information about these differences and the effect that these differences have on the life-styles of individuals.

Everyone is a member of an ethnic group. Yet, little is known about one's own and others' ethnicity. One needs to know and understand the facts about how ethnic experiences affect one's behavioral patterns, value systems, expectations and aspirations, learning styles, or self-identity. One needs to realize that culture is the foundation of one's total identity and that one's identity is shown through: words used to communicate; ways of using time, space, and material; exhibited actions, postures, gestures, tones of voice, and facial expressions; and ways of working, playing, expressing love, and defending oneself (Hall, 1977). In addition, culture imposes order and meaning on all experiences. Individuals from other cultures are compared with one's own and evaluated by one's cultural standards. One's own culture is automatically seen as innate (Gollnick & Chinn, 1986), that is, possessed at birth. Culture, then, is the lens through which one judges the world.

Sumner (1940) described the viewing of other cultures in reference to one's own as *ethnocen-*

trism. So strong are the feelings of ethnocentrism that one's own cultural traits are viewed as natural, correct, and superior to those of another culture whose traits are perceived as odd, amusing, inferior, or immoral (Yetman & Steele, 1975).

Participants and Setting

The following activity may be used with groups of students varying in age and/or grade level. The level of information presented and the expected student outcomes may be altered according to the group's ability level. For example, the expected outcomes would be different for a second-grade group than for an eighth-grade group. Second graders may be expected to "Tell about . . ." or to "Make sentences about . . ." some multicultural concept. Eighth graders, however, may be required to write a short paragraph or an essay, or to share and discuss various multicultural issues. Finally, the eighth graders could be challenged to develop a class notebook of interesting multicultural-related facts, stories, or traditions that could be placed in the school's library or duplicated and shared with class peers.

Intervention

Schools, as socializing agencies, should prepare students to accept cultural and ethnic diversity as a norm in American society. This means learning and developing positive attitudes about a variety of ethnic groups, including their histories, cultural heritages, life-styles, and value systems (Gay, 1977b). In addition, students must learn not only that certain ethnic groups in U.S. society are subjected to discrimination, racism, stereotyping, isolation, and stigmatization, but also that some individuals are treated unequally based upon their religious beliefs or gender. Therefore, students need to learn about concepts such as racism, sexism, prejudice, discrimination, oppression, powerlessness/power, inequality/equality, and stereotypes. The following activity, "Who am I? Who are we?", is an example of the type of activity that will enhance attitudes toward the history, cultural heritage, life-styles, and value systems of different ethnic groups (adapted from Kamp & Chinn [1982, pp. 8–9, 24–26] and M. Ortiz & Travieso [1977, p. 125–126]). In selecting and/or developing other activities to teach multicultural concepts, see Banks (1982); "Curriculum Guidelines for Multiethnic Education" (1976); Gay (1975); Gollnick and Chinn (1986); Grant and Grant (1977); Kamp and Chinn (1982); and Pasternak (1979).

Sample Activity: "Who am I? Who are we?"

Students need to understand who they are by studying their family's heritage. With this information they have a basis for comparing similarities and differences within and between ethnic groups. This activity gives students opportunities to better understand their families and the families of their classmates. Also, parental assistance may be necessary to complete this activity, an admirable objective in and of itself.

Objectives At the end of this activity students will:

1. Identify and list components determining their own heritage.
2. Discuss the characteristics that put them in an ethnic group.
3. Become aware that being a member of an ethnic group is just one aspect of their identity.
4. Gain respect and/or pride for their family and their heritage.
5. Gain an understanding of similarities and differences among and within families of different cultures.
6. Gain an understanding of family and the life-styles of their family and other families.
7. Relate interesting facts, stories, and traditions about their families.

Task Activities

1. Ask the students to develop a family tree. The students should be able to answer questions about the family tree such as:

a. How is the family like a tree?

b. How do the members in the family tree differ?

c. How did names change for some members of the family tree?

d. How did people get their names years ago?

e. How do family trees grow?

2. Request that students interview their mother and/or father, one of their uncles or aunts, and one of their grandparents to obtain stories about the activities they enjoyed when they were growing up. After the interview, the students should develop a written story to be displayed on the class bulletin board or in the hallway. Also, students could share their stories with other class members through oral presentations or by developing a book for all class members. A book can be placed in the classroom's library and/or in the school's main library.

3. Students can develop a list of family traditions, including a list of activities that have become a traditional way of celebrating holidays by the family. These lists can be discussed in class and differences noted according to ethnicity. Lists can be typed and disseminated to class members.

4. Have students interview two members of the family tree (e.g., father and grandfather; father and uncle on mother's side; mother and grandmother) to obtain information on their beliefs on an issue. Get their rationale for their beliefs. Compare and contrast their responses and the basis for their beliefs. Discuss the information in class. List factors that may influence the beliefs of individuals. Discuss the possibility that one factor may have a different impact on individuals within and among families and/or ethnic groups.

5. Ask students to list things they like about their family, including their ancestors; list things they do not understand about a family activity or tradition; list a certain number of things they would like to know more about their family heritage. These lists can be discussed in class and shared in written form.

6. Develop a dictionary of terminology related to the study of heritage, including such terms as the following: heritage, ethnicity, ethnic group, culture, cultural group, ethnocentricism, traditions, language, ancestors, bloodlines, kinship, family, family tree, and customs.

7. Study the countries from which the students' ancestors came and make a list of the countries' customs, food, geography, economic conditions, life-styles, language, hobbies, types of homes, schooling, transportation, jobs and occupations, holidays, recreation, religions, and so forth. Students can draw a map of the countries or make drawings of anything they listed for the countries— clothing, homes, transportation, and so forth. Use these lists and drawings to make class presentations or to share them with parents or friends. Artwork can also be displayed.

Academic activities can be initiated from some of these activities, including activities in mathematics, social studies, reading, writing, history, or politics. The number and type of cognitive-oriented activities depend on the teachers' creativity. Whatever these activities happen to be, they will be relevant and functional for students, for they will be related to their lives.

SUMMARY

As the United States moves forward toward the 21st century, between 25% and 38% (Chinn & Hughes, 1987) of school-age children are culturally and linguistically diverse. An even larger percentage than before of these culturally and linguistically diverse children continues to populate special education classes. For example, in 1978, blacks constituted 23.9% and Hispanics 6.3% of the nation's special education enrollment in public schools (Chinn & Hughes, 1987). In 1984, enrollment of these two ethnic minority groups increased to 32.5% for blacks and 10.6% for Hispanics (Chinn & Hughes, 1987).

The special education child from a culturally and linguistically diverse group is not solely the concern of minority teachers and administrators. Because these children constitute approximately 45% (Chinn & Hughes, 1987) of many special education classes, their education and training should be the concern of *all* educators, regardless of ethnic group status and regardless of their discipline.

Culturally and linguistically diverse students are certainly not new to special education. What is new is the recognition that culturally and linguistically different exceptional children's individual needs and differences should be recognized and addressed in the curriculum. At the present time one can draw inferences from the studies of Hispanic children, and disabled children. From these inferences one can assume, for example, what the characteristics are of learning disabled, Mexican-American children. However, concerted efforts to research the specific characteristics of these various groups of children are needed.

If the intent of PL 94-142's mandate of free and appropriate education is addressed to its fullest extent, then the individual cultural and academic needs of each student will be taken into consideration. The student's ethnic, religious, socioeconomic, and linguistic background, as well as his or her gender, are critical in planning for appropriate instruction and curriculum.

This chapter has presented information on culture, characteristics of students, teacher competencies and skills, and curriculum and instructional strategies estimated to affect not only the students but their teachers as well. Because there is very little information about culturally and linguistically different handicapped children, the ideas and suggestions presented have been derived from the literature about: 1) culturally and linguistically different children, and 2) handicapped children. Care was taken to present suggestions that were based on language development and language learning theory plus the known methodology used in special education.

The "Language Development" activity may be used with handicapped students who are monolingual in their native language. This first activity, as do the remainder of the activities, uses the students' cultural background and the students' language and academic characteristics as a basis for its development. The second and third activities presented concentrated on academic skill development. Mathematics skill development was one of the goals of the second activity while the third activity developed reading skills through writing, an approach consistent with research findings on acquisition of language. The activity for "Teaching Multicultural Concepts" may be varied in difficulty for use with handicapped students of all ages. Its main focus is for students to gain information about themselves, their families, and their heritage. Academic activities may be initiated based on information gathered by students, including mathematics, social studies, and so forth.

The creative teacher, who is not intimidated by the diversity of the student population, has the opportunity to multiculturize many instructional activities. The creative teacher should take every opportunity to integrate students' characteristics into the curriculum. When all educators come to the realization that culturally and linguistically diverse handicapped children are the concern of everyone, then the first giant step will have been made to keep the promise of a free and appropriate education.

STUDY QUESTIONS

1. Distinguish between macro- and microculture. How does each affect one's behavior? How have cultural differences negatively af-

fected the education of ethnic minority students?

2. Tell how the legal system has been used to remedy the problems of inappropriate placement of ethnic minorities into special education classes. Give specific examples.

3. Why is multicultural education proposed as a way to educate all students? Will this educational strategy work with culturally and linguistically different students who are handicapped? How? Under what conditions?

4. Describe the influences of culture on students' values, locus of control, and cognitive style. What are the implications of these differences on the teacher's perception of and the strategies used in educating culturally and linguistically different handicapped students?

5. Tell why the teacher is viewed as key to culturally and linguistically handicapped students' success in school. How can the teacher enhance these students' opportunities for achievement?

6. Describe the characteristics of curriculum and instructional materials that will increase culturally and linguistically different handicapped students' chances of achieving in school. Give specific examples.

REFERENCES

Adkins, P.G. (1970). Relevancy in children's language. *The Reading Teacher, 24* (1), 7–11.

Banks, J.A. (1982). Educating minority youths: An inventory of current theory. *Education and Urban Society, 15* (1) 88–103.

Baptiste, H.P., & Baptiste, M. (1977). Developing multicultural learning activities. In C.A. Grant (Ed.), *Multicultural education: Commitments, issues, and applications* (pp. 105–112). Washington, DC: Association for Supervision and Curriculum Development.

Besvinick, S.L. (1960). An effective daily lesson plan. *The Clearing House, 34* (7), 431–433.

Castañeda, A. (1976). Cultural democracy and the educational needs of Mexican American children. In R.L. Jones (Ed.) *Mainstreaming and the minority child* (pp. 181–194). Reston, VA: The Council for Exceptional Children.

Chall, J. (1967). *Learning to read: The great debate.* New York: McGraw Hill.

Chinn, P.C. (1979). Curriculum development for culturally different exceptional children. *Teacher Education and Special Education, 2* (4), 49–58.

Chinn, P.C. (1987, May 21). *Assimilation or multiculturalism: A challenge for educators in an increasingly pluralistic society.* Keynote address, California State Department National Conference for Personnel Who Work with Culturally and Linguistically Different Students Having Special Needs, Los Angeles.

Chinn, P.C., & Hughes, S. (1987). Representation of minority students in special education classes. *Remedial and Special Education, 8* (4), 41–46.

Chinn, P.C., & Kamp, S.H. (1982). Cultural diversity and exceptionality. In N.G. Haring (Ed.), *Exceptional children and youth* (pp. 371–390). Columbus, OH: Charles E. Merrill.

Chinn, P.C., & Plata, M. (1986). Perspectives and educational implications of Southeast Asian students. In M.K. Kitano &

P.C. Chinn (Eds.), *Exceptional Asian children and youth* (pp. 12–28). Reston, VA: The Council for Exceptional Children.

Chomsky, C. (1972). Write now, read later. In C. Cazden (Ed.), *Language in early childhood education* (pp. 119–126). Washington, DC: National Association for the Education of Young Children.

Coleman, J.S., Campbell, E.Q., Hobson, C.J., McPartland, J., Mood, A.M., Weinfeld, F.D., & York, R.L. (1966). *Equality of educational opportunity.* Washington, DC: Department of Health, Education and Welfare, Office of Education.

Cox, B.G., & Ramirez, M. (1981). Cognitive styles: Implications for multiethnic education. In J.A. Banks (Ed.), *Education in the 80's: Multiethnic education* (pp. 67–70). Washington, DC: National Education Association.

Cummins, J. (1980). The entry and exit fallacy in bilingual education. *NABE Journal, 4* (3), 25–59.

Cummins, J. (1984). Underachievement among minority children. In J. Cummins (Ed.), *Bilingualism and special education: Issues in assessment and pedagogy.* (pp. 93–129). San Diego: College-Hill Press.

Curriculum guidelines for multiethnic education [Special supplement]. (1976). *Social Education.*

Deutch, M. (1965). The role of social class in language development and cognition. *American Journal of Orthopsychiatry, 35,* 78–88.

Development Associates. (1980). *Evaluation of California's educational services to limited and non-English speaking students. Vol. 1.* Report submitted to the office of the Legislative Analyst, California State Legislature, Sacramento, CA.

Diana v. State Board of Education, CA. No. C-70-37 RFP (N.O. Cal, 1970).

Dulay, H., Burt, M., & Kreshen, S. (1982). *Language two.* New York: Oxford University Press.

Dunn, L. (1968). Special education for the mildly retarded: Is much of it justifiable? *Exceptional Children, 7* (35), 5–24.

Elley, W.B. (1981). Why teach a centipede to walk? *Education, 3,* 11–13.

Gallegos, A., Gallegos, R., & Rodriguez, R. (1983). Los inocentes: Considering the *special* need of the Mexican American child. *Contemporary Education, 54* (2), 109–112.

Galloway, C. (1976). *Psychology for learning and teaching.* New York: McGraw-Hill.

Galvan, M.M., & Brodie, J.G. (1977). *Accutrak Texas criterion reference system for oral language: A manual for administering the test* [Draft copy]. San Antonio, TX: Region 20 Education Service Center.

Garcia, R. (1978). The multiethnic dimension of bilingual-bicultural education. *Social Education, 42* (5), 492–494.

Gay, G. (1975). Organizing and designing cultural/pluralistic curriculum. *Educational Leadership, 33* (3), 176–183.

Gay, G. (1977a). Curriculum design for multicultural education. In C.A. Grant (Ed.), *Multicultural education: Commitments, issues, and applications* (pp. 94–104). Washington, DC: Association for Supervision and Curriculum Development.

Gay, G. (1977b). Curriculum for multicultural education. In F.H. Klassen & D.M. Gollnick (Eds.), *Pluralism and the American teacher: Issues and case studies* (pp. 31–62). Washington, DC: American Association of Colleges for Teacher Education.

Gollnick, D.M., & Chinn, P.C. (1986). *Multicultural education in a pluralistic society* (2nd ed.). Columbus, OH: Charles E. Merrill.

Gonzales, P.C. (1981). How to begin language instruction for non-English speaking students. *Language Arts, 58* (2), 175–180.

Good, T.L., & Brophy, J.E. (1971). Analyzing classroom interaction: A more powerful alternative. *Educational Technology, 11,* 36–40.

Goodman, K.S., & Goodman, Y.M. (1977). Learning about psycholinguistic processes by analyzing oral reading: *Harvard Educational Review, 47,* 317–333.

Goodman, Y.M., & Burke, C. (1980). *Reading strategies: Focus on comprehension.* New York: Holt, Rinehart & Winston.

Gough, P.D. (1972). One second of reading. In J.F. Kavanagh & I.G. Mattingly (Eds.), *Language by ear and by eye.* Cambridge, MA: M.I.T. Press.

Grant, C.A., & Grant, C.W. (1977). Instructional materials in multicultural education. In C.A. Grant (Ed.), *Multicultural education: Commitments, issues, and applications* (pp. 113–120). Washington, DC: Association for Supervision and Curriculum Development.

Graves, D.H. (1983). *Writing: Teachers and children at work.* Exeter, NH: Heinemann Educational Books.

Hall, E.T. (1977). *Beyond culture.* Garden City, NY: Anchor Press.

Heller, K.A., Holtzman, W.H., & Messick, S., (1982). *Placement of children in special education: A strategy for equity.* Washington, DC: National Academy Press.

Henderson, R. (1980). Social and emotional needs of culturally diverse children. *Exceptional Children, 46,* 598–605.

Holdaway, D. (1979). *The foundations of literacy.* Sydney, Australia: Ashton Scholastic.

Holdaway, D. (1984). *Stability and change in literacy learning.* Exeter, NH: Heinemann Educational Books.

Kamp, S.H., & Chinn, P.C. (1982). *A multiethnic curriculum for special education students.* Reston, VA: The Council for Exceptional Children.

Kerman, S., Kimball, T., & Martin, M. (1980). *Teacher expectations and student achievement.* Downey, CA: Office of the Los Angeles County Superintendent of Schools.

Kirk, S.A., & Gallagher, J.J. (1983). *Educating exceptional children.* Boston: Houghton Mifflin.

Kreshen, S. (1982). Bilingual education and second language acquisition theory. In California State Department of Education (Ed.), *Schooling and language minority students: A theoretical framework* (pp. 51–79). Los Angeles: Bilingual Education Evaluation, Dissemination, and Assessment Center.

Larry P. v. Riles, 502 F 2d 963 (9th Cir. 1974).

Lau. v. Nichols, 414 U.S. 563 (1974).

Lickona, T. (1977). Creating the just community with children. *Theory into Practice, 16,* 97–104.

Lora v. Board of Education of the City of New York, 456 F. Supp. 1211 (1978).

Lovett, C.J. (1980). Bilingual education: What role for mathematics teaching? *Arithmetic Teacher, 27* (8), 14–17.

Mann, H. (1971). Conducting instruction requires planning. *Teaching Exceptional Children, 3* (2), 87–91.

Manuel, H.T. (1965). *Spanish-speaking children of the Southwest: Their education and the public welfare.* Austin: University of Texas Press.

McDermott, R.P. (1977). The ethnography of speaking and reading. In R. Shuy (Ed.), *Linguistic theory: What can it say about reading?* (pp. 153–185). Newark, DE: International Reading Association.

Mercer, J. (1973). *Labeling the mentally retarded.* Los Angeles: University of California Press.

National Assessment of Educational Progress. (1977). *Hispanic student achievement in five learning areas: 1971–1975.* Washington, DC: U.S. Government Printing Office.

Mercer, J. (1973). *Labeling the mentally retarded.* Los Angeles: University of California Press.

National Assessment of Educational Progress. (1977). *Hispanic student achievement in five learning areas: 1971–1975.* Washington, DC: U.S. Government Printing Office.

National Assessment of Educational Progress. (1981). *Literacy in America: A synopsis of national assessment findings* (No. S4-FL-50). Denver: Education Commission of the States.

Norwick, S., & Strickland, B. (1973). A locus of control scale for children. *Journal of Consulting and Clinical Psychology, 40,* 148–154.

Office of Civil Rights. (1986). *The 1984 elementary and secondary schools civil rights survey.* Washington, DC: U.S. Department of Education.

Ortiz, A.A. (1983). Curriculum and instructional methods for exceptional bilingual children. In Del Green Associates (Eds.), *A review of research affecting educational programming for bilingual handicapped students* (Vol. I, pp. 1–67). (Available from Del Green Associates, Inc., 1030 15th Street, N.W., Suite 1025, Washington, DC 20005)

Ortiz, A.A. (1984). Choosing the language of instruction for exceptional bilingual children. *Teaching Exceptional Children, 16* (3), 208–212.

Ortiz, A.A., & Yates, J.R. (1983). Incidence of exceptionality among Hispanics: Implications for manpower planning. *NABE Journal, 7,* 41–54.

Ortiz, M., & Travieso, L. (1977). Multicultural activities for the classroom teacher. In C.A. Grant (Ed.), *Multicultural education: Commitments, issues, and applications* (pp. 123–126). Washington, DC: Association for Supervision and Curriculum Development.

Pasternak, M.C. (1979). *Helping kids learn multicultural concepts: A handbook of strategies.* Champaign, IL: Research Press.

Piper, D. (1986). Language growth in the multiethnic classroom. *Language Arts, 63* (1), 23–36.

Plata, M. (1986). Instructional planning for limited English proficient students. *Journal of Instructional Psychology, 13* (1), 32–39.

Plata, M., & Cavin, J. (1984). Number skill development in mainstreamed handicapped students. *Teaching Exceptional Children, 16* (2), 131–135.

Plata, M., & Tolliver, J. (1978). Addressing mainstreaming education/Fighting the battle of the gap. *Journal of Instructional Psychology, 5* (1), 8–15.

Ramirez, M., & Castãneda, A. (1974). *Cultural democracy: Bicognitive development and education.* New York: Academic Press.

Rist, R.C. (1970). Student social class and teacher expectations: The self-fulfilling prophecy in ghetto education. *Harvard Educational Review, 40,* 411–451.

Roberts, T., Hutton, J.B., & Plata, M. (1985). Teacher ratings of Hispanic, Black and Anglo students' classroom behavior. *Psychology in the Schools, 22,* 353–356.

Rodriguez, R. (1979). Effectiveness with bicultural children: Approaches for monocultural teachers. *Contemporary Education, 50* (3), 134–137.

Saville-Troike, M. (1978). *A guide to culture in the classroom.* Rosslyn, VA: National Clearinghouse for Bilingual Education.

Saville-Troike, M. (1981). Language diversity in multiethnic education. In J.A. Banks (Ed.), *Education in the 80's: Multiethnic education* (pp. 72–81). Washington, DC: National Education Association.

Saville-Troike, M. (1984). What really matters in second language learning for academic achievement? *TESOL Quarterly, 18* (2), 199–219.

Smith, F. (1978). *Understanding reading* (2nd ed.). New York: Holt, Rinehart & Winston.

Smith, F. (1982). *Writing and the writer.* New York: Holt, Rinehart & Winston.

Sumner, W.G. (1940). *Folkways.* Boston: Ginn.

U.S. Bureau of Labor Statistics. (1984). *Employment and earnings.* Washington, DC: U.S. Government Printing Office.

U.S. Commission on Civil Rights. (1975). *A better chance to learn: Bilingual bicultural education* (Clearinghouse Publication No. 51). Washington, DC: U.S. Government Printing Office.

Vasquez, J. (1978). Locus of control, social class and learning. *Bilingual education paper series.* Los Angeles: National Dissemination and Assessment Center, California State University.

Vasquez, J. (1979). Bilingual education's needed third dimension. *Educational Leadership, 37* (2), 166–168.

Walker, J. (1981). Why do planning? *Industrial Education, 70* (4), 8, 48.

Wallace, G., & Larsen, S.C. (1979). *Educational assessment of learning problems: Testing for teaching.* Boston: Allyn & Bacon.

Williams, L.R., & De Gaetano, Y. (1985). *ALERTA: A multicultural bilingual approach to teaching young children.* Menlo Park, CA: Addison-Wesley.

Yetman, N.R., & Steele, C.H. (Eds.). (1975). *Majority and minority: The dynamics of racial and ethnic relations* (2nd ed.). Boston: Allyn & Bacon.

INNOVATIVE TECHNIQUES IN INTEGRATION

CHAPTER 8

INTEGRATION OPTIONS FOR THE VERY YOUNG CHILD

Marci J. Hanson and Mary Frances Hanline

Young children learn primarily through play and interactions with others. Therefore, social learning activities constitute an important component of a curriculum for young children with special needs. Instructional and developmental goals in areas other than the social behavioral domain also may be achieved in this social context. Because social experiences are so important for the young child, the focus of integration experiences for children with special needs from birth to 5 years of age is on social activities. Integration refers, in this context, to any interactions or contact between children with disabilities and children who are nondisabled. Thus, the model and activities presented in this chapter emphasize the importance of a social learning environment for the young child.

The approach described in this chapter is considered appropriate for children with the full range of disabilities—sensory, motor, communication, affective, and/or cognitive and learning disorders. In addition, many young children have multiple impairments, which may range from severely to mildly involved. Integration activities can be individually tailored for children regardless of the developmental disorder or the severity of the disorder. Further, with the tremendous advances in care in the neonatal intensive care nurseries, more and more infants are surviving though born considerably premature, at very low birth weights, and/or with significant health and developmental risks. Many of these babies require prolonged hos-

pitalization and extraordinary care in the early months and years. Some of these children will recover from the early trauma and some will develop significant disabilities. Regardless of the prognosis, most are considered at risk for developmental delay during the early years and many are provided with special medical and educational services to prevent or ameliorate such delays. Service delivery settings that foster social integration activities may be particularly beneficial for these at-risk children.

The integration of young children who are at risk for developmental delay or who have disabling conditions presents different issues than does integration efforts with school-age children. Not only are developmental, educational, and family involvement needs different at this young age, but the availability of appropriate settings in which integration can be achieved is limited. While an increasing number of states are providing special educational services for children with special needs from birth to 5 years, few furnish publicly funded services for nondisabled children. Therefore, creative options in the local community must be explored in order to provide accessibility to integration opportunities.

UNDERLYING ASSUMPTIONS

The early years represent an ideal time to facilitate social learning. However, the implementation of

In this chapter, "infants and toddlers" refers to children age birth to 3 years, and they are served by "early intervention" programs; "preschool-age" refers to children age 3 to 5 years, and they are served by "preschool" programs.

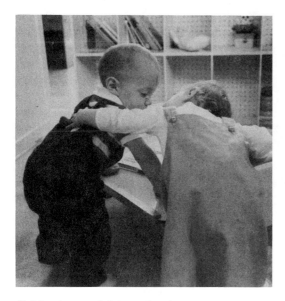

Toddlers in an early intervention program.

social integration activities with the birth-to-5-year age group must be carefully designed around the developmental needs of children of this age. Further, a number of key issues arise that are particular to this group, such as health and safety. These issues influence the degree to which integration activities can or should be implemented as part of an educational curriculum in the infant and toddler (birth to 36 months) or preschool (3 to 5 years) years.

Given the developmental issues that are raised in designing educational interventions (including social integration programs) with children in this age group, several underlying assumptions are presented.

1. Children are social beings and learn from play and social interactions with others. Even the earliest experiences of the young infant involve these social exchanges (Hanson, 1984; Lewis & Rosenblum, 1974, 1975; Peterson, 1987; Tronick, 1982).
2. Any interventions in the early years, particularly during infancy, must focus on the entire family unit—not solely on the child. The family unit may include parents, siblings, extended family members, and other important caregivers. This family environment is the central environment for the young child (Fewell & Vadasy, 1986; Gallagher & Vietze, 1986; Turnbull & Turnbull, 1986).
3. Because the early years are devoted to the child's development of attachment relationships with key caregivers, the child's growing awareness of self, and the child's ability to exercise individuality and to separate for a period of time from caregivers, integration activities must be implemented gradually, be carefully planned, and be attuned to these developmental issues.
4. The degree and type of integration activities provided in the early years most likely will differ from those provided to other age groups. The social skills necessary to participate in and benefit from group-based social integration activities even vary from infancy to preschool age.
5. Developmentally appropriate activities that encourage social exchanges between same-age peers with and without disabilities are beneficial to young children, particularly those of preschool ages. Some benefits that may be derived include advances in communication, attention, social behavior, and learning skills for the less developmentally advanced children. In addition, nondisabled children may begin to accept individual differences at an early age (Guralnick, 1981a, 1981b; Strain & Odom, 1986).

These assumptions establish the theoretical and practical bases for implementing integration activities in the early years. However, such integration efforts must be specifically geared to this very young age group.

SPECIAL CONSIDERATIONS

Due to the specific needs of young children, several key issues must be considered in designing appropriate and effective integration activities. These considerations are discussed briefly below.

1. *Inclusion of the family.* Particularly during infancy, educational intervention activities must be developed to actively involve the child's major caregivers in order to foster the development of mutually satisfying relationships. As the majority of the young child's time is spent in the family environment, this is where the most critical learning occurs in the early years.

2. *Availability of typically developing peers.* Unlike integration opportunities for school-age children, where large numbers of typically developing children are served through compulsory education, few integration opportunities for very young children exist in public education settings. However, many young children do go to day-care facilities and/or participate in early educational programs. Therefore, a range of service delivery options must be considered for integration opportunities with this age group. Such settings may include family day-care homes, day-care centers (both private and public), and both privately and publicly funded preschool programs.

3. *Health and safety issues.* Due to their age and the fact that many infants and young children who are disabled or at risk for developmental delay have medical and health problems, integration activities must be approached cautiously with certain health and safety factors in mind. When young children begin group-care experiences, they commonly develop a number of illnesses due to their increased exposure (Sells & Paeth, 1987). For children with significant medical or health risks, such exposure can be dangerous. Further, babies who were born considerably prematurely or at great medical risk due to other factors often cannot physiologically tolerate the amount of stimulation they would receive in a group-care environment.

4. *Staff training.* Caregivers and teachers who work with children in integrated settings must have training both in typical and atypical child development. Unfortunately, few formal training programs offer such experiences and traditional staff members in day-care and preschool programs have been trained exclusively either in typical child development or in special education. With the current emphasis on integrated early childhood programs, training that combines both areas of knowledge is needed.

In summary, integration activities for the very young child from birth to age 5 necessitate flexible, family, and child-centered social activities. Such activities will be implemented in a variety of service delivery settings.

EDUCATIONAL MODEL

Infants are born social beings and shortly after birth come to recognize and prefer their significant caregivers, typically their parents. The early years are also a time for developing social awareness and the ability to learn from others in the environment. Therefore, integration efforts must consider the young child's *development* of social skills. If the child is disabled or at significant risk for developing delays, social development may proceed more slowly if the impairment affects the child's ability to process or glean information from the environment.

Table 1 outlines the typical course of social development in the first 5 years (Cohen & Gross, 1979; Hanson & Hanline, 1984). Table 2 presents the stages and adaptations in the development of the parent-infant relationship (Sander, 1962). These brief summaries of normal developmental processes underscore the great developmental shifts or changes that occur during the early years. Further, they emphasize the young child's struggle from dependency and attachment to critical caregivers to the development of a sense of self and the

Table 1.   Social development milestones

Birth–6 months	Recognizes familiar persons Smiles Makes social response to self in mirror
6–12 months	Cooperates in "games" with adult
12–24 months	Reaches for and demands attention from significant others Explores environment constantly Plays contentedly if near adults Begins to initiate own play activities
24–36 months	Watches other children play Engages in parallel play (e.g., plays near other children) Briefly joins play of other children Defends own possessions Begins to engage in simple dramatic play (e.g., plays "house" pretending to be adult) Begins to use objects symbolically Constructs with blocks, art materials, and so forth, showing pleasure in whatever is constructed Participates in simple group activities (e.g., story telling, rhyme games)
36–48 months	Shares toys, begins to ask permission to use the toys of other children Takes turns with assistance Spontaneously joins in play with other children Engages in simple and short social interactions with other children Begins to engage in more complex dramatic play by acting out whole scenes that have themes (e.g., going to the grocery store) and by wanting an appropriate prop (e.g., hat or gloves) Plays interactive games (e.g., tag) Creates imaginary characters Enjoys puppet play, singing, chanting
48–60 months	Participates in socially interactive play Plays dress-up and other dramatic play with great attention to detail and with a variety of props Shows interest in exploring sex differences Begins to be critical of own workmanship on art projects, block constructions, and so forth Enjoys hide-and-seek games and hunting for hidden treasures Prefers playing with children of same sex Shows concern for playmates in distress Plays well with one other child without supervision, but may find it difficult to adjust to additional child Prefers playing with other children to playing alone Is alternately aggressive and cooperative with friends

Adapted from Cohen and Gross (1979) and Hanson and Hanline (1984).

ability to separate from the caregivers and achieve identification as an individual. It is in this final "stage" that the young child can begin to benefit fully from peer interactions.

As can be seen, the need for and ability of the child to benefit from integration activities varies across the first 5 years. In infancy, children are dependent upon their caregivers, and also begin learning and becoming aware of themselves. Little or no actual interaction with peers occurs until

Table 2. Stages and adaptations in the parent-infant relationship

Initial regulation (1–3 months)
Caregivers and infants are faced with regulation of biological processes, such as feeding and sleeping, and with states of excitement for social interaction.

Reciprocal exchange (4–6 months)
Reciprocal coordination of caregiving activities and social play. Infants smiling and motor and vocal involvement in back-and-forth exchanges with caregivers.

Initiative (7–9 months)
Development of intentionality on part of infants. Infants more active in getting what they want from caregivers and environment. Infants develop understanding of means-end relationships.

Focalization (10–13 months)
Infants through own locomotion can establish proximity to the caregiver. Make demands on caregivers, particularly mothers.

Self-assertion (14–20 months)
Infants widen range of activities, as determined by themselves. May be in face of maternal opposition. Infants develop sense of selves as individuals.

Adapted from Sander (1962).

toddlerhood (18–24 months). Early integration activities, thus, may focus on family concerns (e.g., the provision of parenting classes dealing with common issues such as feeding, child care, and discipline). In the toddler and preschool years, as children become aware of other children and begin to engage in interactions with peers, social integration activities can be beneficial.

The following discussion presents elements essential to an optimal educational model for early integration. These elements include a range of program options, staff development and training, opportunities for appropriate social interactions, curricular adaptations, and family involvement.

Full Range of Program Models

Differences among community agencies providing integration opportunities, as well as the variable needs of young children who are disabled, require the availability of diverse educational models that can be used to provide opportunities for children to learn and play in integrated settings. Models range from fully mainstreamed programs to programs that utilize reverse mainstreaming. For example, Ipsa and Matz (1978) successfully integrated children with disabilities full time into a regular preschool program that implemented a cognitively oriented curriculum. Project STIP (Supported Transition to Integrated Preschools) (Hanline, 1987) provides support for regular and special education staff so that children attending self-contained special education preschool classrooms in public schools can be integrated (as part of their individualized education programs) into local school district state-subsidized child-care and development programs. Klein and Sheehan (1987) utilize a dual-service model, the Technical Assistance Project (TAP). This model combines the benefits of special education with the benefits available through integration in community day-care centers. The part-time integration is viewed as an addition to the child's more specialized primary educational placement in an early intervention program. Reverse mainstreaming, whereby nondisabled peers are mainstreamed into the special education classroom, is another model used to provide opportunities for integration (Apolloni & Cooke, 1978).

No one model of integration at the early childhood level is supported by the research or literature as being appropriate for every child. The amount, degree, and kind of contact with nondisabled peers must be determined based on each child's individual and family needs and specified in clearly articulated goals and objectives (Safford & Rosen, 1981; Winton, Turnbull, & Blacher, 1984). In addition, the integration should be structured so that both nondisabled children and children with disabilities benefit through social interactions and appropriate learning activities (Meisels, 1977). Integration experiences can be successfully executed in a variety of settings. Key components for optimal experiences are described in the following discussion.

Staff Development and Training

Research and experience have identified teacher attitudes, competence, preparation, and special education support as being major factors that contribute to the success of preschool integration (Guralnick, 1982). A vehicle for developing accepting attitudes toward children with disabilities and their integration into regular education programs, as well as the skills required in teaching young children with disabilities, is staff development (Salend, 1984; Wang, Vaughan, & Dytman, 1985). Staff development activities can provide support and information to regular education staff through a variety of methods, including: ongoing inservice workshops, on-site demonstrations, direct observation with support feedback, discussions during staff meetings, individual consultation, and written materials (Klein & Sheehan, 1987).

To be most effective, the information and service should be provided in a way that is ongoing and responsive to the needs and interests of individual program staff members. Further, such services should address day-to-day implementation problems and occur in the context of the daily work setting (Wang et al., 1985). Hanline (1987) found that, at the preschool level, information about the developmental patterns of children with disabilities, behavior management strategies, and appropriate instruction techniques was identified by regular education staff as being extremely important. In addition, the regular educators felt opportunities to consult on an ongoing basis with special education professionals about the needs of the children being integrated and about appropriate classroom adaptations were equally important to them when integrating children with disabilities. Additional topics of importance for staff development activities are health and safety issues, working with parents, and effective methods for encouraging reciprocal social interactions between children with disabilities and their nondisabled peers.

Preservice training for both regular and special educators should also address integration issues. Like the inservice training methods just described, early childhood teacher training programs must concentrate on training appropriate techniques for the achievement of successful integration efforts in the early years. The passage of PL 99-457 (Education of the Handicapped Act Amendments of 1986), which provides discretionary grant programs for serving infants who are at risk or who are disabled, and which mandates services for preschoolers with special needs to be served in the least restrictive environment, underscores the importance of this training.

Opportunities for Appropriate Social Interactions

Although most social interactions for infants occur within the context of the family, at about 2 years of age children show increasing enthusiasm for playing and interacting with peers. These peer-peer social interactions make a powerful contribution to the young child's development. Through the interactions, children learn to modulate aggressive behavior and learn to engage in appropriate prosocial behaviors, such as sharing, cooperating, and respecting the property of others. In addition, through interactions with others, young children develop a self-concept, formulate moral values, and establish cultural and sex role identities (Hartup, 1978). In integrated settings, the opportunity for nondisabled children and children with disabilities to engage in positive and reciprocal social interactions is critical, as the cross-group social interactions are necessary in order for the children to profit from friendship formation, attitude change, and observational learning (Guralnick, 1981a). In addition, these interactions provide the child who is disabled with the opportunity to learn age-appropriate social skills through experience with naturally reinforcing events in the environment.

In the early years, play is an ideal way to pro-

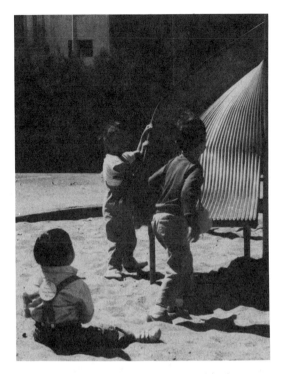

Preschool children at play in an integrated setting.

because they may not spontaneously engage in play behaviors. Further, verbal, sensory, or motor difficulties may interfere with play and communication. These difficulties, however, do not preclude the integration of children with disabilities with their nondisabled peers. Rather, they require that the physical and social environment be structured so that positive and reciprocal social interactions, as well as constructive play behavior, are encouraged.

Social interactions can be encouraged by carefully selecting activities and materials, grouping children, and providing appropriate teacher attention (Guralnick, 1982; Hanline, 1985; Strain & Odom, 1986). Toys such as vehicles, doll houses, and blocks promote social interaction. Dramatic play activities (e.g., playing "house") and equipment requiring two or more children to cooperate (e.g., using rocking boats) also encourage positive social interaction. Structuring activities that require sharing and/or a group effort increases opportunities for social interaction. For instance, activities such as painting a mural or requiring children to share one tub of paste encourage more socially interactive behaviors than do individual art projects or giving each child his or her own dish of paste. Social interaction can be increased by:

1. Limiting the number of children participating in an activity, the size of the play area, and the amount of materials available

2. Forming small instructional and play groups with consideration of the personal characteristics, preferences, and skills of each child

3. Monitoring the effects of varying the ratio of children with disabilities to nondisabled children, varying the match between developmental levels of the children, and varying the size of the groups

Interventions utilizing either teachers or nondisabled peers as change agents also are effective methods for increasing socially interactive behavior. For example, nondisabled peers can be

mote positive social interactions, as well as help children develop and refine communication, cognitive, and motor skills (McHale & Olley, 1982). Play is vital to a young child's development and has been referred to as "the principal business of childhood" (Bruner, 1975, p. 83). Social interactions among young nondisabled children at play occur with varying degrees of sophistication and often include nonverbal as well as verbal communication. Many play activities require minimal skills, making it possible for a child with a limited behavioral repertoire, due to the disabling condition, to take an active part in play.

However, social interactions may be difficult for children with disabilities and thus they may be socially isolated from their nondisabled peers (Cooper & Holt, 1982; Guralnick, 1981b). Difficulties arise because these children often lack age-appropriate play and social interaction skills and taught to make social initiations toward and engage in cooperative play with their classmates who are disabled (Guralnick, 1976; Strain, 1977). Teacher prompting and reinforcing of desired social behaviors also results in increases in socially interactive play (Fredericks et al., 1978; Strain & Timm, 1974). In addition, teachers can individually teach the child who is disabled the appropriate use of materials and peer interaction and then promote generalization of these skills to the integrated preschool classroom (Cooper & Holt, 1982). In this way, the children with disabilities can be seen as competent by their nondisabled peers, further promoting positive and reciprocal cross-group social interactions.

Curricular Adaptations

For several reasons, few modifications to the curricula of programs for young children are needed to accommodate children with disabilities. First, during the preschool years, nondisabled children exhibit a great deal of individual variation in their development, requiring a curriculum that can respond to children at different developmental levels and with differing educational needs. Further, activities and materials for young children frequently require a minimal amount of skill and can be used at varying skill levels. Also the delays and differences in the development of the children who are disabled as compared to their nondisabled peers often are smaller and less obvious than when the children are older. In addition, young children with disabilities usually follow the same sequence of development as nondisabled children, although they may develop at a slower rate. These developmental and curricular factors make the usual learning and play activities of a regular education preschool appropriate for children with disabilities.

However, adaptations may have to be made in order to allow the child who is disabled to participate actively in the activities of a regular early childhood education program. Children with sen-

sory impairments and physical disabilities, as well as children with multiple handicapping conditions, may require adaptations and special equipment. For example, a child with motor problems may need to use large crayons or large paint brushes and have his or her paper taped to the table top during art activities. To encourage independent behavior of a child with a hearing impairment, visual signals (e.g., flashing the overhead lights to signal a transition period) may need to be incorporated into the daily classroom routine. Further, children with behavior and learning problems may need environmental contingencies that are more consistent and structured than are those typically found in early childhood programs. The adaptations needed by each child and each program must be determined on an individual basis in consultation with regular education staff, special educators, and parents. The adaptations should allow the child who is disabled to be as independent and as fully participating as possible, while maintaining appropriate health and safety standards. In addition, care must be exercised so that the adaptations do not socially isolate or negatively stigmatize the child.

Family Involvement

The degree and type of family participation needed for successful integration experiences sets this age group (birth to 5 years) apart from others. As was previously discussed, the young infant spends a majority of her or his time in the home environment and the family members are the most important persons in the young child's life. Children cannot be involved in and benefit from group experiences until they are able to separate from their caregivers and achieve their own individuality. In addition, the first few years of the child's life are a time of change for the family to accommodate the new family member and a time for concentration on the inner workings of the family (Olson et al., 1983). These issues are as applicable to families with nondisabled members as they are to those with a child with a disability. Thus, an early childhood special education program must take these family issues into account.

Unlike the parents of typically developing children, however, parents of children with disabilities must explore a number of early service options for their children and make decisions surrounding issues such as teacher qualifications and attitudes, type of class, size of class, least restrictive environment, and quality of instruction (Winton et al., 1984). For these reasons, many families expect to be and are actively involved in their children's education programs. Further, PL 99-457 mandates the parents' options for participation.

As with the development of appropriate education programs for children, activities for family participation must be individualized to accommodate the particular needs of each family. Though many parents demand active involvement in their child's program, some do not wish to participate so actively. Winton and Turnbull (1981), for instance, found that about one fifth of the parents participating in a special education preschool program desired not to participate in direct services for their youngsters. Further, the type of participation must be individualized: Some parents may prefer informal contact, while others may prefer formal or structured contacts (Blacher-Dixon, Leonard, & Turnbull, 1981).

Summary

To be maximally effective and appropriate, integration activities for young children should be carefully planned, individually tailored to the child and family, and attuned to the child's developmental and health status. Components of an effective model include the provision of a range of program options, staff development and training, opportunities for appropriate social interactions among children, curricular adaptations, and family involvement. The following activities demonstrate the incorporation of these components in activities typically utilized in early intervention and preschool settings.

INTEGRATION ACTIVITIES

Parent Discussion Groups

Rationale

Parents of young children with disabilities have many of the same needs and interests as do parents of children who are developing normally. For example, all share concerns regarding feeding, discipline, child care, and appropriate play activities. Further, from the beginning of the child's life, the young child with disabilities and his or her family should be able to partake of family-oriented community activities without feeling isolated. Discussion groups that integrate parents of children with and without disabilities can ameliorate such isolation.

Participants

The activity described here is appropriate for all families—regardless of whether the children are disabled or not, and regardless of the type or degree of the child's disability.

Setting and Materials

Any community facility or home setting is appropriate. No special materials are needed other than those that may be utilized as part of a discussion around a particular topic. Child care should be available to allow parents to attend.

Intervention

Sponsor a parent information class. Advertise the class widely and in places where parents of children with disabilities are likely to see it (e.g., special newsletters, schools, health and disability service agencies). It is recommended that a series of weekly presentations be given around a topic area. Topic areas should be highly practical in nature and ample time for discussion and questions should be allowed during each presentation. Areas of interest to parents of young children may include:

Basic caregiving—bathing, feeding, dressing, basic hygiene

Feeding difficulties—selection of age-appropriate foods, utensils, positioning,

Growth and development of the young child—typical milestones from birth to 6 months, 6–12 months, 12–24 months, 24–36 months, 3–5 years

Time management—how to get everything done and still have time for yourself

Child care—what options are available, what to look for in a good facility or good caregiver

Play activities—developmentally appropriate and fun activities for the young child from birth to 5 years, including: games, books, songs, finger plays

Helping the child learn—teaching strategies that are useful for the very young child

Discipline—how to, when to

Toilet training—strategies, when to start, how to follow through

Recreational activities—swimming programs, gymnastics for young children, places to hike in the area, playgrounds

Toy making—toys and play equipment easy to make from materials found at home

Additional topics can be derived from a needs assessment once the group of parents has been identified. The most appropriate times and places to facilitate parent participation also can be determined from the needs assessment. Again, it must be emphasized that a key variable in the success of any parent group is the availability of child-care services during the parent meetings.

Adaptations

No adaptations are needed. Parents of children with and without disabilities are likely to have more rather than less in common with one another. However, the individual leading the group should have knowledge of atypical development so that questions pertaining to the children with special needs can be answered. Further, special efforts should be made to encourage parents of children

with special needs to participate so they are able to establish valuable support networks and information resources, and so they will not feel isolated from typical activities in the community.

Reverse Mainstreaming for Toddlers

Rationale

Most toddlers with disabilities are served in early intervention programs for children with special needs because of the availability of specially trained personnel in these programs and because few other appropriate public education options exist for this age group. Therefore, one strategy for creating integration opportunities for the very young child is reverse mainstreaming. In this model several typically developing children are integrated into the education program with the children with disabilities.

Participants

The use of reverse mainstreaming is appropriate for any group of children with disabilities regardless of the disability or the severity of the disorder. Children in the age group of 18–36 months will benefit from this procedure, as will children from 3 to 5 years of age. Several considerations are important in the selection of the typically developing peers, however. Children and families should be interviewed and only those who are genuinely open to and interested in participating should be selected. Typical children for whom reverse mainstreaming works best are in the low end of the age range for the children being served. That is, an 18-month-old nondisabled child may best be reverse mainstreamed into a classroom of 18- to 36-month-old children with disabilities. Further, success will be enhanced by eliminating children from the selection process who are overly aggressive or unruly. Since the major purpose of the early intervention program is to provide special services to young children with disabilities and their families, the addition of typically developing children to the program should enhance the provision of services, not detract from the needs of the target children.

Setting and Materials

Any early intervention program for young children would be appropriate provided an ample teacher-child ratio (e.g., 1:3 or 1:4) can be maintained.

Intervention

Typically developing peers can be integrated into all activities of the early intervention regimen: circle time, large group activities, snack time, and small group activities. Two such activities are described here: circle time and a small group learning task.

Circle Time   Circle time is often conducted at the beginning and end of a session to provide children the opportunity to get to know one another, learn simple songs and finger games, enhance communication and social skills, and provide children with a consistent beginning and closing activity each day.

To enhance interactions and communication skills, pair children with disabilities next to typically developing children in a semicircle around the "teacher" (adult leading the circle-time activities). Encourage the typical peers to demonstrate the finger game or sing the songs (e.g., "Itsy Bitsy Spider," "Wheels on the Bus," "Where is Thumbkin"). Other games include placing a bucket full of hand puppets on the floor and encouraging children one by one to get a puppet. The puppets can be used to sing songs; to shake hands in a greeting song naming each child; to "talk" to other puppets; and to demonstrate concepts, such as up and down or over and under. Once again the typical peers can serve as models for the activity.

Small Group Learning Task to Teach Children to Identify Common Objects   Gather a number of objects that are commonly found around the house and that the children will likely utilize in their play, feeding, and self-care activities (e.g., combs, brushes, toothbrushes, shoes, cups, spoons and forks, books, balls, ap-

ples, bananas). Also gather some "distractor" objects, such as boxes, bowls, and toy cars. Seat two to three children in a semicircle or at a small table. Position children so that they are stable and able to reach and manipulate the materials. Place two to three objects on the table: one target object (e.g., brush) and one or two distractor objects (e.g., small box, letter). Give each child a turn and ask the child to "find the brush." Later, you can make the task more difficult by identifying the function of the object (e.g., "What do you use for your hair?"). If the activity is new to the children, the normal peer model could be used to demonstrate the activity if she or he knows the concept. Different children can be given different objects so that the activity can be individually tailored to each child's level and needs.

Adaptations

Ensure that children with motor difficulties are properly positioned so that they feel stable and comfortable and can manipulate the objects. For children who are unable to reach and touch the object, they may point with their finger or eyes. In addition to the peer model, prompting from the teacher may be needed to teach the response pattern.

Obstacle Courses

Rationale

Obstacle courses provide opportunities for young children to socialize with peers, to improve gross motor skills and muscle strength, to learn to follow directions, and to practice imitating other children. Communication and cognitive development also may be enhanced through appropriate teacher input and peer modeling. In addition, because young children with disabilities may not have delays or may have only mild delays in gross motor skills (e.g., children with hearing impairments, speech and language delays, behavior disorders), this activity allows the child with a disability to be seen by nondisabled children as competent, thus encouraging equity in social exchanges and friendships.

Participants

The activity described is appropriate for most preschool children who have mild to moderate disabilities. However, activities selected to be part of the obstacle course should be chosen with consideration for the children's individual abilities and needs. Adaptations may have to be made for children with physical or visual impairments.

Setting and Materials

An obstacle course may be set up indoors or outdoors, utilizing equipment that is readily available at the preschool site. Playground equipment, tables, chairs, tires, cloth tunnels, and so forth can be used to construct an obstacle course.

Intervention

Set up a simple obstacle course. Be sure that all equipment is in good repair and that adequate staff are available to supervise the children. If the obstacle course is to be conducted outdoors, check the play area for glass, rocks, and holes in the ground that may be dangerous. If climbing activities are included, be sure that the surface underneath is covered with impact-absorbing materials such as mats, bark mulch, and so forth.

Examples of activities to include in the course are:

Crawling under a table
Sitting on a chair
Stepping over a pillow
Crawling through a tunnel
Jumping down from a high place
Throwing a bean bag at a target
Walking on a balance beam
Stepping into rubber tires or hoops
Rocking in a rocking boat
Walking up steps
Jumping on a small trampoline
Swinging on a swing
Bouncing a ball

Sliding down a slide
Pushing a box
Climbing into a carton
Walking on a line
Jumping across a line
Hanging from a bar

Before beginning, state the rules of the activity to the children and have a child demonstrate how to go through the obstacle course. Allow the children with disabilities to have a turn demonstrating the obstacle course to the other children. Be sure the children know what they are expected to do while waiting their turn and after they have completed the obstacle course. Be prepared to slow down children who get reckless or overexcited and to pace the children so they are not pushing each other.

Encourage the children to practice various movement patterns as they move between activities. For example, have them march, walk heel to toe, tiptoe, walk backwards, jump, and hop on one foot from one activity to the other.

Use this time to improve language skills. Prompt the children to tell you what they are doing. In addition, provide input that emphasizes age-appropriate concepts. For example: Sit *on* the chair. *Push* the box. Crawl *through* the tunnel.

To promote social interactions between the children with disabilities and the nondisabled children, alternate the order of children with disabilities and nondisabled children. That is, do not have all the children with disabilities go last or all the nondisabled children go last. Having the children go through the obstacle course in pairs, by pairing the child who is disabled with a nondisabled peer, also encourages cross-group interactions. Encourage the children to watch and imitate each other. Praise these behaviors.

Adaptations

Watch for signs of fatigue or overexertion in children who have activity-limiting health impairments. Children with balance difficulties or other physical coordination problems should be closely supervised. Children with physical disabilities and severe visual impairments may need adult assistance to complete certain activities. Allow the children who may have difficulty with the obstacle course to practice a few times alone with adult supervision and instruction. Invite the occupational therapist, physical therapist, and/or vision specialist to conduct therapy within the framework of the obstacle course.

Housekeeping and Dress-Up

Rationale

Playing "house" provides children with the opportunity to learn and practice communication skills, as well as social skills such as sharing and cooperating. "Dress-up" clothes allow children to practice self-help dressing skills. Playing "house" and "dress-up" are particularily appropriate for integrated settings, as these activities tend to promote social interaction and children at a variety of developmental levels can participate together.

Participants

Young children with a variety of disabling conditions and a range of abilities can participate in this activity without major adaptations.

Setting and Materials

A corner of the classroom should be set up for this activity. Child-size tables, chairs, sink, refrigerator, and stove (along with play food, utensils, dishes, pots, and pans) allow the children to play "house" within a kitchen setting. A variety of dress-up clothes, including hats, shoes, jewelry, purses, vests, and shirts, should also be available. Choose dress-up clothes that are easy to put on, but that have different types of fasteners (e.g., zippers, buttons, snaps).

Intervention

Limit the number of children playing together in this area of the classroom to three or four. This allows each child to participate fully, increases posi-

tive social interactions, and reduces the possibility of inappropriate behavior. Encourage the children to engage in activities that require cooperation. For example, encourage the children to set the table and have a tea party together. Model appropriate activities (e.g., show the children how to wake up the doll from a nap) and encourage the children with disabilities to imitate their nondisabled peers (e.g., have both children put on hats and carry purses). Prompt the children to adopt adult roles and pretend to engage in activities that are relevant to their lives. As children become more engrossed in their play, quietly withdraw from active involvement.

Intervene from time to time to provide language input ("You should put the milk in the refrigerator"), to reinforce appropriate imitative behavior and social interactions, and to help the children expand on their play activities or play sequences. For example, in addition to baking a cake, also have the children blow out pretend birthday candles on the cake or assist the children to add shoes and jewelry to their dress-up ensemble.

Adaptations

Be sure there is ample room for children with disabilities who use braces or walkers to move freely and independently throughout the play area. If children are nonambulatory, seat them in a position that will allow for social interactions and active participation—A table is often the center of activity even in a real kitchen. If children with hearing impairments are playing, encourage the nondisabled children to get their attention before attempting to communicate. Children with behavior disorders may need close supervision and extensive assistance to learn to play cooperatively.

Cooking

Rationale

A group cooking activity, such as making a fruit salad, helps children learn to sequence, follow directions, take turns, and learn from each other in a group setting. This type of activity also provides the opportunity to improve language, cognitive, and fine motor skills, and also provides the opportunity for social interaction.

Participants

The activity described is appropriate for all pre-school-age children, regardless of disabling condition.

Setting and Materials

Conduct this activity while four children are seated around a small table. Be sure to seat nondisabled children next to the children who are disabled. The contents of the fruit salad and dressing will vary, depending on the recipes used. Cooking utensils such as blunt knives, a small chopping board, a bowl, and mixing spoons will be needed.

Intervention

Collect all fruit salad and dressing ingredients and cooking utensils. Seat the children around a small table, being sure that you are able to assist all the children and that they can see you. Explain the activity to the children. Have the children label all salad ingredients and cooking utensils, allowing nondisabled children to do the labeling when appropriate.

Chop one fruit at a time. Place the fruit on the small cutting board and demonstrate how the children are to cut the fruit. Allow each child to have a turn. Encourage social interactions by having each child pass the cutting board and fruit to the next child. Allow the children to put the chopped fruit into the bowl. Continue until all the fruit is chopped. Mix ingredients of the dressing together, providing the opportunity for the children to pour and mix the ingredients. Have a child pour the dressing over the salad, and give each child a chance to mix the salad.

Be sure to talk to the children about what they are doing and encourage them to tell you what they are doing by asking appropriate questions. Emphasize concepts in your discussions. For ex-

ample: "Put the apples *in* the bowl." "Push *down* to chop the banana." Use words such as *next* and *now* to help children sequence activities. Encourage the children to watch and imitate each other.

Make sure that all children help clean up the cooking area. Provide an opportunity for the children to eat the salad and share it with other class members.

Adaptations

The activity just described is an excellent time to introduce simple signs to hearing children if the children with disabilities are communicating with signs. Children with physical disabilities may need assistance with chopping and stirring. Be sure these children are positioned so that they can independently accomplish as much as possible during the activity. Allow children with visual impairments to smell, touch, and taste the ingredients.

Turn-Taking

Rationale

The ability to take turns is a basic social skill required throughout childhood in a variety of play situations. Because it is a skill necessary for peer-peer interactions, it is most appropriate to learn the skill with peers. A nondisabled peer model/playmate may serve to motivate the child who is disabled.

Participants

The activity described is appropriate for any child who has not yet learned to take turns in play situations, but is designed specifically for the young child with severe cognitive delays or for children with multiply handicapping conditions.

Setting and Materials

Use a quiet area of the classroom for this activity. Provide a seating arrangement appropriate for the instructional materials that are being used and for the needs of the children. For example, some children will be able to sit on the floor without support. Other children may need to be supported in a seated position at a table. Suggestions for specific toys are provided below.

Intervention

Select several toys that lend themselves to turn-taking activities. Examples of turn-taking activities include stacking blocks, lining up blocks on the floor, placing rings on a stacking post, playing a drum or xylophone, rolling a ball, putting pegs into pegboards, stringing beads, and hammering pegs into pegboards.

Choose a nondisabled child and a child with a disability to participate in this activity. Position the children so that they are able to see and communicate with each other and can reach the toys easily. Explain to the children that you would like them to play together and take turns while they play. Allow the nondisabled child to have the first turn (e.g., put one peg into the pegboard or put one ring on the stacking post) so that he or she can act as a model for the child who is disabled. Encourage the child who is disabled to watch. When appropriate, tell the child who is disabled that it is her or his turn. Help her or him respond correctly. Then tell the nondisabled child it is his or her turn again. Repeat the process as needed. Be certain that the child who is disabled has the opportunity to initiate the appropriate behavior when it is his or her turn. That is, fade out the verbal and physical prompts as soon as possible.

Teach the nondisabled child to encourage and assist the child who is disabled to take a turn. As the nondisabled child becomes more competent "leading" the activity, remove yourself from the activity and allow the children to play together alone.

Adaptations

Selecting toys that will successfully accommodate specific disabilities is the only required adaptation. For example, choose large objects for children with motor impairments, objects that make sounds for children with visual impairments, visually intriguing objects for children with hearing impairments, and so forth.

Conclusion

All the play and learning activities just presented are representative of typical curricula in early intervention and preschool programs. Because young children learn best through play and interactions with others, the activities capitalize on these goals. All areas of skill development, particularly cognitive, social, and communication, can be facilitated using these procedures. Typically developing peers can be easily involved in all phases of the activities and can provide the model needed to "get an activity going" or motivate another child.

SUMMARY

Young children learn primarily through social interactions. Thus, early integration experiences can be beneficial to children with disabilities by providing them with opportunities to play with children who may be developmentally more advanced and able to model social, communication, and cognitive skills. However, integration experiences must be attuned to the developmental readiness and educational needs of the children, as well as to individual health and family needs. Without consideration of these needs, children with disabilities may be socially isolated in integrated settings, unable to benefit from interactions with their nondisabled peers, and may not receive the intervention needed to promote optimal development. In addition, without adequate concern for health issues, children may not receive the care required to maintain and support good health. Further, without individualized family involvement, neither the family nor the child will derive the full range of benefits from integrated early childhood programs.

Thus, as with integration experiences with other age groups, integration opportunities should be carefully planned and supported by well-trained personnel so that individual child and family needs can be met. The provision of early integration activities, when well planned, can enhance the development of young children (both disabled and nondisabled) through naturally occurring reciprocal social interactions.

STUDY QUESTIONS

1. What are some different service delivery models that can be used to provide opportunities for young nondisabled children and children with disabilities to socially interact?

2. Why are social interactions important in early childhood settings?

3. What can be done to promote social interactions between young children in integrated settings?

4. What are the assumptions underlying providing services to young children with special needs?

5. Why is training of regular educators important to the success of integration? How can this training best be conducted so that it promotes successful integration of young children?

6. What are three issues that must be considered in designing integration opportunities for this young age group?

REFERENCES

Apolloni, T., & Cooke, T.P. (1978). Integrated programming at the infant, toddler, and preschool levels. In M.J. Guralnick (Ed.), *Early intervention and the integration of handicapped and nonhandicapped children* (pp. 147–166). Baltimore: University Park Press.

Blacher-Dixon, J., Leonard, J., & Turnbull, A.P. (1981). Mainstreaming at the early childhood level: Current and future perspectives. *Mental Retardation, 19*(5), 235–241.

Bruner, J.S. (1975). Play is serious business. *Psychology Today, 8*(5), 80–83.

Cohen, M.A., & Gross, P.J. (1979). *The developmental resource: Behavioral sequences for assessment and program planning.* New York: Grune & Stratton.

Cooper, A.Y., & Holt, W.J. (1982). Development of social skills and the management of common problems. In K.E. Allen & E.M. Goetz (Eds.), *Early childhood education: Special problems, special solutions* (pp. 105–128). Rockville, MD: Aspen Systems.

Fewell, R.R., & Vadasy, P.F. (Eds.). (1986). *Families of handicapped children.* Austin, TX: PRO-ED.

Fredericks, H.D., Baldwin, V., Grove, D., Moore, W., Riggs, C., & Lyons, B. (1978). Integrating moderately and severely handicapped preschool children into a normal day care center. M.J. Guralnick (Ed.), *Early intervention and the integration of handicapped and nonhandicapped children* (pp. 191–206). Baltimore: University Park Press.

Gallagher, J.J., & Vietze, P.M. (Eds.). (1986). *Families of handicapped persons.* Baltimore: Paul H. Brookes Publishing Co.

Guralnick, M.J. (1976). The value of integrating handicapped and nonhandicapped preschool children. *American Journal of Orthopsychiatry, 46*(2), 236–245.

Guralnick, M.J. (1981a). The efficacy of integrating handicapped children in early childhood settings: Research implications. *Topics in Early Childhood Special Education, 1*(1), 57–71.

Guralnick, M.J. (1981b). The social behavior of preschool children at different developmental levels: Effects of group composition. *American Journal of Child Psychology, 31*(1), 115–130.

Guralnick, M.J. (1982). Programmatic factors affecting child-child social interactions in mainstreamed preschool programs. In P.S. Strain (Ed.), *Social development of exceptional children* (pp. 71–92). Rockville, MD: Aspen Systems.

Hanline, M.F. (1985). Integrating disabled children. *Young Children, 40*(2), 45–48.

Hanline, M.F. (1987). *Supported transition to integrated preschools* (Grant No. G008530068). Washington, DC: U.S. Office of Education.

Hanson, M.J. (Ed.). (1984). *Atypical infant development.* Austin, TX: PRO-ED.

Hanson, M.J., & Hanline, M.F. (1984). Behavioral competencies and outcomes: The effects of disorders. In M.J. Hanson (Ed.), *Atypical infant development* (pp. 109–177). Austin, TX: PRO-ED.

Hartup, W.W. (1978). Peer interaction and the processes of socialization. In M.J. Guralnick (Ed.), *Early intervention and the integration of handicapped and nonhandicapped children* (pp. 27–52). Baltimore: University Park Press.

Ipsa, J., & Matz, R.D. (1978). Integrating handicapped preschool children within a cognitively oriented program. In M.J. Guralnick (Ed.), *Early intervention and the integration of handicapped and nonhandicapped children* (pp. 167–190). Baltimore: University Park Press.

Klein, N., & Sheehan, R. (1987). Staff development: A key

issue in meeting the needs of young handicapped children in day care settings. *Topics in Early Childhood Special Education, 7*(1), 13–27.

Lewis, M., & Rosenblum, L.A. (Ed.). (1974). *The effect of the infant on its caregiver.* New York: John Wiley & Sons.

Lewis, M., & Rosenblum, L.A. (Ed.). (1975). *Friendship and peer relations.* New York: John Wiley & Sons.

McHale, S.M., & Olley, J.G. (1982). Using play to facilitate the social development of handicapped children. *Topics in Early Childhood Special Education, 2*(3), 76–86.

Meisels, S.J. (1977). First steps in mainstreaming: Some questions and answers. *Young Children, 33*(1), 4–13.

Olson, D.H., McCubbin, H.I., Barnes, H., Larsen, A., Muxen, M., & Wilson, M. (1983). *Families: What makes them work.* Beverly Hills: Sage Publications.

Peterson, N.L. (1987). *Early intervention for handicapped and at-risk children.* Denver: Love.

Safford, P.L., & Rosen, L.A. (1981). Mainstreaming: Application of a philosophical perspective in an integrated kindergarten program. *Topics in Early Childhood Special Education, 1*(1), 1–16.

Salend, S.J. (1984). Factors contributing to the development of successful mainstreaming programs. *Exceptional Children, 5*(50), 409–416.

Sander, L.W. (1962). Issues in early mother-child interaction. *Journal of the American Academy of Child Psychiatry, 1,* 141–166.

Sells, C.J., & Paeth, S. (1987). Health and safety in day care. *Topics in Early Childhood Special Education, 7*(1), 61–72.

Strain, P.S. (1977). An experimental analysis of peer social initiations on the behavior of withdrawn preschool children: Some training and generalization effects. *Journal of Abnormal Child Psychology, 5*(4), 445–455.

Strain, P.S., & Odom, S.L. (1986). Peer social initiations: Effective intervention for social skills development of exceptional children. *Exceptional Children, 52*(6), 543–551.

Strain, P.S., & Timm, M.A. (1974). An experimental analysis of social interaction between a behaviorally disordered preschool child and her classroom peers. *Journal of Abnormal Behavior Analysis, 7,* 583–590.

Tronick, E.Z. (Ed.). (1982). *Social interchange in infancy.* Baltimore: University Park Press.

Turnbull, A.P., & Turnbull, H.R. (1986). *Families, professionals, and exceptionality: A special partnership.* Columbus, OH: Charles E. Merrill.

Wang, M.C., Vaughan, E.D., & Dytman, J.A. (1985). Staff development: A key ingredient of effective mainstreaming. *Teaching Exceptional Children, 17*(2), 112–121.

Winton, P.J., & Turnbull, A.P. (1981). Parent involvement as viewed by parents of preschool handicapped children. *Topics in Early Childhood Special Education, 1,* 11–19.

Winton, P.J., Turnbull, A.P., & Blacher, J. (1984). *Selecting a preschool: A guide for parents of handicapped children.* Austin, TX: PRO-ED.

CHAPTER 9

VOCATIONAL INTEGRATION FOR PERSONS WITH HANDICAPS

Robert Gaylord-Ross

Vocational education attempts to prepare persons with handicaps for gainful employment as adults. The best way to accomplish this goal is to focus on the skills needed in subsequent work environments. These skills may include working on task for considerable periods of time or socializing with co-workers at break-times and while working. When these real work skills have been identified, a teacher may include them, or approximations of them, in the educational curriculum. Unfortunately, too many teachers of students with handicaps have followed developmental or academic models of instruction that focus too heavily on teaching basic academic skills (e.g., the three Rs), and give little attention to preparation for community living and employment. The failure to offer longitudinal career planning, from the primary grades through adulthood, has probably led to the exceedingly high (70%) unemployment rates among disabled adults. (U.S. Bureau of the Census, 1982).

In the past, most disabled persons were judged to be lacking in work potential. At best, they could be placed in a sheltered workshop with other handicapped workers. During recent years there have been substantial changes in vocational education for students with handicaps. Initially, students with the mildest handicaps were mainstreamed into regular vocational education courses, such as automotive mechanics, that served nonhandicapped students. Often, a special

education teacher would serve as a resource specialist to the vocational educator in assisting in the integration of the handicapped student. In addition to classroom mainstreaming, a number of mildly handicapped students were placed in work experiences in real employment settings. For example, working as a food-store checker or a carpenter's assistant helped orient the student toward work and taught him or her many important general work behaviors such as following supervision, being punctual, and staying on task. Although some of these work experiences resulted in permanent jobs, most mildly handicapped persons secured employment through friends and family contacts (Hasazi, Gordon, & Roe, 1985).

Depending on the employment conditions of a region, only about 60% of mildly handicapped adults were obtaining employment (Mithaug, Horiuchi, & Fanning, 1985). Thus, although substantive efforts were made by some school districts in occupational training and work experiences, there was not the follow-along placement and on-the-job support necessary to obtain and maintain employment for persons with mild handicaps. Furthermore, although the Education for All Handicapped Children Act (PL 94-142) strongly suggests that every special education student have at least one vocational objective on his or her individualized education program (IEP), there was no mandate that this be done. Thus, there is much variation from school district to school district in the quality of vocational education services provided. In many districts the extent of vocational education may be to conduct a vocational assessment during adolescence. Many times a teacher may have a student do tasks that appear to be vocational, such as sorting nuts and bolts, without any thought as to how they relate to preparation for employment. In this chapter, as in others in the book, particular activities are described in relation to an overall educational plan.

Vocational education has advanced in recent years to serve students with more severe handicaps. A movement toward community-based training (Brown et al., 1979) developed under the premise that it was necessary to instruct students in actual residential, community, or work settings. Otherwise, little learning would transfer from the classroom to the criterion setting (Horner, McDonnell, & Bellamy, 1986; Horner, Sprague, & Wilcox, 1982). With regard to vocational preparation, it was felt that the student must participate in a number of experiences at real work sites (Gaylord-Ross, Forte, Storey, Gaylord-Ross, & Jameson, 1987). Work atmospheres could not be simulated in classrooms, and the kinds of work skills needed in employment settings could not always be approximated in schools. Thus, a community vocational training movement developed that had severely handicapped students spend increasingly more of their time in real work settings as they advanced through school (Wilcox & Bellamy, 1982; Gaylord-Ross et al., 1987; Sailor et al., 1986). Interestingly, the series of work experiences serves as a useful vocational assessment of the types of jobs for which the student is well suited and the types of jobs the student prefers. Then, when the student is about to leave school, it should be possible to pool this assessment information and make a judicious placement into adult employment.

The newest development in vocational education has occurred in the transition phase of leaving school. In 1984, Congress passed PL 98-199 to promote the development of transitional services for disabled youth. The transition phase roughly spans the years just preceding and just following the finishing of school (16–24). The U.S. Department of Education model of transition (Will, 1984) focuses on providing vocational training, placement, and follow-along services in order to provide nonsheltered work for handicapped persons. Besides providing direct educational services (e.g., on-the-job teaching of job skills), transitional services entail the linkage of school and adult services to provide coordinated transition planning and service delivery. For example, a secondary school work-experience program could coordinate its training with a community college, which may continue vocational training or place the student in a real job.

Another relatively new program model called "supported work" is serving adults with serious vocational handicaps. Supported work (Rusch, 1986; Wehman, 1981) is a model that finds jobs for the individual; provides intensive, on-the-job instruction during the initial period of employment; and provides ongoing support in maintaining or re-placing the handicapped employee. Wehman (1981) has demonstrated a 67% retention rate for individuals served by their supported employment program. Another survey conducted in Virginia (Wehman et al., 1985) showed only a 12% rate of employment among persons with moderate and severe handicaps who have not received employment services.

COMPONENTS IN A MODEL OF VOCATIONAL EDUCATION

A comprehensive vocational education model has a number of components, including the following:

1. The vocational education program should have a *philosophy* that advocates life-span career education. The philosophy should also articulate the relationship of vocational training with instruction in independent living and

community living skills (Brolin, 1982; Halpern, 1985).

2. *Career awareness* (Brolin, 1978, 1982) activities should begin in the primary grades and continue throughout the secondary years. Career awareness entails informing the student about the many career options available. Through films, lectures, books, guest speakers, and other media the student learns about different occupations and the skills needed to fulfill them. Career awareness may also entail counseling the individual and family about career opportunities and commitments.

3. *Career exploration* (Brolin, 1978, 1982) begins in the middle school and continues through high school. Career exploration activities permit the student to get brief exposures to the experience of work. Career exploration activities may include field trips to work sites and job shadowing. In job shadowing a student goes to a work site for one day, follows an individual worker, and participates in some of the job activities. This lets the student get a cursory feel of a particular occupation while working in a factory, in an office, or outdoors. A more intensive career exploration activity is to have the student engage in brief work experiences at the school site. For example, the student could work along with the janitor for 30 minutes, 2 days a week.

4. *Vocational assessment* should be conducted at particular times and on an ongoing basis (cf. Irvin, 1988). Typically, a student receives a comprehensive vocational assessment during the early secondary years (age 14–16). Assessment findings may then be used to plan individualized education programs. Often standardized vocational assessment instruments are pitched too high for students with severe handicaps, and are therefore not appropriate. More professionals are turning to formative or ongoing assessments that repeatedly (i.e., weekly or daily) measure pupil performance in vocational settings.

5. *Occupational training* teaches the secondary student the skills for a particular job, such as a computer keypuncher or a welder. Occupational training has traditionally meant mainstreaming handicapped students into regular vocational education classes. With advances in instructional technology and the emphasis on transition, one might see more occupational training for specific jobs with more severely handicapped students.

6. *Community vocational training* entails placing the student in a series of work experiences at real job sites. The work experiences may be closely supervised by an on-site instructor or the student may work solely under coworker supervision at the job site. Work experiences may result in permanent jobs but their primary purpose is to teach general work behaviors.

7. *Transition programs* attempt to place students leaving school in permanent employment. The transition program may provide direct services such as:
   a. Teaching mildly handicapped students to identify, interview for, and procure employment through Job Club (Azrin & Besalel, 1980; Jones & Azrin, 1975).
   b. Developing jobs for the less capable student and matching individual abilities with job requirements.
   c. Providing initial, on-the-job training and follow-along services through a supported work model.
   d. Offering career counseling and support to the individual and the family.

The notion of career ladders should be introduced so the first job out of school is viewed as a starting point in a progression of upward career mobility. Besides providing direct services, transition programs must also develop interagency linkages with adult service providers. This could involve developing a follow-up monitoring system for school leavers, referring graduates to appropriate adult services, and coordinating community living and employment services.

VOCATIONAL INTEGRATION ACTIVITIES

Career Awareness through Role Modeling

Rationale

Few handicapped adults (30%) are currently employed (U.S. Bureau of Census, 1982). As a result of this, people typically have expectations that children with handicaps will not be employed when they grow up. Most important, the handicapped child may assume that he or she will not work. This expectation is enhanced when the child views adults with similar handicaps who are not working. Sometimes the same family may have two or more generations of persons with no one who has been substantially employed. Psychologists (e.g., Bandura, 1986) have documented the powerful effects of role modeling on human behavior. One learns most of one's behavior patterns from imitating others. Such social imitation is not random, though. One tends to imitate persons with characteristics similar to one's own. For the child with disabilities who only views unemployed adults with similar disabilities, it is likely that he or she will set expectations for similar career failure. It is possible for lectures and other presentations by educators to motivate children with disabilities. Yet, a much more powerful motivation is for them to see or experience a successful, working adult with a similar disability. Such direct experiences may truly motivate the student to strive for career goals.

Career awareness activities (Brolin, 1978, 1982) attempt to give the student information and motivation for a variety of occupations. Career awareness begins in the primary school and continues throughout the secondary years. A main career awareness activity is to have the student experience an individual with a similar disability. The role-model experience may occur through a personal appearance, viewing a film or videocassette, reading a book, or hearing a lecture from a teacher.

Participants and Setting

Vasily is a communication handicapped student at an inner-city elementary school. He is 10 years old, and he is in a fourth-grade class for about 70% of the day. For the other 30%, he attends a resource specialist class for students with communication and learning handicaps. The teacher, Mr. Fontenot, designed a career education program for the students. A career awareness program was planned so that the students would read about and directly experience competent adults with handicaps. Mr. Fontenot hoped that they would learn about a wide range of possible occupations and be motivated to work toward career success.

Intervention

The career awareness program consists of a lecture series conducted by disabled adults, and the reading and discussing of examples of such successful individuals. The lecture series is described here.

Mr. Fontenot identified four individuals from the community who would speak to the resource class of 32 students (who move in and out of the class throughout the day). Research has shown that social imitation is maximized when the role model has the identical characteristics of the observers (Bandura, 1977). Therefore, Mr. Fontenot identified individuals who are black or Hispanic, male, and have had learning disabilities or communication handicaps. Out of his 32 students, 28 fell into this category. This does not mean that other types of role models would not be useful. A career awareness program should have a majority of role models, though, who match the characteristics of the majority of the observers. Psychological research has also shown that role models have a more powerful effect when they are perceived to be reinforced (Bandura, 1986). Thus, individuals who are highly successful in their careers should be selected. Mr. Fontenot contacted and received a positive response from the following individuals:

1. Anthony Jones, 31, is a chemical technician in a research laboratory. Mr. Jones is dyslexic and black.
2. Marcos Guitierrez, 28, is a well-known radio announcer on a local radio station. Mr. Guitierrez was in a bilingual special education program and was a low achiever in school.
3. Cicily Davis, 42, and black, is a practicing nurse in the city hospital. Mrs. Davis was diagnosed as learning disabled and placed in a special education class for most of her school career.
4. Lester Hayes is a defensive back for the city's professional football team. Mr. Hayes was a severe stutterer whose speech has greatly improved through speech therapy.

Each speaker gave his or her presentation in a different quarter of the year, to two different groups of students. Thus, they were at the school for about 2 hours. The speaker was told to bring any materials (e.g., a lab coat) that would illustrate different aspects of his or her occupation. Some speakers invited Mr. Fontenot to bring a group of students on a field trip to their places of business.

Mr. Fontenot asked the speakers to talk for about 45 minutes each, and to address the following points:

1. Give a description of their occupation and some of the day-to-day activities they conduct.
2. Describe their experiences in progressing through school. Note problems they faced related to their disability.
3. Describe their major career and personal problems and how they overcame them.
4. Make suggestions for what the students might do to perform well in school, prepare themselves for a vocation, and gain life satisfaction.

For example, Mrs. Davis described some of her early experiences in growing up black and poor. She described the difficulties she faced in reading and math, and told of being placed in a special education class. Mrs. Davis shared the stigma she felt of being in a separate class all of the time. She told of an aunt who had been a nurse's aide in a hospital, and who had spoken fondly of working in a hospital and serving patients. By middle school, Cicily Davis thought seriously about entering the nursing profession. She was made aware by her counselors that she would have to take considerable coursework in order to become a licensed practical nurse. She worked hard to improve her academic performance, and by high school she began to be mainstreamed into regular classes. She went on to describe how she graduated, entered nursing school, and ultimately became a nurse.

Mrs. Davis then described her two major roadblocks to success. She told how she was hurt by the special education label. Many persons thought she was "dumb" and would never amount to anything. At times, Cicily Davis started believing this about herself. Ultimately, she developed a strong self-belief in her abilities and potential. She told how she was encouraged by three particular teachers and friends. Such encouragement made her feel that she was not alone.

Cicily Davis then went on to give specific recommendations to the students for career success. She told them to work hard in school, to obey their parents, and to read as much as possible. She told the students to set personal goals and to try to identify a likely occupation. Most important, she told the students that there would be times when they would get depressed—everything would appear to be going wrong. Mrs. Davis said this is just the time to try harder and not give up. She quoted Amos of Famous Amos's Cookies who said: "Every time someone said 'no,' he couldn't do it, it meant there was a yes somewhere else."

During her talk students were encouraged to raise questions or make comments. For example, in answering a question, Mrs. Davis told a student how to set up a leisure reading program. Before leaving she told the student to call or visit her any time to have a chat or discuss problems.

Summary and Conclusion

Career awareness, role-modeling activities may prove invaluable in motivating students. Successful role models who have similar ethnic and disability status should be particularly helpful. Live presentations are likely to be the most effective, but they should be complemented with readings, films, and discussions of other role models.

Because of their inspirational nature, role-modeling experiences are somewhat difficult to evaluate. It might be possible to develop a pretest-posttest evaluation of career awareness. Information could be gathered through teacher interview of the student or paper-and-pencil measurement. The instrument could have the students list the occupations in which they are interested, provide information about the jobs, and what kind of training is needed to enter those fields.

Establishing Community Training Sites

Rationale

Vocational experience in real work sites is one of the best ways to prepare an individual for adult employment. General work behaviors can be most efficiently taught in real work settings, as it is difficult to simulate most aspects of the work milieu in the classroom. For example, in the work setting the person must interact with nonhandicapped adults who are peers—not teachers or authority figures. Therefore, there has been a large-scale movement to provide individuals with a series of community vocational training experiences (Gaylord-Ross et al., 1987; Sailor et al., 1986; Wilcox & Bellamy, 1982). Initially, work experiences were established for mildly handicapped students. The student primarily learned the job from the co-workers and supervisors at the site, with little instruction from an educator. More recently, students with more serious vocational handicaps are being served. These students initially or permanently require the presence of an educational instructor.

Although there is a growing trend to develop community vocational training, it takes a considerable amount of knowledge and energy to establish such a program. Many teachers are accustomed to teaching in the classroom and are intimidated by having to go off the school campus. In a sense, the role of the teacher is being redefined as one who contacts employers, instructs in nonschool settings, and works alongside employees. Fortunately, there are guidelines to follow in setting up work experience programs for secondary students.

Program Establishment

A number of steps must be taken in setting up one or more community vocational training sites. The first step is to design the characteristics of your program. It is often good to start small, and this might mean establishing one work site to serve two or three students. Your design should include how the program will be staffed and what kind of other resources will be needed. Your program may be included within existing work experience programs for handicapped or nonhandicapped students. Such an addendum would certainly make your job easier. This chapter describes the case where you are starting a program from scratch (cf. Wershing, Gaylord-Ross, & Gaylord-Ross, 1986).

When you have sketched out a design of your program, you should write it out in a two- or three-page proposal. The proposal should describe the start-up and later phases of the program, and explain the program's ultimate goals. References should be cited of other school districts that have established similar community vocational programs (e.g., Wilcox & Bellamy, 1982).

When the proposal is completed it should be submitted to your administrative superior. You *must* get administrative support for off-campus activities. Sometimes, the administrator may be quite enthusiastic about such a program, and establish a district-wide policy to develop community vocational training. In this case, the additional resources and policy support provided will be quite helpful.

Administrators often have a number of questions about the feasibility of such programs. Showing them alternatives or having them visit other programs may often be helpful. One issue that may come up is the health and accident insurance of students when they are off school grounds. If the students are not employed by a company, the school district insurance policy would cover them just as if they were on a field trip or some other off-campus, school-related activity. If your program results in the employment of a student, then the employer's insurance policy would cover the individual just as it would any other employee.

Another issue that may arise is who will supervise students at the work site. The design of the program should attempt to gradually fade out the degree of supervision on the part of an educator and turn supervision over to a co-worker(s). Therefore, an instructor is likely to work in close proximity to 2 to 5 students. Over a semester, the students should be spread out over the workplace, with the educator spending less and less time in direct contact.

Some school administrators require a credentialed teacher to continuously supervise the student at the work site. This narrow interpretation of supervision requirements will usually curtail the implementation of your program. In fact, most state education codes do not require constant supervision by a credentialed teacher. They do require responsible supervision in an IEP that was designed by a credentialed teacher. Thus, many mildly handicapped students, like their nonhandicapped peers, participate in work-experience programs in which no educator supervises them at the site. Likewise, some students with severe handicaps may not require any educator supervision at the work site. For other students, however, an instructor may be required all or part of the time. The instructor does not necessarily have to be a credentialed teacher. Most likely, a paraprofessional may supervise the student(s) if the teacher does not. In some cases, school districts have used nonhandicapped peer tutors or community volunteers (e.g., parents) to supervise and instruct handicapped students at the workplace.

After administrative approval has been obtained, the teacher must contact employers in order to obtain the first training site. A number of methods may be used to make employer contacts. It would be useful at first to contact existing work-experience or job-development programs in the community. They may be able to provide useful leads to employers. The next, and most likely, step is to walk up to companies, knock on the door, and introduce yourself. If you cannot get access to the employer or the personnel director, try to set up an interview for a later time. You may also call an employer in advance and ask to set up a time to meet.

Work sites should be contacted with some idea of the types of vocational skills that can be learned there. Most places offer the chance to do maintenance and janitorial activities. Restaurants offer the development of food service skills. Offices enable training for clerical skills. You must know your students' vocational abilities and project to future employment possibilities. An adult placement specialist must match up an individual's abilities with the requirements of an appropriate job. Similarly, a teacher must select work-training sites that are going to offer the learning of important general work behaviors and give the individual a try at an occupation that may ultimately lead to permanent employment.

When meeting an employer, you should give an overall description of your special education program and the characteristics of the handicapped students being served. Then, you should describe the design of the community vocational training program. You should state the number of students to be served, how they will be supervised, the hours of their attendance, and what kind of resources the employer needs to provide. The employer might take you on a tour of the facility and you might continue to discuss insurance liability, and whether the students are to be paid and/or ultimately hired. Most community classroom experiences include students who work at a slow rate. It is likely that they will be unpaid, or that an educational stipend will cover their wage. Most community classrooms run for a semester or a year and serve as a training experience where the student's abilities and interests may be assessed. In some cases, the community classroom may result in permanent employment. The training and employment expectations of your program must be clearly explained to the employer. During your tour you might discuss particular work stations and tasks in which the students might engage. Employers are likely to be most concerned with how the program is going to: infringe on space, result in slowed production, or present safety hazards to the students or others. These concerns should be briefly addressed. It is likely that the employer will want to think about participating in the program before giving you a definite decision. You should agree on when you will contact one another in the future.

When an employer has committed to being a training site, and the site is deemed appropriate, it is time to start organizing for implementation. The first thing that is necessary is to visit the work site. During the visitation you should observe and interview workers with the objective of identifying a set of jobs or tasks for the students. When possible, it is useful for a handicapped student to pair up and work alongside a co-worker. This pairing system is likely to evolve once you have been on the site for awhile. After identifying tasks that can be engaged, the teacher should learn how to do them before bringing students to the site. After practicing the tasks the teacher can write detailed task analyses and instructional programs (cf. Gaylord-Ross and Holvoet, 1985) that may be implemented with the students.

Next, arrangements must be made for transporting students to the work site. In some cases, the site may be within walking distance. In most cases, however, public transportation will have to be taken. This can provide a good opportunity to train your students in the use of public transportation—the absence of this skill could limit the future employment opportunities of your students with handicaps. If public transportation is not feasible, it may be necessary to use a school bus to transport students to the work site. An instructor may need to use her or his own car to transport students, although liability and insurance policies should be carefully checked out before proceeding.

When a small group of students is taken out of the classroom with a staff member, a plan must be made for the total staffing of the class. For example, a class may have 12 students, one teacher, and two aides. This results in a 4:1 student-staff ratio. If a paraprofessional took three students off-campus, then two staff members must instruct the remaining nine students. This results in a slightly larger than 4:1 ratio. The teacher may supplement her or his staff resources through peer tutoring and volunteer programs, as well as by mainstreaming students into other educational or community experiences. Also, over time students should require less supervision at the work site. Then, one staff person might rotate to supervise four or more students at a work site.

The next and major step is to bring the students to the site for instruction. The author of this chapter recommends that there be at least three training sessions per week, of at least 2 hours in duration. Yet, some community vocational training is better than none. Therefore, if only one session per week can be managed, then that should be done. Over time, you should plan to expand the program to develop more sites and serve more students.

At first, things will undoubtedly go wrong with transportation, scheduling, task training, and so forth. Yet, with experience, the program will begin to run smoothly. You will also discover that many persons will come forth to offer support. Employers and co-workers have been found to be quite generous in offering materials, apparel, money, and social support in facilitating community vocational training. The true rewards of such programs really come a couple of years down the road when the participants successfully transition to permanent adult employment.

Increasing Production Rate

Rationale

One of the major problems for handicapped persons in retaining their jobs is that they work too slowly (Rusch & Schutz, 1981; Rusch, Schutz, & Agran, 1982). In school, teachers have tended to focus on the learning of new skills; little attention is given to improving the rate of performance of already-learned skills. Since many jobs that handicapped adults obtain are at entry level, rapid and repeated performance is usually required (e.g., assembling parts in a factory line). It is important that teachers work on production-rate objectives throughout the school years. Fortunately, techniques exist that improve production rate. The example provided next occurred in a work setting.

Setting and Participants

A group of four severely handicapped students are being trained in a community classroom model at a nursing home. The students function at the moderate and severe level of mental retardation. Three of the students are ambulatory but one student, Eli, can only get around in a wheelchair. The group is at the nursing home for 3 hours in the morning, 3 days per week. The students perform different tasks such as sweeping floors, doing laundry, and socializing with the clients. Eli's main task is folding towels in the laundry room.

The community classroom instructor, Ms. Forte, collected social validity data on two of the regular workers and found that they folded approximately 100 towels in a 30-minute period. After Eli was taught to fold towels in an accurate manner, he was folding them at the rate of 30 per half-hour period. While Ms. Forte did not feel that Eli had to perform as rapidly as a regular worker, she felt there was much room for improvement in his production rate.

To better analyze Eli's production problem, Ms. Forte observed him for a full 30-minute period on 2 different days. She noticed that Eli performed at two different rates. At times, for 5–10-minute periods, Eli would fold towels at a fairly rapid rate (two per minute). Then he would "drift off" for 1–3-minute periods where he would stare into space and fold at the rate of one third towel per minute.

To increase Eli's rate, Ms. Forte set up a simple "verbal prompting" program. That is, whenever he stared into space and slowed or stopped folding, she would verbally prompt him to "keep folding" or "continue working." Upon receiving one verbal prompt, Eli usually got back to his higher rate for a period of at least 1 minute. If he slacked

off again, the instructor would verbally prompt him to work faster. Figure 1 shows the graph of Eli's rate in baseline (after acquisition training) and during the verbal prompt procedure. It can be seen that the average rate improved from one third to two towels per minute across the two phases.

Although the program proved to be successful, it still was limited because it required the instructor to work one to one with Eli for the full 30-minute period. Ms. Forte then implemented a "co-worker prompting" program. Ms. Forte noticed that there was usually at least one co-worker in the laundry room when Eli was folding towels. Ms. Forte explained to two of the employees about Eli's disability and vocational development. She described his production rate problem and the success of the verbal prompting procedure. She stressed the importance of Eli's working independently from a teacher, and asked the co-workers to become involved in Eli's vocational education. The two employees agreed to verbally prompt Eli whenever he "spaced out" and stopped working. Ms. Forte then stayed out of the laundry room for a 30-minute period. She returned at the end of the period to count the number of towels Eli had folded and to calculate his rate per minute by dividing the number of towels folded by 30.

Figure 1 shows that the co-worker prompt program was successful since Eli's rate averaged almost two towels per minute. There was a slight drop in rate from that of the teacher prompting procedure, because the co-workers could not always be vigilant enough to prompt Eli as soon as he drifted off. (Obviously, the co-workers had their own work to perform.)

The intervention package should be deemed successful because it maintained the treatment gains of the artificial, teacher prompt program. Also, it motivated the student to perform independently with a natural type of assistance.

The notion of co-worker prompting could be extended to school settings, where a handicapped or nonhandicapped person could prompt pupil performance. Peer prompting, whether done by a co-worker or student, has the dual advantage of im-

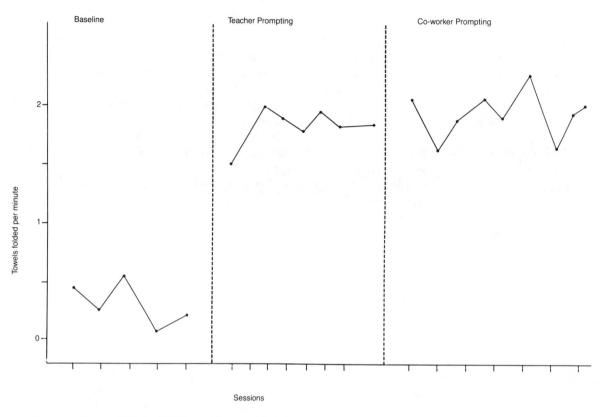

Figure 1.   Graph of Eli's towel-folding performance. Baseline = .3 per minute, teacher prompting = 2.0 per minute, co-worker prompting = 1.8 per minute.

proving production rate and facilitating social interaction.

Social Skill Development

Rationale

One of the main benefits of integration is that it enables handicapped persons to learn normal social behaviors through being in proximity to and imitating nonhandicapped persons. Social interactions may occur while working or at breaktime. For a person to be successful and accepted at work, he must emit a minimum number of socially appropriate behaviors. With regard to vocational preparation, it is important for handicapped youth to be exposed to the types of social interactions that occur in workplaces. The kinds of social inter-

actions that take place in work settings cannot be well simulated in school settings. Therefore, community vocational training becomes critical in exposing handicapped persons to adult supervisors and co-workers.

Although some social behaviors may be learned by observation and imitation, often handicapped persons must be explicitly taught a particular social skill for it to be acquired (Fredericks, Moore, & Baldwin, 1978). Social skill training may be taught in actual situations where the particular skill must be performed (e.g., the playground). More commonly, however, a set of social behaviors is rehearsed through role playing in a similar situation, and then it is noted if the behaviors generalize to the actual social situation. For example, Breen, Haring, Pitts-Conway, and Gaylord-

Ross (1985) had three autistic youth role play conversation at breaktime with their nonhandicapped high school peers. As the autistic students were participating in community vocational training at a nursing home, the training was done in an empty cafeteria there. After the students had learned the conversational skills in the simulated setting, it was noted that the social behaviors generalized to the same cafeteria setting during an actual breaktime in that the autistic students conversed with their nonhandicapped co-workers.

Setting and Participants

Melanie, a 12-year-old moderately mentally retarded student with Down syndrome, participated in a brief work experience at her middle school. For 5 months, 4 days per week, she cleaned and loaded empty trays in a cafeteria line at lunch. Although she performed the job fairly well, it was noticed that she engaged in little conversation with her nonhandicapped peer co-workers. When she did talk, she tended to repeat the same conversation about Sesame Street characters (Haring, Roger, Lee, Breen, & Gaylord-Ross, 1986).

Intervention

Melanie's teacher, Mrs. Roger, observed her behavior and decided to set up a social skills training intervention. Mrs. Roger first conducted an ecological inventory of the types of topics about which the nonhandicapped students conversed both around school and while working on the cafeteria line. The ecological inventory was completed by listening to and interviewing the nonhandicapped students. Next, simulated social skills training was held in the classroom between Melanie and a nonhandicapped peer. The teacher told Melanie and the student to pretend they were working in the cafeteria line. Then, Mrs. Roger prompted Melanie to begin a conversation with the peer on one of the ecologically valid topics (e.g., a TV show). The peer then responded to Melanie's invitation and a conversation ensued.

Table 1 lists the social interaction sequence of different conversations. Social interactions may

Table 1. Training scripts for nonhandicapped peer and autistic student

Autistic student (AS)	Nonhandicapped peer (NP)
Pacman	
1. "Hi."	
	2. "Hi, _____, how are you doing?"
3. "Fine."	
4. "Want to play Pacman?"	
	5. "Sure (yeah, great)" or "No, thanks."
6. Turns on game.	
7. Hands game to NP.	
	8. Plays game until it is over.
	9. Hands game to AS.
10. Reads score.	
11. Turns game off and then on and plays.	
	12. Watches while AS plays; encourages him or her when AS plays well.
13. Reads his or her own score at the end of the game.	
14. Offers game to NP.	
	15. Plays game or says "No thanks, got to go, bye."
16. Says "bye."	
Walkman	
1. "Hi."	
	2. "Hi, how are you?"
3. "Fine."	
4. "Want to listen?"	
	5. "Sure" or "No, thanks."

(continued)

Table 1.   *(continued)*

6. Turns on
    Walkman.
7. Sets volume to 6.
8. Hands head-
    phones to NP.

        9. Puts on head-
            phones.

10. Turns to rock 'n'
    roll station.

       11. Listens or tells
           students to
           change station
           and then listens.

12. "Bye."

Gum

1. "Hi."

       2. "Hi."

3. "What are you
    doing?"

       4. "Just sitting
           around, (not
           much, waiting for
           someone)."

5. "Want some
    gum?"

       6. "Sure (yeah)."

7. Hands stick to
    NP.

       8. Takes stick of
           gum and says
           "thanks."

9. "Sure."
10. Chews gum.

       11. Talks to student.
           Asks him "What
           did you do yes-
           terday? What are
           you doing after
           school?"

12. Responds to
    questions from
    NP.

       13. Hangs out for 1–
           3 minutes.
       14. "Bye."

15. "Bye."

be analyzed into three phases: initiation, elaboration, and termination. Initiation involves one person greeting the other through a verbalization or gesture. The second part of the initiation is when the other person responds to the greeting. Next, one person may elaborate the interaction by beginning to talk about some topic. Then a series of turn taking occurs until the conversation is complete. Finally, each person terminates the interaction through a verbal or nonverbal gesture.

With respect to Melanie, after the first trial of conversation was complete, Mrs. Roger gave feedback about the good or bad aspects of the interaction. After a pause of about a minute, Mrs. Roger asked the two students to begin another trial of social interaction simulation of the cafeteria line. After the students interacted for 30–180 seconds, Mrs. Roger gave them feedback. She told them whether the conversation was on a topic valued by middle school students, and whether the topic was different from one emitted in previous trials.

Praise is given for appropriate and different topics. In the case of an inappropriate topic, students are told it was wrong and given an example of an appropriate topic not practiced in previous trials. When the topic had been rehearsed in previous trials, the teacher tells them so, then gives an example of an appropriate topic that is novel for that session. Thus, the intervention attempts to get the students to vary the themes of their conversations and to stick to normative topics. Daily sessions last no more than 10 minutes as the two students rehearse about six trials. Learning criterion is two consecutive sessions of perfect performance (six out of six trials). A correct trial consists of an appropriate and new topic.

Mrs. Roger also made observations of Melanie during her actual work activity in the cafeteria line. After Melanie reached criterion during simulation, it was noticed that she gradually began to initiate and vary appropriate topics while working. Thus, there was successful generalization from simulated rehearsal to natural performance.

Summary

The case of Melanie presents one example of social skills training. It is possible to develop your own social skills programs by following a sequence of operations. First, identify a social deficit through observation, interview, or data collection. Second, identify the normative social behaviors for that setting. Third, implement a social skills training program. The program could prompt and reinforce the targeted behavior in the criterion setting (e.g., breaktime at a workplace), or it might involve simulated rehearsal with expected generalization to the natural setting (e.g., the case of Melanie). Finally, record whether the simulated social skills training generalizes to the natural setting.

Job Procurement

Rationale

An important yet imposing skill is the ability to find a job. Many handicapped persons lack the cognitive or verbal skills to seek out and secure a job. In these cases, a supported employment program may have to do a job search and match the individual's abilities to an available job. Many more capable persons with handicaps may be quite able to learn the skills necessary to identify jobs and interview for them. Azrin and Besalel (1980) developed a Job Club procedure that teaches handicapped and disadvantaged individuals these skills. The Job Club approach does not view the learning of job procurement as a one-time affair. Rather, after finding a job, the person may use job-procurement skills at some future time in order to find another job after being terminated, or to improve one's position. Job Club is a behaviorally oriented training procedure. It teaches the person to repeatedly track down leads for jobs from different sources. The person continues to seek leads in a nonstop fashion until one or more job interviews is lined up. Job Club also trains the person through social simulation to interview effectively for a job. Research data have shown Job Club to be a successful training procedure (Jones & Azrin, 1975). It is now widely used as a vocational preparation and transition technique.

Setting and Participants

Milt is a mildly handicapped youth who lives in a poor neighborhood in a large city. He is a senior at a large high school, and is participating in a transition program. During the last semester of the senior year, the transition program offers a Job Club program. The class meets daily for one period a day, for a 1-month period; the class of 10 students is taught by a vocational special education instructor.

Intervention

The teacher, Mrs. Griner, explained the purpose of the program to the students on their first day: It would teach students how to obtain and interview for jobs. She stated that they would practice these skills and that it was hoped that all of the students would find a job by the end of the course. (Some students may only want summer jobs; others may want full-time, permanent positions that will define their career; still others will go on to postsecondary education and wish to have part-time jobs while attending school.)

Mrs. Griner also explained the concept of career ladder. That is, the job the student obtains may be a permanent position for life, with promotions within that firm. More likely, the first postschool job would set the stage for better paying, higher status, and more rewarding positions. The importance of establishing a résumé without long gaps of unemployment was stressed. Also, the students were told that fine on-the-job performance would lead to good letters of recommendation from supervisors, which should set the stage for career ladder mobility.

Throughout the class, students were individually counseled. Mrs. Griner focused on what kinds of jobs the students would like, what kinds of jobs they were capable of performing, and the types of jobs available. She attempted to coordinate these variables so that the best type of placement was made.

Job-finding and interviewing skills were worked on simultaneously, at different times of the week or class. Students were told that there are different ways to find out about jobs. One can read the newspaper ads or go to employment agency offices such as the Department of Rehabilitation. Most jobs, it was explained, are obtained through family or friends. This job-finding strategy was described as sitting by the phone and making as many calls as possible for possible leads. The student should call potentially helpful family members and friends, and should read the want ads and call up employers for positions that seem to be of interest. Leads from agencies or other periodicals may also be called.

When calling employers, the students were told to identify themselves and state their interest in a particular position. The students were told to expect to be transferred and have to repeat the message. The students were told to be clear, firm, and brief. If there is a possibility for a job, the student should request that an interview be scheduled. Table 2 summarizes the content of the phone con-

Table 2. Calling employer to set up job interview: role play for Job Club

Student	Employer-Receptionist
1. Dials number.	
	2. "Hello, Macy's." (receptionist)
3. "Hello, I would like to speak to someone in Personnel."	
	4. "OK, I'll transfer you."
	5. "Hello, Personnel." (personnel receptionist)
6. "Hello, I would like to speak to someone about a job."	

(continued)

Table 2. *(continued)*

Student	Employer-Receptionist
	7. "OK, you can speak to Mr. Kelly."
	8. "Hello." (Mr. Kelly)
9. "Hello, I'm Milt Wright."	
	10. "Hi."
11. "I was calling to see if you have any jobs open now."	
	12. "As a matter of fact we have two positions in stock inventory."
13. "Oh, that's great. May I apply for them?"	
	14. "I suspect so. Do you have any previous work experience?"
15. "Yes, I've had two jobs in the past doing clerical and maintenance work."	
	16. "Good, well why don't you come down to Macy's tomorrow to fill out an application."
17. "Terrific, should I ask for you?"	
	18. "Yes, but first see Mr. Clark in personnel."
19. "Fine, I'll be there at about 10 in the morning."	
	20. "Very good, I will see you then."
21. "Fine, it's been nice talking to you."	
	22. "You too, I'll see you then."
23. "Good-bye."	
	24. "Good-bye."

tact. Before making actual calls, Mrs. Griner had students role play the phone exchange. One student played him or herself and the other student (or teacher) played the employer. Students were praised by the teacher for good behaviors. Students were also given corrective feedback for errors. A common error is to talk too long on the phone about themselves or the job. The students were told that the main objective of the phone contact is to briefly find out if a job is available and to set up an interview when there is a job that seems appropriate. The student callers were also told to have a notepad, pen, and calender to write down any important details such as the time and place of the appointment, or further leads.

Once Milt satisfactorily mastered the phone-call behaviors in the role plays, Mrs. Griner set him up to make actual calls. In the original Job Club approach, Azrin and Besalel (1982) had individuals keep calling all day, or on a succession of days, until enough contacts were made. In a modified Job Club, Mrs. Griner had Milt make calls throughout the 45-minute class period and for 2-hour homework sessions after school. Within a week, Milt had succeeded in setting up three job interviews.

The second aspect of job-procurement training prepares the student for conducting job interviews. This training may begin soon after job-finding training. The training again relies on simulated role plays. In the role plays the student plays him or herself. Another student (or the teacher) plays the employer. A general format is set where both players are told of the type of job and company in which the interview takes place. The student is given the preinstructions that he or she should make a friendly greeting to the interviewer as he or she states his or her name. The student should then succinctly state in what job he or she is interested. It is likely that the interviewer will lead most of the discussion. The student must therefore be prepared to answer questions related to:

1. General background information about past schooling and work experiences

2. Characteristics of the job in question and one's own qualifcations for the job

3. Discussions of other topics such as hobbies, events in the news, or common friends or acquaintances

If the interviewer does not provide the information, the student must be prepared to ask about: benefits, wages, and job expectations. Preinstructions tell the student to present a professional image and show that he or she is really motivated to get the job.

When the above pre-instructions were completed, Mrs. Griner had Milt begin a role play with another student. Two role plays were conducted each day, three times per week, until Milt reached the behavioral criteria for interviewing. Mrs. Griner developed a recording sheet that listed the following interviewing behaviors:

1. Greetings and introductions

2. Providing background information

3. Presenting qualifications for the job

4. Obtaining information about the job's characteristics (e.g., benefits)

5. Conducting "small talk" about peripheral matters

6. Projecting a professional image and motivation to obtain the job

Mrs. Griner rated each of these items from one to five after the role play was over. At this time she gave corrective feedback on Milt's performance. She pointed out what he did well and where there was need for improvement. For example, she told Milt that he answered questions about his job qualifications very well. She pointed out that he did not show enough enthusiasm for wanting to get the job. Mrs. Griner then modeled a few statements for indicating a desire for the job. She pointed out that tone of voice and facial expression are key to demonstrating enthusiasm.

Feedback may be shared in other ways, too. The role play may be videotaped and played back with the instructor pointing out strengths and weaknesses. Besides the teacher rating student performance, the student may rate him or herself.

The teacher and self-ratings may then lead to a useful discussion of interview behavior.

Finally, the instructor must set a criterion for when the training is successful. Mrs. Griner's criterion for Milt was two consecutive trials of perfect (all fives on the six items) performance.

When the training is completed the students are ready to go out on their interviews. They are given additional information about being well groomed and being on time for the interview. Practice and assistance might also be given for filling out application forms. When the student has completed the interview, the teacher should discuss how it went. If the student did not get the job, it may be possible for the teacher to call the employer and find out how the student interviewed, and if there were any factors that could be rectified to permit the hiring of the student.

Conclusion

Obtaining job-procurement skills is very important. They train the person to independently obtain jobs. An assumption of job-procurement training is that it will not only help the person get a job at the time of training, but that the procurement skills will maintain over time. Such maintenance will enable the person to obtain other and better jobs at future points in his or her career.

SUMMARY

Five activities for promoting vocational integration have been described. They provide a wide sample of activities that will prepare handicapped students for nonsheltered employment. Of course, there are many other activities that may be conducted to reach this goal. Some of these include doing job shadowing and running a job fair. Although this chapter has stressed training students in real work sites, much valuable vocational education may take place at the school. Vocational ed-

ucation classes to learn specific occupations can be quite effective if the classes are keyed to jobs that actually exist in the marketplace. Simulated training of work situations in school can be valuable if it complements community training (Horner, McDonnell, & Bellamy, 1986). The contemporary educator must develop a well-rounded vocational curriculum that teaches specific occupational skills and general work behaviors, and that consequently results in the successful employment of persons with handicaps.

STUDY QUESTIONS

1. Why is community-based vocational training so important to students with disabilities? Describe some examples of job tasks that could be performed in real work sites.
2. What do career awareness activities attempt to accomplish? Illustrate how a role model with a disability could be used in a career awareness activity.
3. How would you design a program to increase the vocational production of a person with disabilities? What kinds of cues and reinforcers would you use? What criteria would you apply to evaluate whether the instructional program was successful?
4. Describe the main components of a social skills training program (e.g., role playing). Provide an example of a script of a social exchange that could be practiced by a disabled and a nondisabled person.
5. What is the strategy of Job Club to enable persons to get jobs? What specific contact behaviors are taught to set up job interviews? What kinds of social behaviors need to be displayed during a job interview?
6. Define the terms transition and supported employment. What information can be offered to employers to make them interested in hiring persons with disabilities?

REFERENCES

Azrin, N.H., & Besalel, V.A. (1980). *Job Club counselor's manual: A behavioral approach to vocational counseling.* Baltimore: University Park Press.

Bandura, A. (1977). *Social learning theory.* Englewood Cliffs, N.J.: Prentice-Hall.

Bandura, A. (1986). *Social foundations of thought and action: A social cognitive approach.* Englewood Cliffs, N.J.: Prentice Hall.

Breen, C., Haring, T.G., Pitts-Conway, V., & Gaylord-Ross, R. (1985). The training and generalization of social interaction during breaktime at two job sites in the natural environment. *Journal of the Association for Persons with Severe Handicaps, 10,* 41–50.

Brolin, D. (1982). *Vocational preparation of persons with handicaps.* Columbus, OH: Bell & Howell.

Brolin, D. (1978). *Life centered career education: A competency based approach.* Reston, VA: Council for Exceptional Children.

Brown, L., Branston, M., Hamre-Nietupski, S., Pumpian, I., Certo, N., & Gruenwald, L. (1979). A strategy for developing chronological age-appropriate and functional curricular content for severely handicapped adolescents and young adults. *Journal of Special Education, 13,* 81–90.

Fredericks, H.D.B., Baldwin, V., Grove, D., Moore, W., Riggs, C., & Lyons, B. (1978). Integrating the moderately and severely handicapped preschool child into a normal day care setting. In M.J. Guralnick (Ed.), *Early intervention and the integrating of handicapped and nonhandicapped children.* Baltimore: University Park Press.

Gaylord-Ross, R., Forte, J., Storey, K., Gaylord-Ross, C., & Jameson, D. (1987). Community-referenced instruction in technological work settings. *Exceptional Children, 54,* 112–120.

Gaylord-Ross, R., & Holvoet, J. (1985). *Strategies for educating students with severe handicaps.* Boston: Little, Brown.

Halpern, A. (1985). Transition: A look at the foundations. *Exceptional Children, 51,* 479–486.

Haring, T.G., Roger, B., Lee, M., Breen, C., & Gaylord-Ross, R. (1986). Teaching social language to moderately handicapped students. *Journal of Applied Behavior Analysis, 19,* 159–171.

Hasazi, S.B., Gordon, L.R., & Roe, C.A. (1985). Factors associated with the employment status of handicapped youth exiting high school from 1979 to 1983. *Exceptional Children, 51* (6), 455–469.

Horner, R.H., McDonnell, J.J., & Bellamy, G.T. (1986). Teaching generalized skills: General case instruction in simulation and community settings. In R.H. Horner, L.H. Meyer, & H.D.B. Fredericks (Eds.), *Education of learners with severe handicaps: Exemplary service strategies* (pp. 289–314). Baltimore: Paul H. Brookes Publishing Co.

Horner, R.H., Sprague, J., & Wilcox, B. (1982). General case programming for community activities. In B. Wilcox & G.T. Bellamy, *Design of high school programs for severely handicapped students* (pp. 61–98). Baltimore: Paul H. Brookes Publishing Co.

Irvin, L. (1988). Vocational assessment in school and rehabilitation programs. In R. Gaylord-Ross (Ed.), *Vocational education for persons with handicaps* (pp. 111–141). Mountain View, CA: Mayfield Publishing Co.

Jones, R.J. & Azrin, N.H. (1975). *Behavioral Research and Therapy, 13,* 17–27.

Mithaug, D., Horiuchi, C., & Fanning, P. (1985). A report on the Colorado statewide follow-up survey of special education students. *Exceptional Children, 51,* 397–404.

Rusch, F.R. (1986). *Supported employment.* Baltimore: Paul H. Brookes Publishing Co.

Rusch, F.R. & Schutz, R.P. (1981). Vocational and social behavior research: An evaluative review. In J.L. Matson and J.R. McCartney (Eds.), *Handbook of Behavior Modification* (pp. 247–280). New York: Plenum Press.

Rusch, F.R., Schutz, R.P., & Agran, M. (1982). Validating entry-level survival skills for service occupations. Implications for curriculum development. *Journal of the Association for Persons with Severe Handicaps, 7,* 32–41.

Sailor, W., Halvorsen, A., Anderson, J., Goetz, L., Gee, K., Doering, K., & Hunt, P. (1986). Community intensive instruction. In R.H. Horner, L.H. Meyer, and H.D.B. Fredericks (Eds.), *Education of learners with severe handicaps: Exemplary service strategies* (pp. 251–288). Baltimore: Paul H. Brookes Publishing Co.

U.S. Bureau of the Census. (1982). *Labor force status and other characteristics of persons with a work disability.* Washington, DC: Author.

Wehman, P. (1981). *Competitive employment: New horizons for severely disabled individuals.* Baltimore: Paul H. Brookes Publishing Co.

Wehman, P., Hill, M., Goodall, P., Cleveland, P., Brooke, V., & Pentecost, H.H. (1982). Job placement follow-up of moderately and severely handicapped individuals after three years. *Journal of the Association for Persons with Severe Handicaps, 7,* 5–16.

Wershing, A., Gaylord-Ross, C., & Gaylord-Ross, R. (1986). Implementing a community vocational training model: A process for systems change. *Education and Training of the Mentally Retarded, 21,* 130–137.

Wilcox, B., & Bellamy, G.T. (1982). Design of high school programs for severely handicapped students. Baltimore: Paul H. Brookes Publishing Co.

Will, M. (1984). *OSERS programming for the transition of youth with disabilities: Bridges from school to working life.* Washington, DC: Office of Special Education and Rehabilitative Services.

CHAPTER 10

SOCIAL SKILLS TRAINING AS AN INTEGRATION STRATEGY

Michael P. Brady and Mary A. McEvoy

Numerous people have written about the various rationales for integrating handicapped and non-handicapped children. Many people focus on legal bases for integration, including the least restrictive environment (LRE) mandate of PL 94-142 (Brady, McDougall, & Dennis, in press). Others stress the societal and humanitarian reasons, citing the history of neglect for people who are separated from the mainstream of society (Biklen, 1977). Still others see integration as necessary for preparing future generations of Americans to accept individual differences (Brown et al., 1983).

As important as these rationales are, the rationale that most affects teachers of handicapped and nonhandicapped children involves *what children will learn* as a result of integrated programs. As every teacher in the United States can attest, socialization is an extremely important part of every child's education. And, there is now sufficient evidence from educational researchers that the *opportunities* for children to learn social skills are far greater in heterogeneous, integrated settings than they are in homogeneous environments (Strain, 1983).

THE IMPORTANCE OF PEER INTERACTION

Educators, psychologists, human development specialists, and even "front line" staff such as school bus drivers have theories on the importance and nature of child socialization. Some argue that socialization is necessary for ego development, role definition, and personality growth. Others cite the relationship of socialization to citizenship, responsibility, sexual development, and vocational competence.

Socialization can be defined broadly as a judgment of general competence within society (see Gresham, 1986). However, teachers are given the task of identifying, teaching, and being accountable for children's specific educational progress. General concepts such as "competence" not only are difficult to judge and measure, but they are also difficult to teach. There is a central aspect to socialization that contains a teachable, measurable content for teachers. This "common denominator" was described by Strain and Shores (1977) as "social reciprocity" or reciprocal peer interactions. Reciprocal peer interactions occur when two or more children actually "exchange" social interactions with one another. Students share toys, ideas, or even test answers. Students play kickball, darts, or word games. One child "transforms" into a machine that builds or destroys another child's fort. This child-to-child interaction is central to learning social skills that last a lifetime (Hartup, 1978).

This chapter was supported in part by a grant from the U.S. Department of Education, Office of Special Education Programs. The authors wish to thank Bob Williams and Jacquie Hawkins for their reviews and input on this chapter, and Tracy Lilly for her assistance with the manuscript.

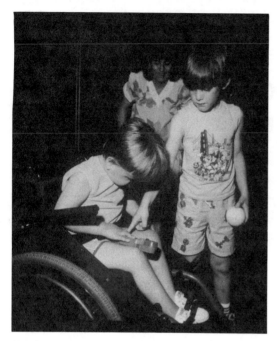

Peer interactions are of primary importance in social skills training.

DIFFICULTIES SOME CHILDREN HAVE INTERACTING WITH PEERS

All children have some difficulty with their social behavior as they grow up. Fortunately, most parents, teachers, and other adults are fairly adept at managing and redirecting temporary problems. Some children, however, seem to have social behavior problems that become serious due to the intensity, persistence, or high rate of the problem. Some of the most common problems that interfere with peer interactions are described in the following paragraphs.

Aggression

Teachers see forms of student aggression daily. As Kauffman (1985, p. 210) reminds, "perfectly normal, emotionally healthy children perform aggressive behaviors, including temper tantrums, verbal assaults, hitting, teasing," and a host of other actions. Aggression interferes with peer interactions when one of two things occurs: 1) the rate of aggression increases instead of decreases as the child grows older; or 2) the intensity of the aggression, as well as the situations in which it is displayed, increases.

Withdrawal

Social withdrawal is fairly common among many children. Most teachers have had students who could sit in class for an entire school year and never volunteer to answer a question, raise their hand, or write on the board. Some children will not even answer a direct question. These children often are just as withdrawn (sometimes more so) in unstructured settings, such as on the playground or during class changes. Often these children miss a tremendous number of socialization opportunities with their peers. Some students with more serious handicaps, such as students with autism, are very socially withdrawn. Some of these children not only withdraw from social interactions but avoid people altogether. Some go to great efforts to try to escape social demands.

Nonresponsiveness

One form of social isolation that mirrors withdrawal in many ways is nonresponsiveness. This includes children who may not initially avoid situations with peers, but who do not respond at all or do not respond appropriately to their peers. Nonresponsive youngsters typically withdraw from peers who invite them to interact. They might shy away from peer activities or they might respond in some inappropriate or negative fashion, such as making disparaging comments, or acting aloof, superior, or bored. Many times, moderately and severely handicapped youngsters do not respond to peer interactions. In the authors' research, they found that severely handicapped autistic children rarely responded to the social bids of nonhandicapped students until they had been *taught* to do so (Brady, Shores, McEvoy, Ellis, & Fox, 1987).

Poor Quality of Interactions

Some children do interact with their peers but the quality of these interactions preclude enjoyment and/or beneficial outcomes. Oftentimes socially immature children lack the skill to stick with a peer activity for more than just a few seconds. These children go from peer to peer and activity to activity, never completing a game or conversation. Sometimes the activities are not only of poor quality but may be socially stigmatizing. For example, many adolescents with mental retardation are overly affectionate toward others. Others may use toys or games that are not appropriate for persons of their own age. Stigmatizing materials and activities promote a child-like image of handicapped people (Brady & Cunningham, 1985).

Generalization Problems

A problem that increasingly has received the attention of researchers in special education relates to students who do not automatically generalize their social skills to novel settings and/or peers. This is most evident with students who play with only one friend, cooperate with only one study group, or behave acceptably in class but not on the playground. Also, many children learn quite sophisticated uses of social behavior (e.g., monitoring their own anger, requesting assistance from other peers) but fail to maintain these behaviors over time. These generalization difficulties are present in many handicapped students but often are present in nonhandicapped children as well.

EDUCATIONAL MODEL FOR SOCIAL SKILLS TRAINING

The benefits of integrating handicapped and nonhandicapped children will likely depend on specific programming variables (Ensher, Blatt, & Winschel, 1977; Guralnick, 1981; Peck & Cooke, 1983; Snyder, Apolloni, & Cooke, 1977). For many children with handicaps, social interaction

does not occur spontaneously. Specific procedures for teaching social interaction must be implemented. Teachers who develop goals and objectives and then teach toward those goals and objectives will increase the likelihood of improving students' social interactions, and thus their competence. Opportunities for social interaction training are numerous. For example, children may need to learn to interact in free-play or recess settings, during lunch periods, during classroom activities, or while participating in school assemblies. Specific procedures for choosing activities for social interaction training are discussed in detail later in this chapter.

The purpose of this section is to present a transdisciplinary model for promoting social integration. The model is a hierarchical model. *Social integration* is clearly the overall goal for all youngsters. This integration depends on the *social interaction skills* that youngsters learn throughout their school years. Finally, interaction is the result of *social skills training*, a teaching-learning process at the heart of public education. Regular and special education teachers, administrators, and nonhandicapped children must work together to assure that social interaction occurs in integrated settings. The underlying philosophy of the model is that social integration is not a "special education" issue, but a school-wide, *general education* issue. Thus, all participants in the school can assist in assuring that social integration works to promote the training and development of social interaction skills. Brady, McEvoy, Gunter, Shores, and Fox (1984) have outlined the roles of students, teachers, and administrators in integrating schools. What follows is a brief description of the roles these people play in the process of integration. (The reader is referred to Brady, McEvoy, et al. [1984] for a complete review.)

Roles of Children

Peers are very important in the social integration process. Peers can serve a number of roles. Oftentimes nonhandicapped peers can serve as "training agents." Peers are especially effective in this role because teachers may not always be available to train social interaction, and peer training promotes both across-setting and across-person generalization (Brady et al., 1987; Strain, Cooke, & Apolloni, 1976). In addition, peers can serve as helpers, "special friends" (Voeltz, 1982), or just "plain" (but important) friends and social contacts (Johnson & Meyer, 1985). Nonhandicapped peers can assist by being receptive to and accepting of handicapped children in integrated settings. Most of all, the roles of children are to experience, learn, and enjoy their social contacts throughout their school years.

Roles of Special Education Teachers

The special education teacher has some very obvious roles. First, the special education teacher will most likely have the responsibility for working with a team in designing goals and objectives for social interaction. In addition, the special education teacher ultimately will be responsible for seeing that the objectives are implemented and evaluated. Hamre-Nietupski and Nietupski (1981) have suggested that special education teachers serve as integration coordinators. They would assist in planning activities to promote integration, including teaching sessions for handicapped and nonhandicapped children. That is, the special education teacher can serve as a consultant to the regular education teacher regarding ways to promote integration, thus assuring opportunities for social interaction training.

Roles of Regular Education Teachers

Regular education teachers can promote social skill development by accepting handicapped children into the classroom, encouraging their students to get to know handicapped youngsters in their school, providing times for student "get togethers," and most of all, setting a positive tone for accepting children's differences. The regular education teacher can take the lead and plan activities that promote interaction between handicapped

and nonhandicapped children (Johnson & Johnson, 1982; Rynders, Johnson, Johnson, & Schmidt, 1980). A number of commercially available multimedia awareness activities are available to teachers to educate nonhandicapped children about children with handicaps. Many regular education teachers have incorporated these or similar activities into units on citizenship, health, family planning, or social studies. Finally, regular educators can work closely with special education teachers to design and implement goals and objectives for the development of social interaction skills in integrated settings.

Roles of Administrators

Perhaps one of the most crucial roles in the integration process is that of the school administrator. If social skills *training* ultimately is to result in social *integration*, handicapped and nonhandicapped students should be included in all regular school settings. The school administrator can help assure integration by scheduling lunch periods, recess times, gym periods, regular class placements, and so forth at times when handicapped and nonhandicapped children can be integrated. In addition, special school-wide activities (e.g., assemblies, field trips) should include participation by both handicapped and nonhandicapped individuals. School administrators can also help promote the positive child-child social integration process by integrating regular and special education faculty. For example, classrooms for children with and without handicaps can be dispersed throughout the building, and all teachers (regardless of specialty) can attend faculty meetings, share the same lounge area, serve on joint committees, and so forth. Regular education teachers can assist in supervising some special education functions (e.g., bus loading) and special education teachers can assist in regular playground duty. Finally, the school administrator can oversee a committee on integration that comprises faculty members, parents, and community personnel to assist in identifying opportunities for integration in school and community settings.

Outcomes

Once the roles in school integration are clear, the process of developing interaction skills becomes easier. The ultimate goal of training social interaction skills is to provide handicapped and nonhandicapped students with the behaviors that promote interactions and, ultimately, integration. Assuming that many of the children in regular schools have never been around a student who is extremely withdrawn, aggressive, or nonresponsive, it is not surprising that many nonhandicapped children do not know how to react to children with such problems. In addition, it is equally unsurprising that handicapped children may not know how to interact with nonhandicapped children. Teachers should understand that training social interaction skills will result in positive changes, for both handicapped and nonhandicapped students. But what are the changes that can be expected? What are the goals and objectives for social interaction training?

The first change may involve adjustments in attitudes and actions. As a result of social interaction training, one would like to see improvements in the attitudes of the nonhandicapped children about children with handicaps. How will it be known if there are changes in attitudes? One way is to assess attitudes. Ask the children, prior to and after training, what they think about children with handicaps. Unfortunately, there is not always a relationship between what people say and what they do (Deno, Mirkin, Robinson, & Evans, 1980). Thus, it is important to look for other indications that attitudinal change has occurred.

There are several ways that teachers can assess changes in the attitudes of nonhandicapped children. Do they include the children with handicaps in school-wide activities? Does interaction between the children with handicaps and the nonhandicapped children occur in the halls between class changes, in the lunchroom, or on the playground? Have children with handicaps been included in any of the various social circles (formal or informal) that exist in schools? Do the nonhandicapped children react to negative statements about the children with handicaps? Are the nonhandicapped children willing to participate in integration activities? These positive actions are an important and often overlooked measure of attitudinal change. If interaction activities are a positive experience for nonhandicapped children, teachers should see important changes in their behavior.

In addition to these attitude changes, changes in the social interaction behaviors of the students with and without handicaps are also of interest, specifically the frequency and types of their initiations, responses to initiations, and the duration of their interactions. These components are discussed in detail below.

Successful Initiations One of the first skills that a teacher should assess is the frequency of initiations. Do the children with handicaps initiate to nonhandicapped children and vice versa? An initiation is a social bid from one child to another for the purposes of starting an interaction. An initiation may be a "Hi!" Or, it may be handing the ball to another child, and saying "Let's play!!" Or it might be asking "Do you have the new Michael Jackson tape?" An important goal in social interaction training is to increase the initiations of both the handicapped and nonhandicapped children. Tremblay, Strain, Hendrickson, and Shores (1981) observed 60 preschool children during free-play activities. They identified several types of initiations to which peers were likely to respond. These included rough and tumble play, sharing, offering assistance, organizing play, asking questions, and offering affection. This information is helpful in designing goals and objectives to increase initiations.

Responding to Initiations It is important that children learn to respond to initiations. A response is an answer to an initiation for the purpose of continuing an interaction. Many handicapped children do not know how to respond to initiations. Often they respond, but in a negative manner. Other times they may not respond at all. Teachers should help handicapped children identify times to respond as well as an appropriate

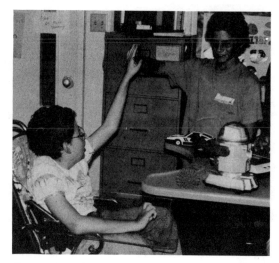

Responding to initiations is an important skill for handicapped children to learn.

manner in which to respond. Likewise, nonhandicapped peers often must be trained to recognize and respond appropriately to the initiations of children with handicaps. Sometimes the initiations may be very subtle. At other times, the initiations may be easy to recognize. However, if an initiation receives either no response or a negative response, it is less likely to occur again than if it receives a positive response. Examples of positive responses include saying "Hi" and showing an interest when someone says "Hi," catching a ball that is thrown, joining in an activity when asked, and so forth. Both handicapped and nonhandicapped children need to learn to recognize and respond to the initiations of peers.

Continuing Interactions   Another outcome of social interaction training is to increase students' ongoing interactions. Once children initiate and respond, it is desired that they continue initiating and responding over longer and longer periods of time. This is known as interaction. Interactions may involve playing cooperatively in a game, working together on a class project, helping each other with school work, and so forth. Longer and more frequent interactions are important outcomes of social interaction training.

Promoting Generalization and Maintenance

It is important that if one teaches a handicapped child to initiate, respond, or interact she or he will do so in a number of settings with a number of children. This is called *generalization*. Often it is not enough to hope that generalization will occur. Teachers must include specific procedures in their social interaction activities to help promote generalization. Briefly, these procedures may include training in several (but not all) settings, training children to interact with different handicapped children, or using materials during training that are likely to be found elsewhere (e.g., the same toys, books, activities). Including procedures to promote generalization is an important part of the social interaction training process.

Another important consideration for training social interaction skills is the development of procedures that increase the likelihood that the children will continue to interact when training is no longer occurring. It is easy to see the importance of this. Often children will attend different schools from year to year; certainly, they will have different teachers. It is hoped that it would not be necessary to train and retrain the same skills every year. Thus, it is important to design training procedures that teach skills that are durable and long-lasting. This is called *maintenance* of training. Using peers in training is an excellent way to help promote maintenance. Even when the teachers are no longer present, the peer group remains fairly stable. The interventions described in the next section include the use of peers as an important maintenance strategy.

HOW TO TEACH SOCIAL ACTIVITIES

Experience and research show that some children do not automatically learn the social skills necessary for social integration. Two ingredients are necessary: *opportunities* and *instruction*. As has been seen in dozens of schools throughout the country, hundreds of hours of instruction, even top-quality instruction, will not result in social integration if students do not have regular opportunities to be social with their peers. Likewise, opportunities alone may not result in skilled behavior. Teaching activities often are necessary.

Teaching social skills is no different from teaching other curriculum areas, such as reading, math, or language arts. For effective instruction, a teacher should state the objective of the lesson, consider the materials, and line up the teaching strategy. To make instruction easier, this section includes a sample social activity plan sheet (Form 1) and instructions for its use. Next there are eight social activities adapted for use with handicapped

as well as nonhandicapped students. Finally, recommendations follow on how to select materials, activities, and peers. (Part of this information has been adapted from Shores et al. [1985]. The reader is referred to this reference for a further description of the training procedures.)

Social Activities

The social activity plan sheets that follow provide activities and effective strategies for teaching social skills. Each activity is based on research findings and is adapted for use by teachers. Information about each section on the sheet is discussed below.

FORM 1

SOCIAL ACTIVITY

Target Children:

Who Else Will Participate:

Goals and Objectives   (*indicates target behavior):
   Initiations   Responses   **Continued Interactions**
   Acquisition   Generalization   **Maintenance**

When and Where the Activity Will Occur:

Age-Appropriate Materials and Activities:

Teaching Procedure:

Activity Description:

Activity and Target Children

The teaching activity is listed in the center at the top of the sheet. Following this is the heading "Target Children." The target children are those students whom the teacher wants to benefit most from the activity. In the social activities that follow, target children include young children with mild handicaps, adolescents who are *not* handicapped, and others.

Who Else Will Participate

The next heading on the activity sheet identifies who else will participate in the activity. These participants will also benefit from the social activity but, unlike the target children, the activity is not designed to increase their social interaction skills.

Some suggestions for selecting the specific "other" children to participate include:

1. Is the student willing to participate?
2. Does the student have a good school attendance record?
3. Does the student follow directions?
4. Does the student enjoy interacting with others?

The social activity presented in Form 2 is designed to target students with mild to moderate handicaps, but uses play activities common to young children without handicaps. The activity of "Farmer in the Dell" is but one of many games employed in the affection research pursued by McEvoy et al. (1988) and Twardosz, Nordquist, Simon, and Botkin (1983). Affection activities, such as patting one another's hands, jointly petting animals, or exchanging hugs, increasingly are being advocated as a means for teaching young children to interact.

Goals and Objectives

Activity goals and objectives are presented next. These outcomes are listed briefly but are not written as formal behavioral objectives. However, they include the specific behavioral responses necessary to make up a social interaction. On each of the eight social activity forms, an asterisk is located next to the outcome that is the intended target behavior for that activity.

A second aspect of this section tells whether the activity is best suited for:

1. Acquisition—initial learning of behavior that the child could not do before
2. Generalization—spreading the child's newly acquired skills to different settings, people, materials, or situations
3. Maintenance—using the new skills across time, particularly after the actual teaching activities have stopped

Again, an asterisk denotes the target for each activity.

In the social activities presented in Forms 3 and 4, the goals and objectives include initiations, responses, continued interactions, acquisition, and generalization. In Form 3 a simple prompt-and-praise activity used by Strain, Shores, and Timm (1977) for acquisition is combined with a generalization strategy (using several peer trainers instead of just one) described by Brady et al. (1987). This activity targets nonhandicapped children, teaching them initiation strategies that are likely to increase responses from handicapped peers. The focus of the social activity in Form 4 is slightly different. While nonhandicapped students still practice initiating, the teacher's focus is on getting the child with handicaps to *respond* to the initiations. Thus, the activities in Forms 3 and 4, in combination, provide direct teaching procedures for children both with and without handicaps.

In addition to the activities provided in this chapter, the teacher may decide to teach social skills using different activities. If so, the teacher must remember to determine the goals and objectives of the activity. Teachers can set these goals for students by briefly assessing what the students currently do. Some questions a teacher should ask while observing the children include:

1. Does the child seek out others with whom to play?

FORM 2

SOCIAL ACTIVITY

Teaching Affection
("Farmer in the Dell")

Target Children:

Mildly to moderately handicapped children ages 3–6.

Who Else Will Participate:

Nonhandicapped age-mate peers.

Goals and Objectives   (*indicates target behavior):

*Initiations	***Responses**	***Continued Interactions**
*Acquisition	***Generalization**	***Maintenance**

When and Where the Activity Will Occur:

Preschool classroom, gym, or playground for 10–15 minutes in small or large groups (e.g., music, good-morning activity).

Age-Appropriate Materials and Activities:

Affection activities are particularly appropriate for young children. Use high-preference games.

Teaching Procedure:

The successful implementation of affection activities is highly dependent on the teacher's ability to keep control of the activity while allowing the children to have fun. The teacher prompts interaction during the course of the activity and praises both prompted and unprompted interactions.

Activity Description:

The teacher and children hold hands forming a circle. The teacher chooses one child (usually a child with handicaps) to be the farmer in the center of the circle. The teacher and children then circle the target child while singing "The Farmer in the Dell." During a second verse, the teacher prompts the handicapped child to choose a friend to join him or her in the center by saying "The farmer hugs (or pats, or gives five) the wife." The target child then exhibits the behavior the teacher has prompted and chooses a child by giving him or her a hug (pat, give five). Teacher praises the handicapped child when he or she demonstrates the affective behavior. The song continues until all children have been chosen to join the target child in the center of the circle.

For more information see McEvoy et al. (1988) and Twardosz, Nordquist, Simon, and Botkin (1983).

2. Does the child respond to others' attempts to include him or her in activities?
3. Does the child continue to interact for any length of time?
4. Is the child smiling appropriately, laughing, or involved with the other person?

When setting goals it is important to remember that each of these behaviors occurs to varying degrees. For example, a child may initiate, but perhaps only to a specific person. The goal for this child might be to initiate to a variety of people. Or a child may respond to initiations, but only during a specific activity. The goal for this child might be to increase responses with different activities. Or a child may interact, but only for brief periods of time. The goal for this child might be to increase the length of time of his or her interactions. Each child's individual goal will be used to plan his or her daily activity.

FORM 3

SOCIAL ACTIVITY

Teaching Nonhandicapped Children to
Initiate to Handicapped Children

Target Children:

Nonhandicapped students (any age).

Who Else Will Participate:

Mildly to severely handicapped age-mate peers.

Goals and Objectives   (*indicates target behavior):

*Initiations	Responses	Continued Interactions
*Acquisition	*Generalization	Maintenance

When and Where the Activity Will Occur:

Daily 20-minute sessions in a gym, playground, or classroom.

Age-appropriate Materials and Activities:

Board games, balls.

Teaching Procedure:

Prior to the activity, the teacher models the use of prompts for handicapped children. Nonhandicapped students practice initiating to the teacher. Initiations include invitation to play ("Let's play"), sharing materials, or giving assistance.

Activity Description:

Nonhandicapped children are prompted by the teacher and praised for sharing materials or organizing activities with their handicapped peers. Increases in peer initiations have been effective in increasing social interactions.

For more information see Brady, Shores, McEvoy, Ellis, and Fox (1987) and Strain, Shores, and Timm (1977).

When and Where the Activity Will Occur

An important decision that a teacher must make is *when* to conduct a social integration activity. In many instances, at least 30 minutes will be needed to conduct a social integration activity. Some of the activities, however, will last only 10–15 minutes. Handicapped and nonhandicapped children must have opportunities to interact at least once per day but should be involved in activities more often. The integration activities should be regarded as a regular lesson and as an important part of the class schedule. Including the activities as part of the class schedule helps assure that the sessions will be conducted, establishes a routine for the students, and provides opportunities for learning to occur.

Many of the social activities provided in this chapter fit the schedule of a standard school day fairly well. For example, the activity outlined in Form 5 (teaching handicapped children to "organize play" as an initiation) was used during regularly scheduled recess-times for younger children (Gunter, Fox, Brady, Shores, & Cavanaugh, 1988) as well as for older teenagers (Fox et al., 1984; Gaylord-Ross, Haring, Breen, & Pitts-Conway, 1984). Other activities take a very different approach. Work by Warrenfeltz et al. (1981) and Kiburz, Miller, and Morrow (1984) included more of a "transition" focus. That is, rather than targeting recess-type interactions, their work taught stu-

---

FORM 4

SOCIAL ACTIVITY

Teaching Handicapped Children to Respond
to Nonhandicapped Students' Initiations

Target Children:

Handicapped students of all ages and abilities.

Who Else Will Participate:

Nonhandicapped children who are "good" social models.

Goals and Objectives   (*indicates target behavior):

Initiations	*Responses	*Continued Interactions
*Acquisition	*Generalization	Maintenance

When and Where the Activity Will Occur:

This activity works well in active or "rough and tumble" games, including playground chase, tickle games, or hide and seek. Limit time to 20 minutes to keep interest high.

Age-Appropriate Materials and Activities:

Materials that are preferred by the handicapped child.

Teaching Procedure:

Prior to the activity, the teacher models initiating for the nonhandicapped students. During the activity, the teacher prompts a handicapped student to respond and encourages a nonhandicapped student to continue initiating.

Activity Description:

By using games and materials that are preferred by the handicapped student, the teacher will increase the likelihood that the handicapped student will get involved. Active games and materials often help.

For more information see Brady, Shores, McEvoy, Ellis, and Fox (1987) and Odom and Strain (1986).

dents skills that would be necessary for successful transitions to nonschool settings, including jobs. While some of the teaching activities took place in class, other activities were carried out "in-the-field." This activity is summarized in Form 6.

When several times for conducting a social interaction training activity have been identified, it is important that the special and regular education teachers coordinate their schedules. Regular education teachers and parents may be unwilling to let their students participate in interaction activities if they are scheduled during academic lessons. Once a time for conducting an interaction activity has been designated, the teacher must identify a place to conduct the activity. A variety of settings are available including the gym, playground, class-

room, and auditorium. It is important that the teacher check on the availability of the chosen area to assure that it will be available every day. It is also important that the area selected is large enough to accommodate the number of children who will be involved in the activity.

Age-Appropriate Materials and Activities

The selection of appropriate materials and activities is crucial to help children meet their goals and objectives as well as to assure that the participants have fun. Table 1 includes several recommendations that Stremel-Campbell, Cambell, and Johnson-Dorn (1985) have made for selecting age-appropriate materials and activities.

SOCIAL ACTIVITY

Teaching Handicapped Children to Initiate
to Nonhandicapped Children
(organizing play and games)

Target Children:
 Handicapped child (any age).

Who Else Will Participate:
 Nonhandicapped age-mate peer.

Goals and Objectives   (*indicates target behavior):

*Initiations	Responses	*Continued Interactions
*Acquisition	*Generalization	Maintenance

When and Where the Activity Will Occur:
 Teacher and two children participate in activity in classroom.

Age-Appropriate Materials and Activities:
 Balls, video games, cassette tapes, other high preference items.

Teaching Procedure:
 The teacher uses a series of prompts (verbal, model, physical) and praise to encourage the handicapped child to initiate "play-organizing" statements and actions to the nonhandicapped peer.

Activity Description:
 The teacher hands materials to the handicapped child. If the handicapped child does not ask the nonhandicapped child to join in an activity, the teacher prompts the child to say "Let's play." If necessary, the teacher models the behavior saying, "Ask Marsha to play like this: 'Marsha, let's play.' " If more help is necessary, the teacher physically prompts the handicapped child to play organize by taking her hands and handing the ball to the peer while saying, "Let's play." All instances of interaction are praised.

For more information see Fox et al. (1984), Gaylord-Ross, Haring, Breen, and Pitts-Conway, (1984), and Gunter, Fox, Brady, Shores, and Cavanaugh (1988).

Student age, interest, willingness, and intellectual sophistication obviously are important when selecting activities and materials. For example, the affection activities presented in Form 2 are excellent activities for young children. For older students, different instructional methods are appropriate. O'Connor (1969), for example, used videotapes and short drama sequences to teach appropriate play. Breen, Haring, Pitts-Conway, and Gaylord-Ross (1985) developed scripts for their participants to follow during skill training. Social activities that include drama sequences and scripting are presented in Forms 7 and 8.

The teacher should vary and rotate the materials and activities to keep the students interested. The most important thing to remember is that the materials and activities should promote interaction. Thus, teachers may have to adapt some materials to allow two or more persons to interact. Four important questions that a teacher should ask about the selection of materials and activities for social interaction activities are:

FORM 6

SOCIAL ACTIVITY

Teaching Positive Responses to Criticism
(self-monitoring and role playing)

Target Children:

Adolescents with conduct problems.

Who Else Will Participate:

Other adolescents who are considered "good" social interactors.

Goals and Objectives   (*indicates target behavior):

Initiations	*Responses	Continued Interactions
Acquisition	*Generalization	Maintenance

When and Where the Activity Will Occur:

In-class activity, particularly useful when preparing adolescents for work or transition activities.

Age-Appropriate Materials and Activities:

Videotapes and monitor.

Teaching Procedure:

Prior to the activity, the teacher prepares short videotaped vignettes.

Activity Description:

Target students identify their problems related to following directions and responding to criticism. With their peers, students view videotaped vignettes of themselves and others responding appropriately. Next, students verbally rehearse appropriate responding. Finally, students role play the activity with all students exchanging roles.

For more information see Kiburz, Miller, and Morrow (1984), Lesbock and Salzberg (1981), and Warrenfeltz et al. (1981).

1. Are the materials safe and durable?
2. Is there adequate space in the play area for the chosen activities and materials?
3. Are the materials and activities well matched to the skill levels and ages of the participants?
4. Are the materials and activities interesting and fun for both the handicapped and nonhandicapped students?

Teaching Procedure

Each of the activities in this chapter can be taught. The teaching strategy is an active one and includes verbal prompting, modeling, guiding, praising, and fading. These tactics are equally effective with both handicapped and nonhandicapped students.

Verbal prompting consists of specific directions by the teacher to a child telling him or her to initiate or respond to a peer. Statements such as "Frank, throw the ball to John," "Bill, give the puppet to Mary," or "Jim, tell Frank he played the game well" are examples of verbal prompts. However, some prompts are less directive. An indirect prompt for a child to respond to a peer's initiation could come in the form of a question, for example, "James, did Brian ask you to play?" Sometimes just saying the student's name is enough to prompt an initiation or response.

Modeling is simply demonstrating the behavior you want the child to perform. The teacher demonstrates while explaining how the child should initiate or respond. When the child performs the behavior, then the teacher praises the child.

Table 1.   Age-appropriate materials and activities

Younger student	Older student
Playing with cars and trucks	Taking turns shooting baskets
Taking turns jumping on a small trampoline	Playing darts on a Velcro dart board
Taking turns rocking on a rocking horse	Making a scrapbook
Playing make-believe kitchen	Cooking
	Painting
Singing	Playing table games (e.g., Sorry, Dominoes)
Dancing	
Making simple snacks	Playing video games
Blowing bubbles	Dancing
Riding/pulling a wagon	Bowling
Playing musical instruments	Playing cards
	Playing Simon
Playing with dolls	Looking at and discussing books or magazines
Playing "dress-up"	
Playing at a sand table	
Playing with Lite Bright	Playing pinball
Playing with puppets	Riding bikes

Adapted from Stremel-Campbell, K., Campbell, R. and Johnson-Dorn, N. (1985). Utilization of integrated settings and activities to develop and expand communication skills. In M.P. Brady and P. Gunter (Eds.), *Integrating moderately and severely handicapped learners: Strategies that work* (p. 200). Springfield, IL: Charles C Thomas; adapted with permission.

Guiding is very useful, particularly in teaching children simple motor behavior, and consists of the teacher manually guiding the student through the desired behavior. For example, the teacher may stand behind a child, guiding both of the child's hands to grasp a ball. The teacher guides the child through the throwing motion, throwing the ball to the peer. The teacher should praise the child even at this stage of teaching. The amount of physical guidance by the teacher is reduced as the child becomes more independent.

Teacher feedback always accompanies these direct teaching tactics. *Praising* is the most common form of feedback in this project. Praising is designed to reinforce interactions between children by expressing your approval. Praise statements

often state the child's name and the specific behavior being praised. Praise should always relate to playing together. "Max, you're having so much fun playing football with Arnold. I like that!" is an example of an appropriate praise statement.

Sometimes, though, praise alone is not effective. More "concrete" feedback was used by Carden Smith and Fowler (1984) who added a token system and a lottery to make sure that positive feedback on students' behavior was obvious to *all* students who were present. Form 9 provides a social activity based on their work.

Finally, teachers should note one caution about praise and other forms of feedback: Too much praise or praise that is too "lavish" can interrupt children's interaction or direct children's attention to the adult. Ultimately, you want interactions between students to occur for their own enjoyment. The solution: Use feedback during instruction, but do so carefully.

Fading or gradual elimination of these direct teaching tactics is used so the students will not become dependent upon your prompts and praise. Once the students begin to interact regularly and enjoy these interactions, you will gradually begin to fade the prompts. For example, if it is necessary for you to use models or verbal prompts in the beginning, look for times when your students will interact without being taught. If they enjoy their interactions together, you could delay a prompt to see if they would begin interacting on their own. Finally, after several teaching sessions you may see interactions simply by arranging the opportunity for students to interact. When this occurs you may be able to change your role from teaching to monitoring.

Developing Other Social Activities

The eight social activities in this chapter are intended to get you started. They are not intended to be your entire social skills curriculum. The sample social activity plan sheet (Form 1) is a blank form. Photocopy and use it, or design your own planning sheet to develop other teaching activities

---

FORM 7

SOCIAL ACTIVITY

Teaching Positive Interactions Through Symbolic Modeling
(videotape drama)

Target Children:
Withdrawn children.

Who Else Will Participate:
Nonhandicapped age-mate peers.

Goals and Objectives   (*indicates target behavior):

Initiations	Responses	*Continued Interactions
*Acquisition	*Generalization	*Maintenance

When and Where the Activity Will Occur:
Training occurs daily for 5 minutes prior to free-play activity. Training occurs in classroom. Free play may be in any appropriate area.

Age-appropriate Materials and Activities:
Videotape of appropriate interaction between students.

Teaching Procedure:
The teacher prepares videotape sequences (approximately 1 minute each) of children playing together appropriately. Examples of sharing, assisting, organizing play, and affection are included. The teacher describes each activity on the videotape. During free play, the teacher praises each instance of interaction.

Activity Description:
Prior to the free-play activity, the withdrawn child views five, 1-minute videotaped samples of children playing appropriately. The child later participates in free-play activity with nonhandicapped students.

For more information see O'Connor (1969).

specific to your own students and your own school settings. Remember, too, that most district, regional, and state education agencies have guides and curricula. Teacher magazines, research journals, and other texts also have suggestions for teaching social skills. A teacher in today's schools has available a vast amount of information. Use it wisely. Identify the students whom you want to teach. Target and then teach toward the intended social outcomes. Select materials and teaching procedures that enhance both learning and having fun. By systematically teaching social interaction skills, teachers have an impact on both handicapped and nonhandicapped learners. Very few

areas of your curriculum have that potential. Just as important, very few areas of your curriculum target having fun as an important outcome of your lesson.

SUMMARY

In this chapter, the premise that social integration can be achieved by teaching social interaction skills to children with and without handicaps was discussed. The authors provided an educational model for social skills training, including roles for

FORM 8

SOCIAL ACTIVITY

Teaching Nonhandicapped Children to Respond
to Handicapped Children
(scripting)

Target Children:

Nonhandicapped adolescents.

Who Else Will Participate:

Handicapped children and adolescents whose initiations are not very noticeable.

Goals and Objectives   (*indicates target behavior):

| Initiations | *Responses | *Continued Interactions |
| *Acquisition | *Generalization | Maintenance |

When and Where the Activity Will Occur:

Any time during the school day. Particularly useful as preparation for work, physical education, or other activities requiring reciprocal exchanges.

Age-Appropriate Materials and Activities:

Most high-preference materials are acceptable.

Teaching Procedure:

This procedure requires rehearsal and practice.
1. The teacher prepares a script and teaches a nonhandicapped student to use a script to respond to initiations.
2. The teacher models various ways handicapped students might initiate, and guides a nonhandicapped student through the responses.
3. The teacher monitors, prompts, and praises a nonhandicapped student for responding to handicapped students' initiations during group or individual activities.

Activity Description:

Scripting can be useful across a variety of activities. The teacher should remember that the script itself is less important than the interactions facilitated by the script.

For more information see Brady, Shores, et al. (1984) and Breen, Haring, Pitts-Conway, and Gaylord-Ross (1985).

educators and intended outcomes for students. They also presented an instructional activity format and eight specific social activities that teachers can adapt for a variety of students. The model and activities are empirically based; that is, they exist because teachers and researchers have joined together to explore ways to promote integration. Just as important, the model and activities are proactive. Learning does not "just happen"— it happens when top-quality instruction is implemented systematically by top-quality teachers. Likewise, social integration must be planned for and taught. To this end, educators play a vital, active role.

FORM 9

SOCIAL ACTIVITY

Teaching Cooperation and Participation
(peer-monitored token economy)

Target Children:

Disruptive children with behavior disorders.

Who Else Will Participate:

Nonhandicapped age-mate peers.

Goals and Objectives   (*indicates target behavior):

Initiations	Responses	***Continued Interactions**
*Acquisition	Generalization	***Maintenance**

When and Where the Activity Will Occur:

During classroom activities in a variety of settings.

Age-appropriate Materials and Activities:

Most high-preference materials; tokens.

Teaching Procedure:

During initial sessions, the teacher describes the token system, and role plays appropriate behavior. The teacher initially awards points for specified appropriate behavior.

Activity Description:

After the children are familiar with the system, the teacher assigns children to teams and selects a team captain. Peers observe teammates, remind them of appropriate behavior, and award points publicly. The team captain changes daily and is chosen by lottery from those team members who receive points for 3 consecutive days.

For more information see Carden Smith and Fowler (1984).

STUDY QUESTIONS

1. What are the difficulties some children have when interacting with their peers?
2. Why are specific teaching activities usually necessary for social integration to occur?
3. What are the similarities and differences among social integration, social interaction and social skills training?
4. What are the three components of a social interaction?
5. What are the differences between changes in attitudes and changes in interaction behavior?
6. Students, regular education teachers, special education teachers, and administrators all play key roles in integrating a school. What specific actions can each of these groups take that would promote social integration?

REFERENCES

Biklen, D. (1977). Exclusion. In B. Blatt, D. Biklen, & R. Bogdan (Eds.), *An alternative textbook in special education* (pp. 135–151). Denver: Love.

Brady, M.P., & Cunningham, J. (1985). Living and learning in segregated environments: An ethnography of normalization outcomes. *Education and Training of the Mentally Retarded, 20,* 241–252.

Brady, M.P., McDougall, D., & Dennis, H.F. (in press). The

schools, the courts and the integration of students with severe handicaps. *Journal of Special Education*.

Brady, M.P., McEvoy, M.A., Gunter, P., Shores, R.E., & Fox,
J.J. (1984). Considerations for socially integrated school environments for severely handicapped students. *Education
and Training of the Mentally Retarded, 19*(4), 246–251.

Brady, M.P., Shores, R.E., Gunter, P., McEvoy, M.A., Fox,
J.J., & White, C. (1984). Generalization of a severely handicapped adolescent's social interaction responses via multiple
peers in a classroom setting. *Journal of the Association for
Persons with Severe Handicaps, 9*, 278–286.

Brady, M.P., Shores, R.E., McEvoy, M.A., Ellis, D., & Fox,
J.J. (1987). Increasing the social interactions of severely
handicapped autistic children. *Journal of Autism and Developmental Disorders, 17*, 375–390.

Breen, C., Haring, T., Pitts-Conway, V., & Gaylord-Ross, R.
(1985). The training and generalization of social interaction
during breaktime at two job sites in the natural environment.
*Journal of the Association for Persons with Severe Handi-
caps, 10*, 41–50.

Brown, L., Ford, A., Nisbet, J., Sweet, M., Donnellan, A., &
Gruenewald, L. (1983). Opportunities available when severely handicapped students attend chronological age appropriate regular schools. *Journal of the Association for the
Severely Handicapped, 8*, 16–24.

Carden Smith, L.K., & Fowler, S.A. (1984). Positive peer
pressure: The effects of peer monitoring of children's disruptive behavior. *Journal of Applied Behavior Analysis, 17*,
213–227.

Deno, S.L., Mirkin, K., Robinson, S., & Evans, P. (1980).
*Relationships among classroom observations of social ad-
justments and sociometric rating scales* (Research report
No. 24). Minneapolis: University of Minnesota, Institute for
Research on Learning Disabilities.

Ensher, G.L., Blatt, B., & Winschel, J.F. (1977). Head Start
for handicapped children: Congressional mandate audit. *Exceptional Children, 43*, 202–210.

Fox, J.J., Gunter, P., Brady, M.P., Bambara, L.M., Spiegel-
McGill, P., & Shores, R.E. (1984). Using multiple peer
examplars to develop generalized social responding of an
autistic girl. In R.B. Rutherford & C.M. Nelson (Eds.),
*Monographs on behavior disorders: Severe behavior disor-
ders of children and youth* (Vol. 7, pp. 17–27). Reston, VA:
Council for Exceptional Children.

Gaylord-Ross, R., Haring, T., Breen, C., & Pitts-Conway, V.
(1984). The training and generalization of social interaction
skills with autistic youth. *Journal of Applied Behavior Analysis, 17*, 229–247.

Gresham, F. (1986). Conceptual issues in the assessment of social competence in children. In P.S. Strain, M.J. Guralnick,
& H.M. Walker (Eds.), *Children's social behavior: Development, assessment, and modification*. Orlando, FL: Academic Press.

Gunter, P., Fox, J.J., Brady, M.P., Shores, R.E., & Cavanaugh, K. (1988). Nonhandicapped peers as multiple ex-
emplars: A generalization tactic for promoting autistic students' social skills. *Behavioral Disorders, 13*, 116–126.

Guralnick, M.J. (1981). Programmatic factors affecting child-
child and social interactions in mainstreamed preschool programs. *Exceptional Education Quarterly, 1*(4), 71–91.

Hamre-Nietupski, S., & Nietupski, J. (1981). Integral involvement of severely handicapped students within regular public
schools. *Journal of the Association for the Severely Handicapped, 6*, 30–39.

Hartup, W. (1978). Peer interaction and the process of socialization. In M.J. Guralnick (Ed.), *Early intervention and the
integration of handicapped and nonhandicapped children*
(pp. 27–51). Baltimore: University Park Press.

Johnson, R., & Johnson, D. (1982). The social structure of
classrooms. In M.C. Reynolds (Ed.), *The future of mainstreaming: Next steps in teacher education* (pp. 26–31).
Minneapolis: University of Minnesota, National Support
Systems Project.

Johnson, R., & Meyer, L. (1985). Program design and research to normalize peer interactions. In M.P. Brady &
P. Gunter (Eds.), *Integrating moderately and severely handicapped learners: Strategies that work* (pp. 79–101). Springfield, IL: Charles C Thomas.

Kauffman, J.M. (1985). *Characteristics of children's behavior
disorders* (3rd ed.). Columbus, OH: Charles E. Merrill.

Kiburz, C.S., Miller, S.R., & Morrow, L.W. (1984). Structured learning using self-monitoring to promote maintenance and generalization of social skills across settings for a
behaviorally disordered adolescent. *Behavioral Disorders,
10*, 47–55.

Lesbock, M.S., & Salzberg, C.L. (1981). The use of role play
and reinforcement procedures in the development of generalized interpersonal behavior with emotionally disturbed,
behavior disordered adolescents in a special education classroom. *Behavioral Disorders, 6*, 150–163.

McEvoy, M.A., Nordquist, V.M., Twardosz, S., Heckaman,
K.A., Wehby, J.H., & Denny, R.K. (1988). Promoting autistic children's peer interaction in integrated early childhood settings using affection activities. *Journal of Applied
Behavior Analysis, 21*, 193–200.

O'Connor, R.D. (1969). Modification of social withdrawal
through symbolic modeling. *Journal of Applied Behavior
Analysis, 2*, 15–22.

Odom, S., & Strain, P.S. (1986). A comparison of peer-initia-
tion and teacher-antecedent interventions for promoting reciprocal social interaction of autistic preschoolers. *Journal
of Applied Behavior Analysis, 19*, 59–71.

Peck, C.A., & Cooke, T.P. (1983). Benefits of mainstreaming
at the early childhood level: How much can we expect?
Analysis and Intervention in Developmental Disabilities, 3,
1–22.

Rynders, J.E., Johnson, R.T., Johnson, D.W., & Schmidt, B.
(1980). Producing positive interaction among Down syndrome and nonhandicapped teenagers through cooperative
goal structuring. *American Journal of Mental Deficiency,
85*, 268–273.

Shores, R.E., McEvoy, M.A., Fox, J.J., Brady, M.P., Denny,
R.K., Heckaman, K., & Wehby, J.H. (1985). *Social integration of severely handicapped children* [training manual].
Nashville, TN: George Peabody College of Vanderbilt University.

Snyder, L., Apolloni, T., & Cooke, T.P. (1977). Integrated settings at the early childhood level? The role of non-retarded
peers. *Exceptional Children, 43*, 262–266.

Strain, P.S. (1983). Generalization of autistic children's social behavior change: Effects of developmentally integrated and segregated settings. *Analysis and Intervention in Developmental Disabilities, 3,* 23–34.

Strain, P.S., Cooke, T.P., & Apolloni, T. (1976). *Teaching exceptional children: Assessing and modifying social behavior.* New York: Academic Press.

Strain, P.S., & Shores, R.E. (1977). Social reciprocity: A review of research and educational implications. *Exceptional Children, 43,* 526–530.

Strain, P.S., Shores, R.E., & Timm, M.A. (1977). Effects of peer social initiations on the behavior of withdrawn preschool children. *Journal of Applied Behavior Analysis, 10,* 289–298.

Stremel-Campbell, K., Campbell, R., & Johnson-Dorn, N. (1985). Utilization of integrated settings and activities to develop and expand communication skills. In M.P. Brady & P. Gunter (Eds.), *Integrating moderately and severely handi-*

capped learners: Strategies that work (pp. 185–213). Springfield, IL: Charles C. Thomas.

Tremblay, A., Strain, P.S., Hendrickson, J.M., & Shores, R.E. (1981). Social interactions of normal preschool children. *Behavior Modification, 5,* 237–253.

Twardosz, S., Nordquist, V.M., Simon, R., & Botkin, D. (1983). The effect of group affection activities on the integration of socially isolated children. *Analysis and Intervention in Developmental Disabilities, 3,* 311–338.

Voeltz, L.M. (1982). Effects of structured interactions with severely handicapped peers on children's attitudes. *American Journal of Mental Deficiency, 86,* 380–390.

Warrenfeltz, R., Kelly, W., Salzberg, C., Beegle, C., Levy, S., Adams, T., & Crouse, T. (1981). Social skills training of behavior disordered adolescents with self-monitoring to promote generalization to a vocational setting. *Behavioral Disorders, 7,* 18–27.

CHAPTER 11

COOPERATIVE LEARNING AND MAINSTREAMING

David W. Johnson and Roger T. Johnson

David hesitates at the door of the classroom but the special education teacher escorts him firmly to the empty desk near the front of the room. He is afraid to look around. "Will the kids like me?" he wonders. "I know I'm not very smart. Will they make fun of me?"

The students who recognize him shake their heads in disbelief. "Not Dumb David! What's he doing in our room?"

Similar scenes with other handicapped children are occurring in regular classrooms all over the country. Often the handicapped students may be anxious and fearful and the nonhandicapped students may regard them with distaste. When handicapped students are placed in the regular classroom it is the beginning of an opportunity to deeply influence their lives by promoting constructive relationships between them and their nonhandicapped peers. Like all opportunities, however, mainstreaming carries the risk of making things worse as well as the possibility of making things better. Handicapped students could be stigmatized, stereotyped, and rejected. Even worse, they might be ignored or treated paternalistically. It is also possible, however, that true friendships and positive relationships will develop between handicapped and nonhandicapped students. The essential question is, "What does the regular classroom teacher do to ensure that constructive, caring, and supportive relationships are developed between handicapped and nonhandicapped students?" The answer to this question goes beyond constructive teacher-student interaction and the providing of students with appropriate instructional materials. The answer is found in how relationships among students are structured.

Mainstreaming is based on the assumption that placing heterogeneous students (in terms of handicapping conditions) in the same school and classroom will facilitate positive relationships and attitudes among the students. Yet there is considerable disagreement as to whether there are conditions under which physical proximity between handicapped and nonhandicapped students will lead to constructive relationships. The lack of theoretical models and the presence of apparently inconsistent research findings have left the impression that mainstreaming may not be working and may not be constructive. One of the key factors identified by the research as determining whether mainstreaming promotes positive or negative relationships among heterogeneous students is whether students cooperate, compete, or work independently on their academic assignments. By structuring positive, negative, or no interdependence among heterogeneous students during academic learning situations, teachers can influence the pattern of interaction among students and the interpersonal attraction that results (Deutsch, 1962; Johnson & F. Johnson, 1987, Johnson & R. Johnson, 1984c; Johnson, Johnson, & Holubec, 1986).

SOCIAL INTERDEPENDENCE IN THE CLASSROOM

"What to do with David?" the teacher thinks. "I can have David compete with the nonhandi-capped students, but he will lose. I can have every student work on their own individually, but then no one will get to know David. Or, I can use cooperative learning groups and have David work with nonhandicapped classmates. But does he know how to work cooperatively with others?"

In any classroom, teachers may structure aca-demic lessons so that students are: 1) engaging in a win-lose struggle to see who is learning best, 2) learning individually on their own without in-teracting with classmates, or 3) working in pairs or small groups to help each other master the as-signed material. In a *competitive* learning situa-tion, students' goal achievements are negatively correlated; that is, when one student achieves his or her goal, all others with whom he or she is com-petitively linked fail to achieve their goals. Stu-dents work against each other to achieve a goal that only one or a few students can attain. Students are graded on a curve, which requires them to work faster and more accurately than their peers to achieve outcomes that are personally beneficial but detrimental to others. They either study hard to do better than their classmates or they take it easy because they do not believe they have a chance to "win."

In an *individualistic* learning situation, stu-dents' goal achievements are independent; the goal achievement of one student is unrelated to the goal achievement of others. Students seek out-comes that are personally beneficial and they ig-nore as irrelevant the goal achievements of their classmates. Teachers structure lessons individu-alistically by requiring students to work by them-selves to accomplish learning goals unrelated to those of their classmates, evaluating students' efforts on a fixed set of standards, and rewarding students on the basis of how their performance

compares with the preset criterion of excellence. Each student has a set of materials and works at his or her own speed, ignoring the other students in the class.

For the past 45 years competitive and individu-alistic goal structures have dominated American education. Students usually come to school with competitive expectations and pressures from their parents. Many teachers have tried to reduce class-room competition by switching from a norm-referenced to a criterion-referenced evaluation system. In both competitive and individualistic learning situations teachers try to keep students away from each other. "Do not copy!" "Move your desks apart!" "I want to see how well you can do, not your neighbor!" are all phrases that teachers commonly use in their classrooms. Students are repeatedly told "Do not care about the other stu-dents in this class. Take care of yourself!"

There is a third option. Teachers can structure lessons cooperatively so that students work to-gether to accomplish shared goals. In a *coopera-tive* learning situation, students' goal achieve-ments are positively correlated; that is, students perceive that they can reach their learning goals if and only if the other students in the learning group also reach their goals. Thus, students seek out-comes that are beneficial to all those with whom they are cooperatively linked. Students are as-signed to small groups and instructed to learn the assigned material and to make sure that the other members of the group also master the assignment. Students discuss material with each other, help one another understand it, and encourage each other to work hard. Individual accountability is checked regularly to ensure all students are learn-ing. A criterion-referenced evaluation system is used.

Cooperative learning is the most important of the three ways of structuring learning situations, yet it is currently the least used. In most schools, class sessions are structured cooperatively only for 7%–20% of the time (Johnson & Johnson, 1983). Cooperative learning, however, should be used whenever teachers want students to learn more, like school better, like each other better, have higher self-esteem, and learn more effective social skills. When handicapped students are being mainstreamed it is especially important that classrooms be dominated by cooperation among students (Johnson & R.T. Johnson, 1986a; Johnson, Johnson, & Maryuama, 1983).

BASIC ELEMENTS OF COOPERATIVE LEARNING

"There are many different ways I can use cooperative learning," the teacher thinks. "When should I have David work cooperatively with others, and how do I structure the cooperative groups to ensure that David is liked and accepted by his classmates?"

There are many ways in which cooperative learning may be used in class, from having pairs involved in 5-minute discussions to create an anticipatory set to multiday curriculum units. Teachers may modify existing lessons and curriculum materials to include cooperative learning. Whenever they do so, certain elements are essential. Johnson and Johnson (1986b, in press) state that cooperation is most effective when:

1. Students clearly perceive their positive interdependence.
2. Students interact face to face.
3. The task is structured so that individual accountability is clear and the efforts of all members are needed for group success.
4. Students have the necessary collaborative skills.
5. Students know how effectively their learning group is functioning.

The first requirement for an effectively structured cooperative lesson is *positive interdependence,* which exists when students perceive that they are linked with others in a way that they cannot succeed unless the other group members also succeed and vice versa. This means that the work of each group member contributes to the success of all other group members. Positive interdependence is a sense of common fate (you succeed or fail together) and mutual causation (both your work and the work of the other group members are required for any one of you to succeed). The first requirement for cooperative learning is that *goal interdependence* be clearly structured by the teacher. Goal interdependence exists when individuals perceive that they can attain their goals if and only if the other individuals with whom they are cooperatively linked attain their goals.

Once goal interdependence is established, it may be supplemented and strengthened by including other types of positive interdependence within the lesson. The supplementary types of positive interdependence (which are overlapping and not independent from each other) are as follows:

1. *Reward interdependence* exists when each group member receives the same reward for successfully completing a joint task. Reward interdependence needs to be structured in a way that ensures that one member's efforts do not make the efforts of other members unnecessary. For example, if the highest score in the group determines the group grade, low-ability members would see their efforts to produce as unnecessary and they might contribute minimally; high-ability members might feel exploited and become demoralized and, therefore, decrease their efforts so as not to provide undeserved rewards for irresponsible and ungrateful "free-riders" (Kerr, 1983).
2. *Resource interdependence* exists when each member has only a portion of the information, resources, or materials neccessary for the task to be completed and members' resources have to be combined in order for the group to achieve its goal.
3. *Role interdependence* exists when each member is assigned complementary and interconnected roles that specify responsibilities that the group needs in order to complete a joint task.

4. *Task interdependence* exists when a division of labor is created so that the actions of one group member have to be completed if the next group member is to complete his or her responsibilities. That is, the overall task is divided into subunits that must be performed in a set order for the task to be completed.

Positive interdependence has numerous effects on individuals' motivation and productivity, not the least of which is to highlight the fact that the efforts of all group members are needed for group success. There are many paths to positive interdependence. Teachers are encouraged never to use only one when two ways are possible. The more ways positive interdependence is structured within a lesson, the clearer the message will be to students that they must be concerned about and take responsibility for both their own and each other's learning.

The second requirement for an effectively structured cooperative lesson is *face-to-face interaction* among group members. Within cooperative lessons, teachers need to maximize the opportunity for students to promote each other's success by helping, assisting, supporting, encouraging, and praising each other's efforts to learn. While positive interdependence in and of itself may have some effect on outcomes, it is the interaction pattern among individuals fostered by the positive interdependence that most powerfully influences productivity, learning, cognitive and social development, and socialization. First, there are cognitive activities and interpersonal dynamics that only occur when students get involved in explaining to each other how the answers to assignments are derived. This includes orally explaining how to solve problems, discussing the nature of the concepts being learned, teaching one's knowledge to classmates, and connecting present with past learning. Second, it is within face-to-face interaction that the opportunity for a wide variety of social influences and patterns emerges. Helping and assisting take place. Accountability to peers, ability to influence each other's reasoning and conclu-

sions, social modeling, social support, and interpersonal rewards all increase as the face-to-face interaction among group members increases. Third, the verbal and nonverbal responses of other group members provide important information concerning a student's performance. To obtain meaningful face-to-face interaction the size of groups needs to be small (from two to six members), as the perception that one's participation and efforts are needed increases as the size of the group decreases. However, as the size of the group increases the amount of pressure peers may place on unmotivated group members increases as well. Whatever the size of the group, the effects of social interaction cannot be achieved through nonsocial substitutes such as instructions and materials.

The third requirement is *individual accountability*, which exists when the performance of each individual student is assessed and the results are given back to the group and the individual. It is important that the group knows who needs more assistance, support, and encouragement in completing the assignment. It is also important that group members know that they cannot "hitchhike" on the work of others. When there is high individual accountability, when it is clear how much effort each member is contributing, when redundant efforts are avoided, when every member is responsible for the final outcome, and when the group is cohesive, then all group members work hard to achieve their goals. The smaller the size of the group, the greater the individual accountability may be. Common ways to structure individual accountability include giving an individual test to each student and randomly selecting one student's product to represent the entire group.

The fourth element of cooperative learning is the appropriate use of *interpersonal and small group skills*. Placing socially unskilled individuals in a group and telling them to cooperate does not guarantee that they are able to do so effectively. Persons must be taught the social skills for high-quality collaboration and be motivated to use them (see Chapter 14). Groups cannot function effectively if students do not have and use the needed collaborative skills. These skills have to be taught just as purposefully and precisely as academic skills. Collaborative skills include leadership, decision-making, trust-building, communication, and conflict-management skills. Procedures and strategies for teaching students social skills may be found in Johnson (1986, 1987), Johnson and F. Johnson (1987), and Johnson et al. (1986).

The final element of good cooperative learning is *group processing,* which exists when group members discuss how well they are achieving their goals and maintaining effective working relationships. Groups need to describe which member actions are helpful and unhelpful and make decisions about which behaviors to continue or change. Such processing enables learning groups to focus on group maintenance, facilitates the learning of collaborative skills, ensures that members receive feedback on their participation, and reminds students to practice collaborative skills consistently. Some of the keys to successful processing are allowing sufficient time for processing to take place, making processing specific rather than vague, maintaining student involvement in processing, reminding students to use their collaborative skills while they process, and ensuring that clear expectations as to the purpose of processing have been communicated (Johnson & F. Johnson, 1987; Johnson & R. Johnson, 1984a).

Each of the five elements contributes to the effective use of cooperative learning.

THE TEACHER'S ROLE IN IMPLEMENTING COOPERATIVE LEARNING

"If I am going to use cooperative learning groups to mainstream David," the teacher muses, "What is my role in doing so? How do I structure and conduct lessons cooperatively? I think I will start with *math.* David is 2 years behind grade level, but I can give him simpler

problems to solve. But whom should he work with? What materials will they need?"

In order to promote effective instruction within cooperative learning situations, the teacher is both an academic expert and a classroom manager. When planning, structuring, and managing cooperative learning activities, teachers must complete the following five activities (Johnson & F. Johnson, 1987; Johnson & R. Johnson, 1984a; Johnson et al., 1986):

1. Specifying the objectives for the lesson
2. Making a number of decisions about placing students in learning groups before the lesson is taught
3. Clearly explaining the task, the positive interdependence, and the learning activity to the students
4. Monitoring the effectiveness of the cooperative learning groups and intervening to teach collaborative skills and to provide assistance in academic learning (such as answering questions and teaching task skills) when it is needed
5. Evaluating the student's achievement and helping students discuss how well they collaborated with each other

Students are taught to look to their peers for assistance, feedback, reinforcement, and support. Students are expected to interact with each other, share ideas and materials, support and encourage each other's academic achievement, orally explain and elaborate the concepts and strategies being learned, and hold each other accountable for learning. A criterion-referenced evaluation system is used.

The following discussion elaborates on these activities and details a procedure for structuring cooperative learning: The subject area discussed is "math." More complete descriptions of how to structure cooperative learning may be found in: *Cooperation in the Classroom* (Johnson & R. Johnson, 1984c), *Learning Together and Alone: Cooperative, Competitive, and Individualistic*

Learning (Johnson & R.T. Johnson, 1987a), *Circles of Learning: Cooperation in the Classroom* (Johnson et al., 1986), and *Structuring Cooperative Learning: The 1987 Handbook* (Johnson & R.T. Johnson, 1987b). Two films are also available that demonstrate the use of cooperative learning procedures (*Belonging* [1980], and *Circles of Learning* [1983]).

Objectives

Two types of objectives need to be specified before the lesson begins: 1) an academic objective specified at the correct level for the students and matched to the right level of instruction, and 2) a collaborative skills objective detailing what interpersonal and small group skills are going to be emphasized during the lesson. A common error many teachers make is to specify only academic objectives and to ignore the collaborative skills objectives needed to train students to cooperate with each other.

Decisions

Deciding on Group Size   Cooperative learning groups tend to range in size from two to six. When students are inexperienced in working cooperatively, when time is short, and when materials are scarce, the size of the group should be two to three. When students become more experienced and skillful, they will be able to manage groups of four or five members. Cooperative learning groups need to be small enough so that every student has to participate actively. A common mistake is to have students work in groups of four, five, and six before the students have the skills to do so competently.

Assigning Students to Groups   Teachers may wish to assign students by ability to heterogeneous or homogeneous learning groups. When working on a specific skill, procedure, or set of facts, homogeneous groups may be useful. When working on problem-solving tasks and on learning basic concepts, heterogeneous groups may be most appropriate. When in doubt, teachers should

use heterogeneous groups where students of different achievement levels in math, ethnic backgrounds, sexes, and social classes work together. Teachers will want to take special care in building a group where students who have special learning problems in math or who are isolated from their peers will be accepted and encouraged to achieve. Random assignment of students to groups is often effective.

Planning How Long Groups will Work Together   The third decision teachers make is how long to keep groups together. Some teachers assign students to groups that last a whole semester or even a whole academic year. Other teachers like to keep a learning group together only long enough to complete a unit or chapter. In some classrooms, student attendance is so unpredictable that teachers form new groups each day. Sooner or later, however, every math student should work with every other classmate. Usually it is preferable to keep groups together for at least 2 or 3 weeks.

Arranging the Room   Members of a learning group should sit close enough to each other that they can share materials and talk to each other quietly and maintain eye contact with all group members. Circles are usually best. The teacher should have clear access lanes to every group. Common mistakes that teachers make in arranging a room are to place students at a rectangular table (where they cannot have eye contact with all other members) or move several desks together (which places students too far apart to communicate quietly with each other and share materials).

Planning Materials   Instructional materials need to be distributed among group members so that all students participate and achieve. Especially when students are inexperienced in cooperating, teachers will want to distribute materials in ways planned to communicate that the assignment is a joint (not an individual) effort and that students are in a "sink-or-swim-together" learning situation. Materials can be arranged like a jigsaw puzzle so that each student has part of the materials needed to complete the task. The step for structuring a jigsaw lesson are to: 1) distribute a set of materials to each group, divide the materials into parts, and give each member one part; 2) assign students the individual tasks of learning and becoming an expert on their part of the material and planning how to teach the material to the other group members; 3) have each student meet with a member of another learning group who is learning the same section of the materials and confer about how best to teach the section to other group members (expert pairs); and 4) have the groups meet and the members teach their area of expertise to the other group members so that all students learn all the assigned material. An alternative to a jigsaw is giving one copy of the materials to a group to ensure that the students will have to work together.

Assigning Roles Cooperative interdependence may also be arranged through the assignment of complementary and interconnected roles to group members. Such roles include a summarizer (who restates the group's major conclusions or answers), a checker (who ensures that all members can explain how to arrive at an answer or conclusion), an accuracy coach (who corrects any mistakes in another member's explanations or summaries), and an elaborator (who asks other members to relate current concepts and strategies to material studied previously). Assigning students such roles is an effective method of teaching them cooperative skills and fostering interdependence.

Academic Task and Cooperative Goal Structure

Explaining the Academic Task Teachers clearly explain the academic task so that students comprehend the assignment and understand the objectives of the lesson. Direct teaching of concepts, principles, and strategies may take place at this point. Teachers may wish to answer any questions students have about the concepts or facts they are to learn or apply in the lesson.

Structuring Positive Goal Interdependence

Teachers communicate to students that they have a group goal and must work collaboratively. This may be done by asking the group to produce a single product or report, arriving at a consensus concerning how assigned problems are solved, providing group rewards, giving bonus points if all members of a group reach a preset criterion of excellence, or picking a student at random to represent the group and explain its conclusions to the class. In a cooperative learning group, students are responsible for learning the assigned material, making sure that all other group members learn the assigned material, and making sure that all other class members learn the assigned material, in that order.

Structuring Individual Accountability The purpose of the learning group is to maximize the learning of each member. Lessons need to be structured so that the level of each student's learning is assessed and that groups provide members with the encouragement and assistance needed to maximize performance. Individual accountability may be structured by having each student individually tested or randomly choosing the work of one member to represent the group as a whole.

Structuring Intergroup Cooperation The positive outcomes found with a cooperative learning group can be extended throughout a whole class by structuring intergroup cooperation. Bonus points may be given if all members of a class reach a preset criterion of excellence. When a group finishes its work, the teacher should encourage the members to go help other groups complete the assignment.

Explaining Criteria for Success Evaluations within cooperatively structured lessons need to be criterion referenced. At the beginning of the lesson teachers need to explain clearly the criterion by which students' work will be evaluated.

Specifying Desired Behaviors The word "cooperative" has many different connotations and uses. Teachers will need to define cooperation operationally by specifying the behaviors that are appropriate and desirable within the learning groups. Beginning behaviors are "stay with your group," "use quiet voices," and "take turns." When groups begin to function effectively, expected behaviors may include having each member explain how to get an answer and asking each member to relate what is being learned to previous learning.

Monitoring and Intervening

Monitoring Students' Behavior The teacher's job begins in earnest when the cooperative learning groups begin working. Much of the teacher's time is spent observing group members to see what problems they are having completing the assignment and working cooperatively. Many teachers also use student observers to gather information on the appropriateness of activities within each group.

Providing Academic Assistance In monitoring the learning groups as they work, teachers will wish to clarify instructions, review important math concepts and strategies, answer questions, and teach academic skills as necessary.

Intervening to Teach Cooperative Skills
While monitoring the learning groups, teachers often find students who do not have the necessary cooperative skills and groups where members are having problems in collaborating. In these cases, the teacher should intervene to suggest more effective procedures for working together and more effective behaviors in which students should engage. Basic interpersonal and small group skills may be directly taught (Johnson, 1986, 1987; Johnson & F. Johnson, 1987).

Providing Closure to Lesson At the end of each lesson, students should be able to summarize what they have learned. Teachers may wish to summarize the major points in the lesson, ask students to recall ideas or give examples, and answer any final questions students have.

Evaluation and Processing

Evaluating Students' Learning Students' work is evaluated, their learning is assessed, and feedback is given as to how their work compares with the criterion of excellence. The quality of students' work as well as the quantity should be addressed.

Assessing How Well the Group Functioned The learning groups assess how well they worked together and plan how to improve their effectiveness in the future. The authors' two favorite questions for doing so are: "What actions helped the group work productively? What actions could be added to make the group even more productive tomorrow?" A common error of many teachers is to provide too brief a time for students to assess the quality of their collaboration.

Summary

Implementing cooperative learning is not easy. Implementing cooperative learning involves a structured, but complex, process. It can take years of practice to become an expert. Teachers may wish to start small by taking one subject area or one class and using cooperative learning procedures they feel comfortable teaching, and then expand into other subject areas or other classes.

IMPACT OF COOPERATIVE EXPERIENCES ON HANDICAPPED AND NONHANDICAPPED STUDENTS

David sits in a group with Frank and Helen. "Will they like me?" he wonders. "What will they do if I make mistakes?"

"Don't worry," the teacher tells him. "Just relax and do your best and everything will be fine."

"We are supposed to make sure everyone in our group learns," thinks Helen. "What if I can't help David learn? What if he refuses to work?"

"Here is the best way to work with David," the teacher tells Helen and Frank. "Ask him to explain how to solve each of his problems. If he does not understand, explain. Encourage him. Praise him when he gets a problem right. Don't criticize him when he does not understand. He will also encourage you and ask you to explain how to solve your problems."

Nearly 500 studies exist documenting the relative efficacy of cooperative, competitive, and individualistic goal structures. This is the oldest existing tradition in American social psychology. There have been 90 years of research on cooperative, competitive, and individualistic efforts. Extensive reviews of this research have been written (Johnson & R. Johnson, 1974, 1978, 1983, in press; Johnson et al., 1983; Johnson, Maruyama, Johnson, Nelson, & Skon, 1981; Sharan, 1980; Slavin, 1983). This section discusses the outcomes of cooperative learning most important for mainstreaming: relationships between handicapped and nonhandicapped students, achievement, self-esteem and psychological health, and social skills.

Relationships between Handicapped and Nonhandicapped Students

There is considerable evidence that cooperative learning experiences, compared with competitive and individualistic ones, promote more positive relationships between handicapped and nonhandicapped students (Johnson & R. Johnson, 1974, 1978, 1983, 1984b, 1985, 1987; Johnson et al., 1983). A recent meta-analysis reviewing all available studies comparing the three types of instructional situations on relationships among students (98 studies conducted between 1944 and 1982) found that these results held among handicapped and nonhandicapped students, students from different ethnic groups, and homogeneous students (Johnson et al., 1983).

The theoretical framework behind the meta-analysis posits the following. Handicapped students are stigmatized and viewed by nonhandicapped peers in negative and prejudicial ways. Physical proximity in and of itself does not change this. Whether the relationships between handicapped and nonhandicapped peers become more negative or more positive depends on how the teacher structures classroom learning. When learning situations are structured cooperatively, and handicapped and nonhandicapped students

work together in the same learning groups, then they: interact in positive ways, feel supported and encouraged to achieve, gain an understanding of each other's perspectives, build a differentiated and realistic view of each other, accept themselves as their peers accept them, feel academically successful, and develop a positive relationship with each other. When learning situations are structured competitively or individualistically, handicapped and nonhandicapped students: do not interact with each other, feel disconnected and rejected by each other, adopt inaccurate perspectives, have monopolistic and oversimplified views of each other, have low self-esteem, are relatively unsuccessful academically, and have negative relationships with each other.

Achievement

Both nonhandicapped and handicapped students achieve more in cooperative than in competitive or individualistic learning situations. A meta-analysis of all the available relevant research studies (122 studies from 1924 to 1981) clearly indicated that cooperative learning experiences result in higher achievement and greater retention of learning than do competitive or individualistic learning experiences (Johnson et al., 1981). In a cooperative learning situation, students at the 50th percentile performed at approximately the 80th percentile of students in competitive and individualistic learning situations. This finding holds true for all age groups, ability levels, subject areas, and learning tasks. Students in cooperative learning situations tend to use higher level thought processes, engage in more higher level oral rehearsal, and discover higher level strategies more frequently than do students in competitive and individualistic learning situations.

Self-esteem and Psychological Health

An important aspect of mainstreaming handicapped students into the regular classroom is the effect it has on their self-esteem. Cooperative learning experiences resulted in higher levels of self-esteem, healthier processes for deriving conclusions about one's self-worth, and greater psychological health than did competitive and individualistic learning experiences (Johnson & R. Johnson, 1974, 1983, 1985, 1987). These findings are true for both handicapped and nonhandicapped students.

Social Skills

Employability rests to a great extent on the ability to work collaboratively with superiors, colleagues, subordinates, and clients. Obviously, students who have had extensive cooperative learning experiences have been found to have more interpersonal and small group skills than did students who have primarily experienced competitive and individualistic learning experiences (Johnson & R. Johnson, 1983). The ability to utilize one's knowledge and resources in collaborative activities with other people in career, family, community, and societal settings was found to be promoted by cooperative learning experiences.

Conclusions

When handicapped students are mainstreamed into the regular classroom, the primary goal is to involve them in constructive relationships with nonhandicapped peers. When cooperative learning is emphasized, that goal is accomplished along with a number of other important instructional outcomes. With the amount of research evidence available, it is surprising that classroom practice is so oriented toward individualistic and competitive learning. It is time for the discrepancy to be reduced between what research indicates is effective and what teachers actually do.

INTEGRATING HANDICAPPED STUDENTS INTO COOPERATIVE LEARNING GROUPS

"The research was right," the teacher thinks. "Frank and Helen sincerely like David. The three of them are working well together. David is happy about being in the regular classroom. Without cooperative learning it may not have worked."

When handicapped students are mainstreamed into cooperative learning groups there are a number of issues that the classroom teacher should consider. The handicapped students may have considerable anxiety about how they will be treated by their nonhandicapped classmates. The nonhandicapped students may be anxious about how to interact with the handicapped students being mainstreamed. The handicapped students may withdraw and be hesitant to interact with their nonhandicapped classmates. In order to create positive and constructive cross-ethnic relationships, handicapped students may be trained in social skills by special education teachers and/or by peers. In addition, nonhandicapped students may need to be trained to be supportive of their handicapped classmates' efforts to achieve and behave appropriately. It will take special arrangements to ensure that the achievement of the academically handicapped students is maximized. Handicapped students may be given academic coaching. Assignments for the handicapped students may be modified and individualized. Careful attention to positive interdependence, individual accountability, collaborative skills, and group processing usually solve such problems. Some suggestions for dealing with such problems follow.

When Handicapped Students are Anxious

Many handicapped students may be fearful and anxious about participating in a cooperative learning group with nonhandicapped peers. Methods of alleviating their anxiety are:

1. Explain the procedures the learning group will follow.
2. Give the handicapped student a structured role so that they understand their responsibilities. Even if a student cannot read, he or

she can listen carefully and summarize what everyone in the group is saying, provide leadership, help to keep the group's work organized, and so forth. There is always some way to facilitate group work, no matter what handicap a student may have.

3. Enlist the aid of a special education teacher to coach the handicapped students in the behaviors and collaborative skills needed within the cooperative group. Pretraining in collaborative skills and periodic sessions to monitor how well the skills are being implemented will increase the handicapped student's confidence.

4. Enlist the aid of a special education teacher to pretrain the handicapped student in the academic skills needed to complete the group's work. Try to give the handicapped student a source of expertise the group will need.

When Nonhandicapped Students are Anxious

Many nonhandicapped students may be concerned that a handicapped student will lower the overall performance of their group. The three major ways of alleviating their concern are:

1. Train nonhandicapped students in helping, tutoring, teaching, and sharing skills. The special education teacher may wish to explain to the group how best to teach the handicapped group members. Many teaching skills, such as the use of praise and prompts, are easily taught to students.

2. Make the academic requirements for the handicapped students reasonable. Ways in which lessons can be adapted so the students at different achievement levels can participate in the same cooperative group are:

   a. Use a different criterion for success for each group member.
   b. Vary the amount each group member is expected to master.
   c. Give group members different assign-

ments, lists, words, or problems, and then use the average percentage worked correctly as the group's score.

   d. Use improvement scores for the handicapped students.

   If it is unclear how to implement these procedures, consult with the special education teacher to decide what is appropriate for the specific handicapped student.

3. Give bonus points to the groups that have handicapped members. This will create a situation in which nonhandicapped students want to work with their handicapped classmates in order to receive the bonus points.

Passive Uninvolvement by Handicapped Students

When handicapped students are turning away from the group, not participating, not paying attention to the group's work, saying little or nothing, showing no enthusiasm, or not bringing their work or materials, the teacher may wish to:

1. Jigsaw materials so that each group member has information the others need. If the passive uninvolved student does not voluntarily contribute his or her information, the other group members will actively involve the student.

2. Divide up roles and assign the passive uninvolved student one that is essential to the group's success.

3. Reward the group with bonus points, grades, or nonacademic rewards on the basis of their average performance, which will encourage other group members to derive strategies for increasing the problem member's involvement.

PROMOTING POSITIVE CROSS-HANDICAPPED RELATIONSHIPS

Two important and interrelated strategies for ensuring mainstreaming success are to train handicapped students in the social skills required for forming friendships and/or to reinforce handicapped students directly for behaving appropriately. In order for handicapped students to use/practice social skills, the teacher must use cooperative learning activities—most social skills are inappropriate during competitive and individualistic learning activities. Further, it takes considerable practice to master interpersonal skills. One or two opportunities a day is not enough. Cooperative learning allows students to practice and be reinforced for using social skills continually throughout the school day. Regular classrooms are better settings for social skills training than are special education classes. In the regular (compared with the special education) classroom there are a greater number of socially skilled peers who can serve as models and coaches for academically and socially handicapped students. Also, the nonhandicapped students may be trained to be supportive of their handicapped classmates' efforts to behave appropriately.

Coaching

Coaching involves directly teaching handicapped students the interpersonal and small group skills they need to interact effectively with their peers. It consists of a three-step procedure:

1. Usually a regular teacher, teacher aide, or special education teacher takes the handicapped student out of the classroom and works one-on-one to teach the handicapped student well-defined social skills.
2. The handicapped student is then given the opportunity to apply the social skills in interactions with nonhandicapped peers while the tutor observes.
3. The tutor then gives the handicapped student feedback on how well he or she enacted the social skills. Further teaching in how to perform the skills is then provided.

This coaching–peer interaction–feedback sequence is repeated several times. Coaching is the most successful of the procedures for teaching social skills. It is difficult to conceive of coaching being used independently from cooperative learning. Heterogeneous cooperative learning groups provide the context within which coaching may take place and social skills may be perfected.

Training in Social Skills

When a new skill, such as "checking" or "encouraging participation," is going to be introduced to the class, the following procedure should be used:

1. Handicapped students may be taken aside by a special education teacher and taught the skill first. They are then prepared to engage in the skill when the group meets, demonstrating expertise in the behaviors being emphasized by the teacher during that session.
2. The teacher may use group contingencies to encourage and reinforce the use of social skills by group members. A group contingency consists of rewarding group members on the basis of the frequency with which group members engage in targeted social skills. This ensures that group members will encourage and cue each other's enactment of the targeted skills. Handicapped students who are pretaught the skills usually earn a number of bonus points for the group, increasing their status with handicapped groupmates.
3. Nonhandicapped students who are socially skilled may serve as models for less skilled handicapped peers, teaching social skills through guided examples. Withdrawn, poorly accepted, or otherwise socially unsuccessful students see, and interact with, peers who successfully engage in appropriate behaviors and are reinforced for doing so.
4. Group processing may be used to ensure that both handicapped and nonhandicapped students engage in the metacognitive thought (thinking about how they are thinking) required to develop self-monitoring (observe

how well they are performing) and self-control. At the end of each group session the teacher has group members evaluate their use of the targeted skills on a checklist and share their self-ratings with the group. By discussing how frequently they and other members demonstrated the targeted skills, students enhance their self-monitoring and self-control.

Training Nonhandicapped Students to be Supportive

When handicapped students are placed in cooperative learning groups with nonhandicapped peers, there is some danger that the nonhandicapped students will be bewildered and puzzled by the handicaps and will not understand how best to help the handicapped students learn. It is often useful for the following to be done:

1. The special education teacher trains the nonhandicapped students in the procedures and skills most effective for teaching their handicapped groupmate. These teaching strategies may be either general or specifically tailored to the handicap of the group member.
2. Nonhandicapped students may be taught how to provide support and encouragement for handicapped groupmates. General training in encouraging participation, praising efforts, and generally serving as a cheering section for handicapped students may ensure that the interaction is constructive.
3. Group identity may be enhanced to create "ingroup feeling." When a high sense of group identity is present, all members will be accepted and supported as "one of the group."

MAXIMIZING HANDICAPPED STUDENTS' ACHIEVEMENT

To maximize handicapped students' achievement in the regular classroom the regular teacher may

wish to ensure periodically that handicapped students are trained to have a special academic expertise, can explain what they have learned both within the group and in subsequent individual situations, and are given assignments appropriate for their ability level.

Giving Handicapped Students Academic Expertise

Constructive relationships between handicapped and nonhandicapped students are facilitated when multidimensional views of each other are present. Such multidimensional interpersonal perceptions are facilitated when handicapped students behave in ways that clearly contradict the stereotyped view of them by their nonhandicapped peers. Thus, if handicapped students are perceived to be academically limited, creating situations in which they have clear academic expertise will help promote more constructive cross-handicap relationships. Procedures for creating academic expertise by handicapped students include the following:

1. The day (or for several days) before a new group assignment is given, a special education teacher or a teacher's aide may tutor the handicapped student in the material to be covered. The handicapped student then becomes the group's expert on the material. If the group is going to discuss a certain reading assignment, for example, the handicapped student can be taught the assignment by a tutor prior to the group meeting.
2. Pair the handicapped student with one of the better (academically) students in the class, and have the pair meet to discuss the assignment and make sure that both members understand the assignment. Then have pairs combine into groups of four and repeat the process. Such preparation pairs are also effective during jigsaw lessons when each pair studies a different aspect of the assignment. When groups report, the rule that each group member must make half of the presentation must be enforced to ensure that the handi-

capped students' expertise is demonstrated and perceived.

Ensuring Handicapped Students Can Explain How to Derive Answers

One of the potential problems with integrating learning disabled and academically handicapped students into cooperative learning groups with nonhandicapped peers is that the handicapped students may fail to understand the material the group is studying. There is some fear that the brighter students will simply tell the handicapped students answers without ensuring that the handicapped students really understand how to complete the assignment. In order to ensure that handicapped students do in fact understand the material they are studying, the teacher should:

1. Emphasize the role of checker to ensure that the handicapped student is able to explain how the answers were obtained or the rationale for the group's conclusions. The checker ensures that *all* group members are able to explain how to complete the assignment. A common mistake made in working with low-achieving students is to have them listen to explanations rather than give explanations. The role of checker is critical to good cooperative learning (especially when academically handicapped students are being mainstreamed) because it requires all members of the group to give explanations.
2. Give the handicapped student a partner who is responsible for ensuring that the handicapped student understands and can explain the work.
3. Emphasize individual accountability and give frequent assessments of how much each member of the group has learned in order to ensure that group members help handicapped students complete the assignments and understand the material being studied.
4. Use improvement scores rather than absolute scores. For the handicapped students, im-

proving over their past performance may be the appropriate way to reward achievement.
5. Encourage nonhandicapped students to give encouragement and support to (i.e., be a cheering section for) handicapped groupmates.

Another concern about the achievement of low-performing, learning disabled, academically handicapped students is whether they can transfer what they learn in cooperative groups to situations in which they are required to demonstrate their knowledge and skills individually, by themselves. This is a matter of positive interdependence and individual accountability, the combination of which requires group members to be concerned with each other's learning. The handicapped students should periodically be: 1) required individually to take tests outside of the group setting to demonstrate their knowledge and skills, and 2) assigned to new groups and be required to teach the nonhandicapped members of the new group what they have learned in their previous group or preparation pair. All group members should be given training in how to "check for understanding," "elaborate," and "explain clearly how to complete the assignment."

Individualizing Material for Diverse Students

One of the problems for teachers is how to ensure that a lesson will be appropriate for all members of the class. Often a lesson directed at students at one achievement level is too difficult or too easy for students at another. This situation can lead to frustration or boredom, respectively, on the part of students at the low or high ends of the academic skills continuum. In turn, these feelings can precipitate behavior problems and lack of motivation to learn. Teachers often feel that: 1) they do not have the special skills needed to effectively construct a lesson for students with learning problems because they have not received special training in these areas; and 2) the time spent in developing such lessons, or in managing the behavior of motivational problems of mainstreamed students, takes time that they should be spending with their other students who are more likely to profit from their efforts. In actual fact, it is usually easier to individualize instruction in a class where cooperative learning dominates than in a class where individualistic learning dominates. Within cooperative groups:

1. Students may be trained by the special education teacher to provide an idiosyncratic teaching program specifically geared to the handicapped member of their group.
2. The quantity and level of work required may be varied within the group as easily as within the entire classroom. Handicapped students may be overwhelmed by the quantity of the work required or by the level of the work required. Thus, the amount of work required, the level of the work required, and the criterion for success may all be adapted to the capacity of the group member. Handicapped students may be required to do less work or to do simpler work and may then be evaluated on the basis of the percentage correct or their improvement scores.

SUMMARY

Whether mainstreaming results in positive or negative outcomes for handicapped and nonhandicapped students depends on how teachers structure classroom learning. If positive cross-handicapped relationships are to be established and the achievement and social development of both handicapped and nonhandicapped students are to be maximized, learning situations should be structured cooperatively, not competitively or individualistically. For cooperative learning to be most effective, positive interdependence, individual accountability, training in collaborative skills, and processing of how effectively the group is working have to occur. The specific procedures teachers need to structure cooperative learning have been specified and validated through numerous research studies. Mainstreaming may be implemented successfully and promote positive cross-handicap relationships, achievement, student self-esteem and psychological health, and social skills, but it probably requires the predominant use of cooperative learning procedures. When handicapped students are mainstreamed into cooperative learning groups there are a number of issues that the classroom teacher should consider. The handicapped students may have considerable anxiety about how they will be treated by their nonhandicapped classmates. The nonhandicapped students may be anxious about how to interact with the handicapped students being mainstreamed. The handicapped students may withdraw and be hesitant to interact with their nonhandicapped classmates. In order to create positive and constructive cross-handicap relationships, handicapped students may be trained in social skills by special education teachers and/or by peers. In addition, nonhandicapped students may need to be trained to be supportive of their handicapped classmates' efforts to achieve and behave appropriately. It will take special arrangements such as academic coaching and individualizing the work required of handicapped students to ensure that the achievement of the academically-handicapped students is maximized.

STUDY QUESTIONS

1. What is the definition of cooperative learning?
2. What are the five basic elements of a well-structured cooperative lesson?
3. Why is cooperative learning an essential component of mainstreaming?
4. What are the steps in the teacher's role for structuring a cooperative lesson?
5. What is the impact of cooperative experiences on handicapped and nonhandicapped students?
6. How may handicapped students be integrated into cooperative learning groups?

REFERENCES

Belonging [16 mm film]. (1980). Edina, MN: Interaction Book Co.

Circles of learning [16 mm film]. (1983). Edina, MN: Interaction Book Co.

Deutsch, M. (1962). Cooperation and trust: Some theoretical notes. In M. Jones (Ed.), *Nebraska symposium on motivation* (pp. 275–319). Lincoln: University of Nebraska Press.

Johnson, D.W. (1986). *Reaching out: Interpersonal effectiveness and self-actualization* (3rd ed.). Englewood Cliffs, NJ: Prentice-Hall.

Johnson, D.W. (1987). *Human relations and your career* (3rd ed.). Englewood Cliffs, NJ: Prentice-Hall.

Johnson, D.W., & Johnson, F. (1987). *Joining together: Group theory and group skills* (3rd ed.). Englewood Cliffs, NJ: Prentice-Hall.

Johnson, D.W., & Johnson, R. (1974). Instructional structure: Cooperative, competitive, or individualistic. *Review of Educational Research, 44,* 213–240.

Johnson, D.W., & Johnson, R. (1978). Cooperative, competitive and individualistic learning. *Journal of Research and Development in Education, 12,* 3–15.

Johnson, D.W., & Johnson, R. (1983). The socialization and achievement crisis: Are cooperative learning experiences the solution? In L. Bickman (Ed.), *Applied social psychology annual 4* (pp. 119–164). Beverly Hills: Sage Publications.

Johnson, D.W., & Johnson, R. (1984a). Building acceptance of differences between handicapped and nonhandicapped students: The effects of cooperative and individualistic problems. *Journal of Social Psychology, 122,* 257–267.

Johnson, D.W., & Johnson, R.T. (1984b). Classroom learning structure and attitudes toward handicapped students in mainstream settings: A theoretical model and research evidence. In R. Jones (Ed.), *Special education in transition: Attitudes toward the handicapped* (pp. 118–142). Reston, VA: The Council for Exceptional Children.

Johnson, D.W., & Johnson, R. (1984c). *Cooperation in the classroom.* Edina, MN: Interaction Book Co.

Johnson, D.W., & Johnson, R.T. (1985). Impact of classroom organization and instructional methods on the effectiveness of mainstreaming. In C.J. Meisel (Ed.), *Mainstreamed handicapped children: Outcomes, controversies and new directions.* New York: Lawrence Erlbaum.

Johnson, D.W., & Johnson, R.T. (1986a). Mainstreaming and cooperative learning strategies. *Exceptional Children, 52*(6), 553–561.

Johnson, D.W., & Johnson, R.T. (1986b). Motivational processes in cooperative, competitive, and individualistic learning situations. In C. Ames & R. Ames (Eds.), *Attitudes and attitude change in special education: Its theory and practice* (pp. 249–286). New York: Academic Press.

Johnson, D.W., & Johnson, R.T. (1987a). *Learning together and alone: Cooperative, competitive, and individualistic learning.* Englewood Cliffs, NJ: Prentice-Hall.

Johnson, D.W., & Johnson, R.T. (1987b). *Structuring cooperative learning: The 1987 handbook.* Edina, MN: Interaction Book Co.

Johnson, D.W., & Johnson, R. (in press). Cooperative learning. In S. Kagan, D.W. Johnson, & R. Johnson (Eds.), *Handbook of cooperative learning methods.*

Johnson, D.W., Johnson, R., & Holubec, E. (1986). *Circles of learning: Cooperation in the classroom* (rev. ed.). Edina, MN: Interaction Book Co.

Johnson, D.W., Johnson, R., & Maruyama, G. (1983). Interdependence and interpersonal attraction among heterogeneous and homogeneous individuals: A theoretical formulation and meta-analysis of the research. *Review of Educational Research, 53,* 5–54.

Johnson, D.W., Maruyama, G., Johnson, R., Nelson, D., & Skon, L. (1981). The effects of cooperative, competitive, and individualistic goal structures on achievement: A meta-analysis. *Psychological Bulletin, 89,* 47–62.

Kerr, N. (1983). The dispensability of member effort and group motivation losses: Free-rider effects. *Journal of Personality and Social Psychology, 44,* 78–94.

Sharan, S. (1980). Cooperative learning in small groups: Recent methods and effects on achievement, attitudes, and ethnic relations. *Review of Educational Research, 50,* 241–271.

Slavin, R. (1983). *Cooperative learning.* New York: Longman.

CHAPTER 12

MICROCOMPUTERS AND NEW TECHNOLOGIES

Peggy B. Wilson,
Vicki R. Casella, and William C. Wilson

Initially, educational computer technology was viewed primarily as a vehicle for accelerating the learning of mathematics and for promoting scientific study. This was accomplished with selected students in a relatively isolated computer laboratory environment. This view of the use of computers in education persisted until two significant advances in computer technology occurred: 1) the introduction of microbased processors (the central processing units utilized in personal computers), and 2) the development of educational software programs that addressed a wide range of curriculum objectives. The advancement of both hardware (computer equipment) and software (instructional programs) has created an explosion in the development of computer technology designed specifically for classroom and curriculum applications.

The emergence of new microtechnology is changing the concept of computer usage from a luxury item with limited accessibility to an everyday tool necessary in today's world. The use of computers in education has had major impact on our educational structure and educational strategies for teaching students with disabilities. The use of computers has reinforced the importance of individualized learning and has broadened opportunities for educators to ensure equal educational opportunities for all children, especially those with special needs.

INDIVIDUALIZATION AND ACCESSIBILITY: FEDERAL LEGISLATION

Although the computer can provide some obvious avenues for addressing individual differences, access to equipment and software has not been as available to special populations as it has been to nondisabled or gifted populations. Thus, equal education opportunity pertaining to the access and use of computers has become an item of discussion for school districts and an implementation problem for many principals.

Section 504 of the Rehabilitation Act of 1973 (PL 93-112) clearly stated that discrimination against handicapped persons was illegal. Thus, all school districts must assure that persons with disabilities are provided the same rights and opportunities to all educational programs as their nondisabled peers. While the law was written long before computers became commonplace in classrooms throughout the United States, the application of the principle is rather simplistic; that is, individuals with disabilities have the same rights and privileges pertaining to the use of computers in educational programs as do nondisabled individuals.

The 1986 amendments to the Rehabilitation Act (PL 99-506) included new language that specifically addressed the emergence of new electronic technological applications. A new section, 508, directed the government to develop guidelines for electronic accessibility. The intention of the guidelines is to reinforce the premise of non-discrimination as delineated in Section 504 and to extend to persons with disabilities the rights to electronic equipment and special peripherals.

Less problematic are new approaches to individualized learning, thus extending the individualized education program (IEP) provisions of the Education for all Handicapped Children Act (PL 94-142) into the world of technology. New software, adaptive devices, and hardware are now included as tools for learning and are written as part of many IEPs. Thus, two important federal mandates, written in the mid-1970s, can serve as standards for the distribution and use of micro-technology in special education and rehabilitation programs. These laws can serve as a force for assisting individuals with disabilities in achieving and maintaining academic, social, and independent living goals in our society.

MICROCOMPUTERS AND THE INTEGRATION OF STUDENTS WITH DISABILITIES

The remainder of this chapter addresses how computers and other technological tools are being used to facilitate the integration of students with special learning needs into the academic mainstream by providing: 1) access to curriculum, 2) opportunity for social interaction, 3) enhancement of communication options, and 4) development of personal productivity skills. These actions are described within the context of an educational model that follows.

EDUCATIONAL MODEL

Historical Model and Resulting Negative Effects

In many instances, the introduction of technology into academic settings has instituted radical changes in educational assessment, planning, implementation, and evaluation. In no area has this change been greater than with students with special needs. When special education developed as a profession, a positive concern for meeting the special needs of students frequently resulted in an isolationist situation. Students' deficit skills were pinpointed, special strategies were developed to remediate those skills, and these plans were implemented in a program that required the student to be relegated to a self-contained special classroom, or periodically pulled out of the regular academic program for remedial work. The structure of pull-out programs or self-contained educational environments may help some students; however, the structure does not serve all students to the best advantage. The disadvantages to this type of program include: 1) problems in teacher scheduling, 2) disruption of students' important academic and social interactions, 3) unrealistic time constraints on students, 4) lack of communication among professionals, 5) ambiguity in purpose, 6) discrepancy in presentation strategies of academic information, 7) stigma attached to "special" status, 8) breakdown in communication between caregivers and professionals, 9) lack of consistency in expectations, and 10) fostering of students' dependency on an exclusive educational environment.

New Service Model

A critical examination of special education policies and practices has resulted in a shift of focus within the delivery structure. Four major elements have emerged in the new educational model for service delivery. These reflect the future direction for special education in that:

1. The integration of the student with special needs into the regular academic setting has become a major emphasis.
2. Special education personnel serve in a consultant or supportive role to the classroom teacher and to the student.
3. Many new strategies and tools have been incorporated to ensure academic and social integration of special needs students.
4. Strategies include a closer examination of

curriculum goals and objectives, cooperative learning groups, peer and cross-age tutoring, and the implementation of microcomputer technology.

Some of the most exciting changes in service delivery have occurred in the use of high technology with the special needs population within the regular classroom environment. The most publicized aspect of this technology has centered around the computer serving as a "voice" for severely disabled, nonoral students. This, however, is only one example of the effectiveness of appropriately utilizing the computer in facilitating the integration of special needs students into the educational mainstream. For many learning disabled students, a carefully selected word processing program with a thesaurus and spelling check system has become a vehicle to produce legible written communication. Students who need many repetitions of a task in order to develop a shorter response time with increased accuracy are finding the computer a far more effective learning tool than the traditional flashcards and ditto worksheets. Visually handicapped students are developing independence in the preparation of reports and written assignments through the use of "talking" word processors on the computer.

In many instances, the technology plays an alternative or supportive role in the integration of students with special needs, such as a writing tool for a learning handicapped student. For others, however, the computer is the very basis or the cornerstone of the integration process, the only viable access to communication and academic information. As the above examples illustrate, effective uses of microcomputer technology can facilitate the academic and social integration of special education students into regular education programs within the context of an appropriate service delivery model.

CONCERNS TO BE ADDRESSED

Although a model is a means to an end, the current model, as it pertains to the educational use of computers for special needs students, cannot be successful without the usual support systems and adequate guidelines for the selection and use of technological advances (i.e., hardware and software). Concerns about computers in education also need to be addressed. Four major areas of concern include: 1) equipment, 2) teacher education, 3) curriculum, and 4) individual student needs. The issues, questions, and answers that follow should provide some practical guidelines for educational personnel utilizing technology to facilitate integration.

Equipment

When microtechnology first became available for education, the major questions centered on hardware. Educators were concerned about which brand of computers would be appropriate, how much memory would be required, what peripheral equipment would be necessary, and which computer would support curriculum goals and objectives. Frequently, however, financial considerations overshadowed the importance of addressing these questions, and educational administrators made purchasing decisions directed by an economic rather than a programmatic basis. Special education programs receiving consideration for computer equipment were limited to those serving academically gifted students. This trend has changed considerably and teachers have become involved in program and purchasing decisions. In addition, a major effort has been expended toward meeting the federal mandates affording access to all students, regardless of handicapping condition.

Teacher Education

Once computers had been purchased and placed in the schools the major concern became one of how to get teachers involved in using the machines in order to implement curriculum goals and objectives. Questions revolved around the types of training necessary to develop expertise and to effect change as well as the attitudinal changes necessary to assure success. The most important question was how to successfully redefine the role of the classroom teacher in order to emphasize the planner/facilitator responsibility rather than the traditional teacher/leader responsibility. Many districts chose to meet this challenge by providing inservice training for teachers and by joining in a cooperative effort with universities to initiate pre-service training for prospective teachers. Technology resource centers were established in many areas to provide on-site support and training. One of the more effective techniques in the redefinition of roles has been the implementation of a teacher-coach training model. In this model, on-site mentor teachers are identified and provide coaching and support for teachers seeking to develop specific skills. The issue of changing negative attitudes toward the use of computers has yet to be addressed effectively. For many teachers, the application of technology has been transitory and its usefulness limited to narrow, hi-tech–related endeavors, such as computer programming or business education applications. However, while the regular education community has viewed the implementation of high-technology education with guarded optimism, special education teachers have been most receptive to incorporating computers into their curriculum.

Curriculum

Utilization of technology in education has greatly affected the content and delivery of the academic curriculum. Answers to the following questions are being sought by teachers, parents, and administrators in order to provide them with information that will facilitate the integration of this technology into the curriculum.

Which areas of the curriculum can be served effectively by the use of a computer?   Initially, math and science were the major curriculum areas most affected by the introduction of technology. Educational computer consortia have contributed to extending the use of technology (primarily computers) into additional curriculum areas. A broad spectrum of skills is now addressed through commercial software. Most recently, the need for software that facilitates the

student in transition has been realized and many vocational/career-related programs are now available. The inclusion of alternative input options in the software and the development of adaptive/assistive devices have assured academic access to all students, even those with severe physical handicaps.

How can use of the computer dictate or initiate changes in the existing curriculum?   At the onset of educational technology, computers were used primarily to complement and implement the existing curriculum. However, when educators began to understand its capabilities, the computer became a tool for radically expanding the learning process. For example, some of the most sought after software programs, such as *Rocky's Boots,* from The Learning Company, and *The Factory,* developed by Sunburst Communications, extend beyond traditional curriculum guidelines and offer simulations that can promote the development of higher order thinking skills. These simulations challenge children to formulate hypotheses, develop strategies, implement a plan, test the results, evaluate the situation, and make modifications based on the evaluation. The strategies children develop using these programs can be useful in resolving problems that occur in other aspects of their academic, personal, social, and vocational environments. The computer and accompanying software has thus removed numerous physical and academic barriers for many handicapped students and has allowed them the same experiences and opportunities as their nonhandicapped peers.

How can schedules and materials be modified to reflect the curriculum changes?   The installation of computers in many school programs has been achieved through the creation of laboratories through which all eligible students are rotated on a regular basis. The manager of the computer lab is generally in control of the schedule and, frequently, even assumes the responsibility of academic programming for the students. In other schools, computers have been placed at the disposal of the classroom teacher who is responsible for determining how they will be used in meeting curriculum goals and what materials need to be purchased or developed to implement given educational objectives. Scheduling and material modifications will only be helpful if the teaching faculty or computer room supervisors are sufficiently well versed in applications that are being presented. Although software is now much easier for the novice to use and apply to learning situations, often inservice training will be the only professional alternative available to teachers who still face the dilemma of having to train themselves, develop lesson plans incorporating the material, and successfully use the software with students having a variety of educational disabilities.

What criteria should be used in the selection of software? Particular attention should be paid to the accuracy of the academic content of the program and to the manner in which it evaluates a student's response. For example, when the program asks a question to which there are several correct responses (e.g., answers to the questions "Who was the first president of the United States?" could be: George Washington, Washington, or G. Washington), it should accept any of the correct alternatives, not simply one specific response. Beyond this, ideally the criteria employed to select software will be dictated by the teaching style of the instructor, the specific needs of the student who will be the end user, and the goals and objectives of the curriculum. Professional journals such as the *Journal of Special Education Technology* (see Test, 1985) and organizations such as the National Council for Teachers of Mathematics (see Heck, Johnson, & Kansky, 1981) have published guidelines for evaluating software in the specific curriculum areas and for specific needs. These guidelines provide a framework from which teachers may select those criteria that are pertinent to their particular teaching situation.

Who is responsible for the selection and evaluation of educational software? Common strategies employed by schools include: 1) a district-wide committee evaluates software and offers a recommended list for the various subjects and grades; 2) the school establishes a software evaluation committee; 3) principals, with or without teacher input, determine software purchases; 4) individual teachers select software for class use; or 5) computer lab managers or computer resource teachers purchase software for school-wide use. The crucial concern should be meeting the needs of all the teachers and students at a particular site. Students with special learning needs must be considered in the selection and evaluation of software.

How would the software be implemented into the curriculum? The determining factors in formulating a response to this question are the physical location of the computers, the attitude of the classroom teacher toward the role of computers in education, the particular subject area being taught, and the teaching strategies employed by the teacher. While many teachers choose to use the computer as an integral part of a unit of study, others choose to develop separate computer activities that enhance a particular subject. On the one hand, if the computers are located in a laboratory setting and the class has access on a scheduled basis, the teacher may choose to introduce a topic, develop classroom activities to ensure that students have a basic understanding, and then use the computer lab time to allow students to practice to mastery. On the other hand, if the teacher has access to a computer in the classroom, a software program may be selected to aid in the introduction of a concept to the entire class, with the teacher using the computer as an extension of the curriculum materials available.

Individual Student Needs

A close examination of these aspects of change led logically to evaluating the student and assessing how the computer could be used to the best advantage to meet the child's academic, social, and emotional needs. The process of meeting an individual student's needs can be broken down into two major areas: 1) the evaluation/placement process, and 2) the provision of services. The renewed thrust toward integrating the special needs student into the regular education program can be greatly enhanced through the use of existing technology in both areas of this process.

TECHNOLOGY IN THE EDUCATIONAL PROCESS

Microtechnology can be used to facilitate the integration of a special needs student into the mainstream education program if professionals involved in the evaluation/placement process and provision of services are aware of the contributions computer hardware and software can make. Personnel responsible for the management of a student's individualized education program (IEP) are required to:

1. Conduct and report a total educational assessment
2. Develop an education program plan
3. Identify a supportive team to realize program goals
4. Participate in the selection of appropriate materials and supplies, including microtechnology hardware and software
5. Conference, consult, and/or train the educational team members, including teachers, parents, and supportive personnel
6. Monitor the student's progress after placement has been made
7. Evaluate the effectiveness of the components of the educational program
8. Recommend modifications to the student's program as necessary

Not only can the computer make a significant contribution to the student's successful integration, but computer technology can have an important function in most aspects of the placement and provision of services process.

Conducting Assessment

Software programs have been developed that help in the educational evaluation of students' performance. These programs can serve as diagnostic tools for analyzing specific problems in various academic areas. For example, *Math Assistant I* and *Math Assistant II,* from Scholastic software, were designed to help diagnose problems and pinpoint the specific place where a student errs as he or she learns the four basic arithmetic operations. These programs also have a feature that monitors and records each student's progress. Some researchers have also found the use of software in the assessment stage to be highly effective in the areas of spelling (Hasselbring & Crossland, 1981) and reading (Mason, 1980). As with most assessment tools, caution must be exercised in interpreting the results. Varnhagen and Gerber (1984) delineate some of the concerns associated with use of the computer in the assessment process.

One of the most important functions the computer can perform in the assessment process is in the preparation of the report. The most frequently used software at this stage is a word processing program; however, there are programs available such as the *WISC-R Computer Report* by Charles Nicholson (1983), from Southern MicroSystems for Educators, that generate reports based upon comparisons of subtest data that the tester inputs.

Developing Individualized Education Program Plan

Software companies have spent considerable time and money in creating programs to assist in the development of an IEP for a student. These programs are available for personal computers and for district-wide mainframe equipment. The typical format of these programs is as follows: 1) biographical information on the student is typed into the program, 2) the scores and/or observational data from the assessment are entered, 3) educational objectives that correlate to the assessment data are selected from the program's data bank of criterion-based objectives, and 4) an education plan is generated for a given student.

The above-listed attributes of computerized IEP software may be helpful to program personnel but may raise questions about "canned" IEPs with generic objectives. Computer software programs become far more useful if: 1) the format of the printout can be customized to correspond to district-mandated forms, 2) the overall goals and objectives can be modified by individual teachers or by district curriculum personnel, 3) teachers or support personnel can selectively choose specific objectives from those displayed by the program for a child, 4) the program allows for update information or record keeping on a student's education plan, 5) statistical information regarding one or more students can be retrieved for developing reports and proposals, and 6) the developers of the program provide ready technical assistance and update information on the software. Programs that offer these components are found in the *Individualized Planning System* and *Curriculum Management System* by Kirk Wilson, from Learning Tools Inc. of Cambridge, Massachusetts.

Some district personnel report that the time and expense involved in developing a computer-based educational planning system is justified because: 1) in the long run, it saves an inordinate amount of professional time in the creation of an IEP; 2) the goals and objectives are specific to their given school program; 3) teachers and other support personnel can be involved in the development and selection of the content, and therefore have a greater understanding of and commitment to the educational goals included; and 4) the use of the program ensures a developmentally sequential education plan for students from year to year.

Identifying Education Team

Within each school district there is a wealth of talent. However, accessing pertinent information about each person whose input might be relevant or critical in a given situation is exceedingly difficult due, in part, to a breakdown of communication among various departments. A central computerized clearinghouse can alleviate this difficulty and greatly simplify the process. A data management program that identifies the person, specifies strengths and talents, indicates schedules and assignments, and contains other relevant information, makes the process of assembling a team a much easier task and ensures that the student's needs are being addressed by the best service personnel in the district.

Selecting Materials and Supplies

Once an individual's education program has been established, it is necessary to determine the role technology will assume in meeting the defined goals and objectives. This step in the process is difficult and time consuming because the more viable decisions concerning the educational use of computers are made by persons who keep abreast of all the current published research and descriptive data concerning the effectiveness of computer applications in education, and who have an in-depth knowledge of available equipment and software. The technology, itself, can play an important part in the gathering of this information. An example of an information network used daily by thousands of educational personnel is SpecialNet, a sophisticated telecommunications network that encompasses various organizations and affords the capability of two-way communication via a modem (telephone access device). SpecialNet is the largest known educational network of "electronic bulletin boards" on a variety of subjects including news items, legislation, jobs, software, and adaptive devices. Users pay a subscription fee and then are able to dial and search through the on-line information to locate the necessary resources quickly. "Special Education Solutions" is an electronic data file on SpecialNet that lists high-technology as well as other resources available to persons with disabilities. This is an on-line data file, maintained by the Apple Computer Corporation and available to anyone using an Apple computer and a modem. The system contains 1,000 entries. Similarly, *Apple Link: Personal Edition* is a nationally available on-line information service that utilizes a question-and-answer format in ord ⁀ to provide users with updated information pertair ng to a number of education technology–related issues. In order to access this network, the consumer purchases a subscription from an Apple dealer and via the modem comes "on-line" with the system. Much of this information for special education needs is also reprinted in *Apple Computer Resources in Special Education and Rehabilitation* (Brightman, 1988).

Conducting Teacher/Parent Inservice Training

Implementing an education program requires the cooperation and commitment of a team of people. The computer can be used as a tool to develop inservice training handouts, generate schedules, and track progress. Several software companies provide videotapes for training on how to use the computer to assist in meeting educational goals. Sunburst Communications has taken a leadership role in developing videotapes that present their computer programs and demonstrate how they can be used in a classroom situation. These include *Bears, Monsters and Frogs: An Approach to Problem Solving* and *Using Databases in the Classroom,* designed by Sunburst Communications and the Bank Street College of Education.

Monitoring Student Progress

Record keeping and reporting is a time-consuming, but vital responsibility that must be undertaken to ensure that a placement decision was accurate and that the student's educational success is being monitored appropriately. Many software programs facilitate this task by providing a record-keeping utility built into the program. Students' records can be saved and printed out so that progress may be determined. Data-management and spreadsheet programs can assist in record keeping and charting for a student. A well-designed gradebook program can show each student's success rate numerically or graphically. Report writing can also be simplified with the use of a word processing program.

Evaluating Effectiveness

The careful selection of software can facilitate this stage of the process. Using the computer to perform statistical calculations on the student's record of performance will help give an objective view of each component of the education program. The computer's ability to analyze errors and recognize error patterns not only assists in the evaluation process, but also provides the teacher with information necessary to design intervention strategies to address critical skill development for each student.

Recommending Modifications

Students' needs constantly change and programs must be modified to address these changing situations. Using the information gathered through the evaluation process, educators can further use the computer to prepare reports and the collected data to justify recommending any modifications in the child's education program.

TECHNOLOGY IN THE INTEGRATION PROCESS

Once the decision regarding the student's placement within the mainstream has been made, the emerging role of the special education teacher dictates a shared responsibility with the regular classroom teacher for the planning and development of the student's integrated education programs, including the introduction and use of the new technology. There are three major steps in this process: 1) determining the role technology will play in the mainstreaming process, 2) assessing the current use of technology in the classroom and curriculum, and 3) developing intervention strategies to integrate the use of computers into the education program.

Role of Technology

The first step is to determine whether the computer or other microprocessor-based technology will serve as a cornerstone in the child's educational placement, or whether it will serve as an adjunct to traditional educational materials.

A Cornerstone   Historically, when a student's handicapping condition precluded his or her full participation, with little or no assistance, in a regular classroom environment, he or she was regulated to a specialized institution or to an isolated education program. This was particularly true for severely physically involved students who were incapable of oral or written communication. A computer with selected assistive/adaptive devices can serve to minimize the effects of the disability on the communication process and provide an avenue for effective integration into the mainstream that would otherwise be more difficult, if not impossible.

Adjunct to Traditional Materials Frequently, the student with special needs has met with failure using traditional educational materials in situations led by teachers using standard teaching techniques. Research studies (Arms, 1984; Bell, 1983; Kleiman, Humphrey, & Lindsay, 1983) have shown that students are greatly motivated by the use of a computer in educational situations. Skillful teaching combined with appropriate use of the computer may help provide a key to effective integration of students into the regular classroom. Strategies developed to use technology that have proven to be effective were those that could be readily incorporated into the existing class structure with minimal disruption.

Current Use in the Classroom and Curriculum

Once it has been determined that the use of technology will be incorporated into the student's integrated education plan, the second step in the process is to ascertain how the technology is currently being used in the schools. Computers may be used by educators: 1) to promote mastery through repetitive drill, 2) in a tutorial/practice mode to augment traditional instruction, 3) to help students develop generalizable problem-solving skills, 4) as supplementary instructional material, 5) to encourage students to incorporate independent learning strategies to achieve increased personal productivity, and 6) to provide access to verbal and written communication through the use of adaptive/assistive computer equipment.

Figure 1 illustrates a hierarchical use of the computer with special needs students, with drill-and-practice software being the most frequently used type of program and communication software being the least often used. The diagram further illustrates the sophistication of use in that the easiest and most common use of the computer for special needs students involves a drill-and-practice format. The most sophisticated and least frequent use of the computer and one that involves the most training is as an augmentative communication aid, with adaptive/assistive devices providing access for physically and communicatively disabled students.

Although only one of the current uses of computer technology by educators is specifically for students with disabilities, all have contributed to the successful integration of these students into the academic mainstream of education. This integration process is more readily accomplished when the teacher has first determined how the computer is to be used to assist all students in achieving educational goals in the classroom, how the technology can complement his or her particular teaching style, and which areas of the curriculum lend themselves to computer-assisted instruction.

When these decisions have been made through a systematic approach to decision making, as illustrated in Figure 2, appropriate intervention strategies that address specific needs of the integrated special learner must be developed. Those strategies that have been most successful have not been developed in isolation, but rather have been an integral part of the decision-making process.

Development of Integration Strategies

The development of specific strategies is the third step in incorporating the use of technology in the planning and development of a student's integrated education program. There are many variables that will influence the development of strategies, including: the location of the computer, the teacher's access to the equipment, available software, and the teacher's commitment to the use of technology. However, the major considerations are

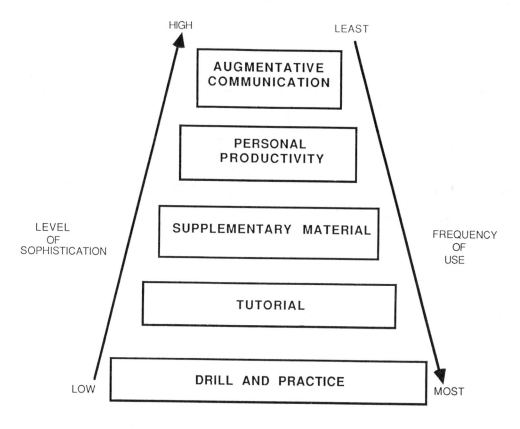

SOFTWARE: USE vs. LEVEL OF SOPHISTICATION

Figure 1. A hierarchical use of computer software with special needs students.

the current use of technology, the educational situation, the needs of the student, and the educational objectives. It is within this context that specific integration strategies are discussed in the next section.

INTEGRATION STRATEGIES

Promoting Mastery through Repetitive Drill

Computer Use

Promoting mastery through repetitive drill is the most common use of computers in education.

Teachers view the software as an alternative or supplement to traditional workbooks or practice sheets. Drill-and-practice software programs do not introduce new material, but can present questions, prompt for answers, evaluate input, and indicate correct or incorrect responses. The purpose of these programs is to promote mastery and to assist the student in developing a rapid response time.

Student Needs

Specific learning characteristics of students should be identified prior to selecting drill-and-practice software. Drill-and-practice software has been used successfully with students who:

Computer Assistance Decision Making Process

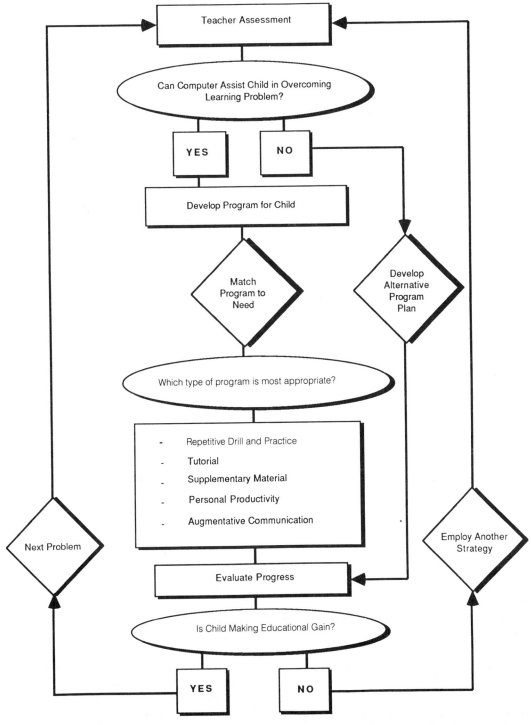

Figure 2. Computer assistance in the decision-making process for helping a child overcome a learning problem.

Fully understand a concept

Need repetitive presentation to achieve mastery

Benefit from immediate feedback for a response

Have repeatedly failed using traditional materials and presentation methods

Want or need an opportunity to practice in private

Can work without constant adult supervision

Intervention

Using the computer for drill and practice has proven to be effective for many students with special needs (Chiang, 1986). Integrating this use of the computer can be achieved through skillful selection of software programs, careful structuring of the classroom schedule, and effective use of volunteers or paraprofessionals. The successful intervention strategies that follow were systematically developed, based on a thorough examination of the existing situation and cooperatively planned objectives for the student.

Situation Leslie, a 10-year-old boy, has been identified as learning handicapped and is in need of remedial work. The student assessment team has determined Leslie's appropriate placement to be in a regular classroom with assistance from a special education resource teacher. Math is the academic area in which he has the most difficulty, but he cannot be scheduled for special assistance during the math time slot in the regular class. Leslie is grouped with the lowest level math group, but cannot compete successfully even in this placement. This situation has resulted in Leslie's exhibiting nonattending behaviors during the math activity, causing a disruption for the other students. In addition to supplemental math material, the regular classroom teacher has a computer in her room and has a small collection of educational software programs.

Objective(s) The regular classroom teacher and the resource specialist worked together to develop a plan for meeting Leslie's needs under the prevailing educational situation. The teachers decided: 1) to provide a viable math activity within the classroom for Leslie even though he could not participate successfully in any of the established

groups, 2) to schedule the math activity on the same timetable as for the other students, 3) to increase Leslie's ability to work independently, and 4) to assist Leslie toward mastery of basic math facts.

Strategies The intervention plan included extensive use of the computer to reach the basic objectives.

1. The classroom computer schedule was arranged so that Leslie was on the computer, working at the appropriate level, while the class was involved in group work that was inappropriate for him.

2. The computer was used to diagnose and remediate specific problem areas so that Leslie could work independently. Two separate software programs were helpful in this step of the plan. The special education resource teacher used *Math Assistant I* and *Math Assistant II*, from Scholastic Software, to provide an item analysis on specific problem areas in Leslie's understanding of the four basic arithmetic operations. Once the problem areas were identified, two drill-and-practice programs were selected for his use in the regular classroom. The series of basic math programs, *Basic Skills In Addition, Basic Skills in Subtraction, Basic Skills in Multiplication,* and *Basic Skills in Division,* from Love Publishing Company, provided the foundation for the use of the computer. These programs give students systematic practice in the four fundamental mathematic functions by: 1) giving the student a placement test, 2) branching to the appropriate skill level determined by the performance on the placement tests and providing tutorial and/or practice at that level, 3) allowing the student to take a self-test to determine whether more practice is needed, and 4) administering a mastery test for the specific level assigned to the student. This program records and stores the scores for this test for teacher use. Both the special resource teacher and the classroom teacher found this

information valuable in developing future lesson plans and targeting specific problem areas. Additional software programs, *Stickybear Math* and *Stickybear Math 2*, produced by Optimum Resource, Inc., were selected to provide a game format for drilling Leslie on basic math facts.

3. Leslie was grouped for computer work with others who functioned at a slightly higher level in math. These students acted as peer tutors around the computer. As he had experienced success on computer-generated math problems prior to working with other students, Leslie felt comfortable in this situation and was able to accept the prompting and modeling provided by his peers. The peer group realized that Leslie, given time and some coaching, was capable of completing the assignments and this transferred into their acceptance of him in their social activities. This peer-tutoring situation gave Leslie an opportunity to develop and practice appropriate social interaction skills in a structured environment, and the skills he learned in one situation were quickly generalized into other social interactions and situations.

4. Arrangements were made for a volunteer to assist Leslie with work on a computer. A high school student doing an independent study project was selected to monitor his progress and to provide input as necessary. This "big brother" situation gave Leslie even more social status in the classroom as well as helping him develop the math skills necessary to accomplish his assignments. The high school student requested a 2-month extension on his assignment in order to stay with Leslie until the end of the school year.

Special Considerations The computer can be a valuable learning tool in this situation if the work presented is at an appropriate level and progress is monitored. Care should be taken not to foster dependency on either individuals or the computer and opportunities should be provided to assure transfer and mastery of skill.

It is critical that students fully understand the concept being practiced prior to using drill-and-practice software or the student will perpetuate errors and become more frustrated in the learning process. If additional or different instruction on the concept is needed, perhaps the more appropriate use of the computer would be in a tutorial/practice mode.

Tutorial/Practice Mode to Augment Traditional Instruction

Computer Use

Tutorial software is a far more sophisticated programming and instructional design task than software developed for drill and practice. While the latter is used to reinforce and enhance learning that was initially introduced, tutorial software is designed to take on the responsibility for actually teaching a new skill or concept. A well-designed tutorial uses text explanations, descriptions, and diagrams and other graphic illustrations to introduce new material; probes for understanding with different question formats; and then, poses various problems for the student to solve. If the student experiences difficulty with a given part of the concept, a quality tutorial program detects the specific problem area; provides an alternative explanation; allows additional practice; and after the student demonstrates understanding, moves on to introduce the next segment of the material.

Student Needs

Frequently students have difficulty grasping a new concept. This difficulty may be due to a myriad of reasons, having nothing to do with the intellectual level of the student or the complexity of the concept. An examination of the problem may reveal that the student has processed some parts of the concept, but has misunderstood others or that more practice is needed on a given area before total understanding can take place. Many times just having the concept explained in a different way will clarify any problems and the student will be able to proceed with no difficulty. Tutorial programs have been helpful to students who:

Need a consistent, systematic presentation of new material

Need prompting through a multistep process, such as manipulation of fractions

Need corrective feedback with explanation of error

Need an alternative to the traditional presentation of material

Need modeling and examples provided

Need guided practice to ensure understanding of new material

Intervention

In every educational situation a teacher must present new information to a disparate group of students, and if all students are to benefit from the presentation, the teacher must adapt the presentation to meet the needs of individual students, provide for significant amounts of student interaction and participation, and test for understanding of the concept. The selection and use of a well-designed tutorial software program can alleviate some of the pressure that comes with providing for the individual needs of students.

Situation Amanda was having difficulty learning long division. The teacher introduced the process to the entire class, worked several examples on the board, and then gave students worksheets to practice. The concept was presented in the textbook and examples were given. After repeated tries at mastering the information and being unsuccessful, Amanda, as well as numerous other students, had become frustrated and discouraged with the classwork and homework assignments. The teacher had tried all the conventional material in her classroom and was interested in trying other approaches.

Objective(s) The classroom teacher and Amanda's parents included objectives in her plan that would assist in maximizing her success. The following intervention plan, which has generic applicability for students facing similar situations,

was developed: 1) to provide additional instruction on the concept; 2) to introduce the process in a systematic presentation; 3) to provide alternative instruction and practice material; 4) to monitor progress carefully; and 5) to allow for private, supervised, individual practice time.

Strategies The objectives, as they were developed, required an inordinate amount of individual attention for each student. The teacher had no additional help in the classroom; therefore, the use of a computer became a vital tool in meeting the objectives. This was accomplished through the selection of tutorial software programs, the use of peer tutors, and effective communication between the school and the parents.

1. Tutorials were selected that:
   a. Provided an introductory component that showed students how to complete the task, step by step
   b. Allowed the students to choose the level of difficulty of the problems and determine the number of digits in the divisor
   c. Prompted the students where to place the next number in each step of working the problem
   d. Displayed the correct answer after two errors were made at any one step and provided a hint as to what should be done
   e. Tutored the students when they asked for help by providing an explanatory sentence with an example
   f. Printed out the students' scores along with a message of encouragement or praise
   g. Presented problems and prompted for solutions in a consistent manner
2. Amanda was scheduled on the computer for individual time and her parents, who had a home computer, were encouraged to provide the same tutorial program for her at home.
3. A computer schedule was generated that placed the students having difficulty at the computer with students who understood the concept. This allowed for peer tutoring and

some supervision for the students who were having problems.

4. Once Amanda had mastered the concept, she became a peer tutor and helped those still having difficulty. Frequently when students with special needs receive intensive individual training on a given concept, they become far more adept at completing the task than those students who understand the concept marginally and try to master the task without the benefit of special instruction. When this situation exists, it is an excellent time to allow the student with special needs to move beyond the role of student and into the realm of tutor. This usually results in tremendous gains in self-esteem for the tutor and a greater acceptance of the special needs student on the part of the person receiving the help. Letting students go through the process of explaining the concept and monitoring another student also reinforces their mastery of the material.

Special Considerations Very few good tutorial software programs are available and currently they are best considered as an instructional tool for a capable educator, rather than as a replacement for traditional instruction (Willis, 1987). In the selection of these programs, teachers must be concerned that: 1) the vocabulary is consistent with class presentation, 2) the reading level is appropriate for students, 3) all steps leading toward understanding are clear and presented with the same consideration for mastery, 4) the presentation is free from gaps in information, and 5) the presentation of the concept is not contradictory to the presentation of information given in class.

Some of the problems encountered in using tutorial software center around the rigidity in the thinking process that these programs can reinforce. Alternative methods are not encouraged. They often give a narrow presentation and the material is devoid of context. One of the most obvious criticisms is that they do not stimulate varied approaches to problem solving, but rather embody the principle that there is only one way that is the right way. There are uses of the computer, however, that actually encourage an exploration-and-discovery approach to problem solving.

Developing Generalizable Problem-Solving Skills

In analyzing research findings and reports, Willis (1987) points out characteristics that differentiate sophisticated thinkers from less skilled thinkers: "the ability to take in information, organize it into meaningful units, extract the essence or principles of truth contained in the information into a set of general rules, and then put it to work solving other problems" (p. 111). Unfortunately, far too little attention is paid in our society to the development of critical-thinking skills, the development of strategies for inquiry, or the ability to think analytically. Recently, however, many schools have included the development of critical-thinking skills and problem-solving strategies in their curricula. Such resource guides as *CompuTHINK* (Hamilton & Saylor, 1986) *Problem Solving Workshop* (Sunburst Communications, 1985) and *Teaching to the Third Power* (Wisenand et al., 1986), provide teachers with a framework, strategies, examples of applications, and computer software integration into problem solving. These guides use generalizable strategies for solving problems that have been identified and taught to students of various ages. Simply stated, given a problem situation where the solution is not obvious, the student must get enough information to understand the problem, organize the information, decide on a strategy or plan, try it out, and then check to see if it worked. Students learn that they can organize the information to make it coherent and useful and that there are logical systems they can use rather than just random guessing. Those approaches that help students to search for and organize information, look for a pattern and develop steps to getting to an answer are called problem-solving strategies. The use of strategies and collaboration to find alternatives are encouraged rather than simply competition to get the answer. These strategies include such generalizable skills as: 1) making an organized list, chart, or table; 2) using simple objects or drawing a picture to represent parts of the problem; 3) simplifying the problem or breaking it into parts; 4) working backwards or re-creating the pattern; and 5) using guess-and-check or trial-and-error. Strategies may be used singly or in combination and help the student to arrange or represent information and use it to test, synthesize, and implement solutions to new problems. Such critical-thinking skills can be used to solve problems in other content areas such as science, mathematics, and language arts. In solving problems students build confidence and flexibility of thinking that transfers to other "real world" experiences.

Computer Use

The computer and the right kind of software can aid in the development of these strategies or tactics of learning in several ways. Specific strategies such as making tables or lists, working backwards, and using a simple model are incorporated in software designed to teach problem solving. Several kinds of programs have been designed to facilitate the acquisition of problem-solving skills: 1) programs that introduce strategies for problem solving, 2) programs that teach processes for solving specific problems, 3) programs that encourage exploration and discovery to address problems, and 4) programs that require the development of multiple approaches for problem solving. The purpose of this type of software is to stimulate divergent thinking, encourage creative approaches to the resolution of problems, and develop systematic approaches to problem situations that may transfer to other personal and academic areas. One of the major advantages to using problem-solving or simulation software is that it lends itself to group presentations and joint efforts. Methods and materials for teachers and analyses of software are now available in *CompuTHINK* (Hamilton & Saylor, 1986) and *Teaching to the Third Power* (Wisenand et al., 1986)

Student Needs

Many students refuse to try to solve a problem unless the strategy and solution are familiar. For those who do try, difficulties in problem solving arise when: 1) the student has developed the attitude that there is only one way to solve every problem, 2) the student does not see the pattern or procedure that makes information coherent or logical, 3) the student does not proceed to seek unknown information and organize the information, and 4) the student exhibits rigidity in thinking and fear of failure that preclude attempts at employing multiple strategies. Software that involves the student in breaking these habits and establishing new patterns has been successful with students who need to develop:

An orderly process to approach any problem
Generalizable strategies for working through new
    situations
Divergent thinking skills
Sufficient self-confidence to undertake risks

Intervention

Effective use of this type of educational software requires considerable planning and preteaching. Programs proven to be most valuable in developing these skills are those that provide initial modeling of the problem-solving routines, instructor-guided practice using the program, and independent or group practice with appropriate feedback. Successful strategies incorporating problem-solving skills through the use of computers have been very effective in facilitating the integration of students with special needs. Students are assigned different roles commonly used in cooperative groups such as: the doer, the prober, the summarizer, the questioner, the praiser, and the recorder. The most popular programs supply teacher support materials for preteaching, student worksheets, and other similar problems for students to do off the computer.

Situation Ryan is a learning disabled seventh-grade student. He has good visual-spatial skills but reads at a third-grade level. He is reluctant to try most classroom tasks if reading is involved because of his history of failure. He is withdrawn and quiet, and never volunteers. Even if he has an idea of what the answer might be he would rather be a nonparticipant than be "wrong" in front of his peers.

Objective(s) The regular classroom teacher would like to assist Ryan in: 1) participating in small and large groups, 2) learning and using problem-solving strategies, 3) building on a strength area to strengthen a need, 4) strengthening organizing and classifying skills, 5) building self-confidence, and 6) strengthening word recognition skills.

Strategies The intervention plan included some preplanning and a range of components, first off the computer and then incorporating it. These included:

1. Grouping the students
2. Developing cooperative working groups
3. Learning and practicing problem-solving vocabulary and strategies
4. Building on a strength
5. Organizing and classifying
6. Word recognition
7. Curriculum application

The regular classroom teacher had already introduced concepts of attributes such as shape, size, color, and direction. Furthermore, she used these attributes in a matrix to show how they could be organized in columns or rows based on an attribute or rule. She then introduced a Venn diagram as another way of organizing by attributes or rules where items may share or combine rules or properties. By showing the properties of two overlapping groups the learners were able to predict the properties of the items where the groups overlapped. Students were thus familiar with attributes and generating rules about combining them.

At the same time, students were put into cooperative learning groups and given practice on working cooperatively within a group. Ryan was assigned roles first as a praiser and then as a doer, each of which gave him important social and task-specific roles. Since he was good at visual-spatial tasks he could usually figure out the answer, but had occasional difficulty with being able to describe his use of rules verbally and frequently was unable to tell how he arrived at his answer. The strategies of using a matrix and/or diagram to organize the attributes were extended into two more projects on classifying; one on endangered species and one on characteristics of their classmates such as height, birth month, hair color, and favorite foods. The students were required to use the proper vocabulary when describing items and their properties. The teacher skillfully gave problems requiring students to find examples of a rule such as "all of the members of a set were brown." Once this was accomplished the students would do the reverse and look at sets to see if they could find a common property or rule based on color, shape, or filling. Once the students could do this task the problem was presented in text form. Ryan worked on the vocabulary, spelling, and comprehension of the text with his resource room teacher. He also did exercises on properties of words and visualizing their meanings.

For the computer application the teacher chose *High Wire Logic,* by Sunburst Communications, Inc., for the major activity. The students were again grouped and new rules of combinations of attributes were presented in paper-and-pencil tasks. The students were given worksheets that contained small matrices that helped them organize the information and look for patterns and combinations rules such as filled and blue. In teams or groups of four they would scan the examples provided by the computer and check those shapes that fit the rules and those that did not. They would then develop rules that fit the sets they were given, type them into the computer, and test their assumptions. Since each problem often had many correct answers they also recorded the answers they had used on a separate steno pad and kept track of the greatest number of rules they had been able to generate.

During this activity Ryan was a fully participating member of his team. He shifted to the different roles on his team easily because of the structure of the program. When entering the attributes for the rules only the first letter of each word was required. To facilitate this the teacher had left a card above the keyboard stating the possible attributes and rules. Ryan was able to use his strengths to help solve the problems; his difficulties with the text had minimal impact—first, because of the structure of the matrix, and second, because only the first letter was required when entering into the computer. When he served as recorder all he had to do was copy the correct rule from the screen. Since he was a contributing member of a high-scoring team, Ryan was valued by his classmates. With each example having more than one correct answer, the students were required to be flexible in their thinking and shift from one attribute or rule to another.

Special Considerations   There was other software available that addressed some of the concepts and skills that the teacher first introduced on the use of matrices. The decision not to use this software was made because: the screens and graphics appealed to a much younger student, it did not use text at all, and it did not lend itself to group participation. For students to generalize a strategy such as using a chart or matrix, it must be used in the content areas of the curriculum in addition to the computer activity. A matrix is particularly useful as an organizing strategy and the attributes are easy to control and observe. The teacher in the above situation asked other teachers to use these strategies in their classes, and also offered awards to students who thought of useful ways of employing the strategies.

As Supplementary Instructional Material

Computer Use

Although this is a relatively new use of computers in education, it is appealing to teachers because it: 1) can provide an alternative way to present curriculum content to the entire class or to a single student; 2) can drastically reduce the amount of time necessary for the preparation of materials; and 3) can allow access to the curriculum for individuals who, prior to the introduction of technology in education, were unable to participate fully or independently. Since this is an area that has not been explored in depth, several different situations illustrating the use of computers as supplementary instructional material are given.

Student Needs

Students with special needs frequently develop an expectation of failure because of previous experience with traditional materials and methods of presentation. The novelty of the computer and the ability of programs to present information in a structured sequence, in small, manageable steps can aid in breaking the "failure cycle." For example, seeing 20 problems on a worksheet may completely overwhelm a student. Those same 20 problems may pose no difficulty if presented 1 at a time on the computer, with intermittent reinforcement for completion. Historically, situations exist where the student with special needs is denied access to classes and information due to health, sensory, or physical access problems. Here again, the computer can aid in alleviating this situation. In general, this use of the computer is effective with students who exhibit one or more of the following conditions:

Need alternative to traditional material
Cannot physically manipulate materials
Sensory impairment makes access impossible
Need organized presentation of materials
Need individualized instructional material generated

Intervention

The integration strategy employed in this use category varies with the situation, the student, and the student's needs. These uses of the technology frequently make more demands initially on the educators involved and require additional training for mastery, on the part of both the teacher and the student; but ultimately, the time and training result in immeasurable benefits.

Situation 1 Christina is an honors high school student with aspirations of attending a major university to obtain a degree in science. She had successfully completed all the academic work undertaken at the high school level and went to her advisor to register for classes for the next semester. Chemistry was one of the curriculum courses recommended for the college-bound students and Christina looked forward to taking the class. The advisor refused to allow Christina to register because she has cerebral palsy, is in a wheelchair, and has limited use of her upper extremities. The chemistry class requires a laboratory and he felt that Christina would pose a hazard to herself and others in that setting. He would not allow her to take the class without the lab and refused to discuss placing her with a lab partner so that she could participate, as an observer, in the experiments.

Objective(s) The special education resource person assigned to monitor Christina's progress has determined that her physical limitations should not limit her educational opportunities. In coordination with the chemistry instructor, a computer programmer, and Christina, the following objectives were developed: 1) that Christina would be registered in the chemistry class with the other 10th-grade students, 2) that a viable alternative would be found for the laboratory component of the class, and 3) that Christina would successfully master the information presented in class and in the lab in order to qualify for college admission.

Strategies The intervention plan included the use of peers, volunteers, and the use of an Apple computer.

1. All students in the lab were assigned partners on a rotating basis so that every 2 weeks the grouping changed. This precluded one student from shouldering the responsibility for conducting all the experiments for the semester. This particular strategy worked so well in Christina's class that the chemistry lab in-

structor decided to structure all the lab situations the same way. They found that much more sharing of responsibility took place and that students were more willing to change their role in the lab when the grouping was constantly changing.

2. A search was launched for a chemistry lab simulation software program that would allow Christina to perform the experiments on the screen, without danger to herself or others. This was the hardest objective to meet. Several programs were tested and parts of each were excellent, but other areas were poor or weak. *Chem Lab,* from Simon and Schuster, was determined to meet most of the needs presented in this situation. This program contains 50 different experiments with thousands of possible combinations of chemicals and was, by far, the most realistic of the chemistry laboratory simulations.

3. A request for a software programmer to assist in the modification of some of the existing software was issued. A student from a local university volunteered to help modify software when possible, and create programs when necessary.

4. The teacher wanted to be sure Christina understood the sequence of specific procedures; therefore, a parent volunteer offered to come during the teacher's planning time and allow Christina to "talk" her through the various steps. The teacher graded her in exactly the same manner the other students were evaluated.

Situation 2 Susan is a fifth-grade student who has severely limited use of her right arm and restricted use of her left. Intellectually, Susan tests above average and she is able to maintain her grades in a regular fifth-grade class. The one difficulty faced by Susan is how to complete written assignments. She is unable to use traditional writing materials and there is an increasing amount of written work required.

Objective(s) Working in conjunction with

the regular educator, the special education supportive services team at the school and Susan's parents developed a plan to ensure that Susan would be able to participate fully in the classroom activities. This plan involved: 1) securing an alternative to traditional writing materials for Susan, 2) not removing Susan from the regular class to generate written assignments, 3) a supportive service team member providing assistance for Susan in learning to operate the alternative material or equipment, and 4) Susan's family taking an active role in her education program.

Strategies All members of the educational team were committed to assisting Susan develop her skills to the point that she could independently manage the required written assignments. The computer, on a portable stand with a printer, was seen as an excellent means to accomplish these objectives.

1. Susan has dependable use of her left hand; therefore, a Dvorak Left-Handed Keyboard modification was added to an Apple IIe computer and a printer was provided.

2. A typing program, *MicroType, The Wonderful World of PAWS* (Haugo, Hausmann, & Jackson; South-Western Publishing Company) was purchased for school and home use. The occupational therapist devoted part of the individual therapy time to developing the fine motor skills necessary for typing. A constant monitoring of Susan's improvement showed that she gained weekly in speed on the keyboard.

3. A word processing program, *MultiScribe,* from Scholastic Software, was selected for her use as a writing tool. This program is simple to operate, yet is a powerful word processing tool.

4. An analysis of the written assignments was done with the regular classroom teacher, and changes were made to accommodate Susan's speed in completing the work. For example, the teacher required the students to write each of the questions at the end of the chapter in the various content areas and then answer them. Entire sentences had to be copied when it was necessary to fill in a blank. To ensure that Susan be able to finish the work in the assigned period, she was given permission to type only the answer rather than the complete question or sentence.

5. Susan's speed on the keyboard, initially, kept her from writing the long creative stories she was able to tell. Rather than lose the creativity in Susan's story writing, a peer who was skilled at the keyboard would act as her secretary and type in the story as Susan told it.

6. Susan's family bought the software programs used in school and set aside time each evening for her to practice the skills learned in school. A unified approach to developing the various strategies for Susan's integration into the regular class proved to be most effective as she is now able to complete her assignments independently.

Situation 3 Cleveland, a fifth-grade student, is in a regular class for every subject area, but requires extensive remedial instruction in all areas of reading and in written language skills. He is highly verbal and can readily understand and recall information that is presented orally. His ability to relate new data to his existing information base is exceptional. In spite of these obvious strengths, Cleveland has limited opportunity to participate in most language arts activities in the classroom and has little respect from his peers. In order to gain status, Cleveland frequently resorts to aggressive and disruptive behaviors in class.

Objective(s) The regular classroom teacher sought assistance from the special education resource specialist and the computer resource teacher in developing a plan that would emphasize Cleveland's skills and allow a more acceptable participatory role in class activities. The plan included: 1) the selection of software that could be used in a group situation, 2) the development of a support team for Cleveland from among his peers,

3) the provision of opportunities for Cleveland to be involved in oral presentations, 4) the development of activities that would allow Cleveland to take a leadership role in verbal discussions, and 5) the use of software that encouraged exploration and discovery to resolve situations.

Strategies Fortunately, just as these plans were being formulated, Tom Snyder Productions released a new genre of software, *Decisions, Decisions,* that allowed opportunities for all of the objectives to be met. This software forms the basis or outline for class/group decision-making activities. The computer presents information, the teacher facilitates class discussions, and students investigate the possibilities and learn group process skills while they attempt to arrive at a decision. The plan to meet the objectives for Cleveland involved:

1. A situation familiar to the entire class was selected from the *Decisions, Decisions* software packages. One of them, *Immigration: Maintaining the Open Door,* from Tom Snyder Productions, was particularly appropriate for this class as the school's population is primarily from ethnic minorities, many of whom are first-generation American-born.
2. A set of activities was conducted to introduce the class to group process skills, such as quality circle, paraphrasing, brainstorming, and so forth. After the concepts were introduced, the class broke up into small groups to practice some of the principles. Cleveland was designated as a group leader and was charged with the responsibility of seeing that the group functioned appropriately.
3. The major questions addressed in the software were introduced to the class and research teams were developed to gather information they felt would be necessary to solve the problem presented in the program. Cleveland was assigned a major responsibility in the group, that of monitoring the progress of each of the members of his team. This allowed him to participate even though much of

the reading material was too difficult for him to understand.

4. The teams met to debrief from their research efforts by giving verbal reports. This provided Cleveland with the content he would need to participate in the class discussions. Cleveland acted as a group facilitator in this debriefing process. Students reminded him when he was too aggressive in his role and he responded appropriately.
5. When the software was used with the entire class Cleveland was given the responsibility of summarizing the information presented from each of the discussions. This allowed him to use his strength of relating new information to his existing information base and to exercise his strong verbal skills. Cleveland's participation was exemplary. He contributed significantly to the discussions and when he spoke out of turn, a gentle reminder from the teacher or one of the students was all that was necessary to get complete cooperation.

Special Considerations Frequently teachers are faced with seemingly impossible situations in terms of access to information by students with special needs. The resolutions of these difficulties can often be found in appropriate use of computer hardware and software. This use, however, takes more planning and a greater time commitment from educators. It is important to keep in mind that ultimately, due to this involvement, the student can develop critical skills that will allow him or her to lead a more independent and productive life.

Achieving Increased Personal Productivity

Computer Use

Productivity initially came from business use of computers. This began with word processing, to which spell checking, and recently thesauruses such as *Bank Street Writer III,* from Scholastic Software, were added. Now personal productivity software includes organization and time and task management (*Pacesetter,* from MindPlay, and *Homeworker,* from Davidson and Associates) and personal budgeting (*Touch Window,* from Personal Touch Corporation). Increasing a student's ability to do more higher quality work in a shorter time by using productivity software has the potential for very significant impact. The ongoing development of computers and software is making it possible to meet the needs of most mildly disabled students.

Student Needs

While all students can benefit from using the type of productivity software listed above, it is of particular importance to students who have problems with any aspect of written expression, including:

Difficulty with penmanship, spelling, or word finding
Problems with elements of sentence structure or paragraph development
Problems with postwriting evaluation and editing
Difficulty organizing or keeping information and relating that to the accomplishment of assignments in the classroom

Situation   Jim is a 15-year-old student with learning disabilities and a long history of problems with writing. He had difficulty with spelling, punctuation, vocabulary, sentence structure, and organizing and sequencing his ideas. While he wrote in sentences, he tended to use the same simple sentence structures repeatedly—active, affirmative, declarative. Jim had difficulty getting his thoughts in order, both verbally and in writing. Paragraphs contained a number of unrelated sentences. He had little variation in vocabulary, tending to use the same terms repeatedly. He still had a high rate of misspelled words and rarely caught his own errors even on short words. His handwriting was barely legible and though he had been asked to skip lines he frequently forgot. This frustrated teachers who wanted to help him. Without the assistance of the resource specialist, Jim had difficulty completing even one assignment.

Objective(s)   Several of Jim's teachers wanted him to use word processing to complete his written assignments. But, as noted above, Jim needed more than just word processing. Any objectives developed for Jim had to be commensurate with the following: 1) Jim needed to have access to software that would address his skill deficits, and 2) he needed to have software that would help him to develop his skills while compensating for his weaknesses.

Strategies   This student had such a wide range of problems with written language that several strategies were required. These had to be planned, integrated, and sequenced in order to have the desired effect. The resource teacher was required to team up with the business education teacher, the English teacher, Jim, and his parents to set the plan in motion. A year-long plan with checkpoints at specified intervals would provide a more comprehensive approach. First, Jim needed to take typing and learn keyboarding, using a typing tutorial to learn typing on a computer, in his business education class. This would provide Jim with the basics to help him find solutions to his other writing problems. Next he would learn word processing. *Bank Street Writer III,* from Scholastic Software, would be a good choice since it meets several needs:

1.   It is easy to learn and use. *Bank Street Writer III* would make use of Jim's strong visual skills by using a "mouse" to move to the part of the screen to be used. The mouse would help him to select simple "pull down" command menus on the screen so that he would not have to learn confusing command codes for such tasks as underlining or moving text.

2.   This word processing program also contains a spell checker. The spell checking software would allow Jim to check any word when he was uncertain; he could also spell check his whole document for both spelling and typographical errors. This would not automatically change words to correct spelling but would select words not found in its "dictio-

nary," highlight them, and suggest correct alternatives that might be put in place of the word in question.

3. The program also has a thesaurus capability. First a word is selected, then the computer checks its lists and a number of synonyms are suggested. As with the spell checker, the computer "looked up" the word but Jim had to decide which word to use.

Jim needed to develop good prewriting skills as well. Jim wanted to write about bicycle racing, a sport in which he is an expert. The English teacher has taught the components of a good composition in class. A prewriting activity using the "clusters" technique was conducted and all of the students developed the components of the information that they will put into an outline before they write their composition. This requires visualization, a strength for Jim. He had lots of good information and was able to construct a well-developed cluster.

The English teacher introduced the *Writer's Helper* (Conduit) program in her class. This software offers a number of different prewriting and writing activities. Each of these was presented in class. Jim selected three: the "Trees" prewriting activity to further organize his ideas, and "Paragraph Writing" and the "Five Paragraph Theme" to help him get his ideas into sentences and properly sequenced paragraphs.

The structure of the *"Five Paragraph Theme"* exercise provided a breakthrough. It began by asking Jim for his point of view on his topic, bicycle racing, and then asked for three topic sentences. The program continues by asking for further information, in sentence form, on each of the topic sentences. When the student is finished supplying the information, the program takes all the sentences and assembles them into a five-paragraph theme. It adds transitions where needed to make sense.

Once the theme was created, it needed editing. Jim saved his document as a file for the *Bank Street Writer III* word processing program, from Scholastic Software. His first task was to use the spell checker on his theme. When his errors were

pointed out by the computer, he corrected them. Next he tried to find as many of his own grammatical errors as possible and made any other editing changes he could. He then printed this draft and showed it to his teacher. More changes were suggested so he used his word processor to do the cutting, pasting, and adding. Finally he used the program's thesaurus to find synonyms for the words that he overused. With those changes in place, he printed up another version of his essay for the teacher's review. He now had a readable paper with complete sentences, properly sequenced flow, correct spelling, and clearly expressed ideas. Later he was able to use his own transition phrases in place of those generated by the computer.

To capitalize on his strengths in art and design, Jim made a diagram for his paper showing various bicycle-riding safety equipment.

Situation 2 A group of high school students in a learning disabilities resource class were having difficulty planning and carrying out assignments in their other classes. Most frequent difficulties were: 1) not being able to clearly describe the task, 2) inability to break the task down into manageable and sequential parts, and 3) inability to "manage" time and the activities to get the task done.

Objective(s) The resource room teacher and the students agreed to implement the following strategies: 1) students will outline their assignments such as a book report or short term paper, and 2) on one assignment they would estimate the time required for each part and schedule themselves on a calendar for each component. They would report their progress to the group twice a week.

Strategies The teacher introduced a new program called *PaceSetter,* by Mindplay. Three of the group decided to use it, while three others used their traditional methods. Those who used *PaceSetter* followed the computer steps through the process. They outlined the steps, described them, and printed out their expanded outline. Next, they scheduled themselves enough time to complete each activity. Third, as they began work on any section of the project they posted their progress in *PaceSetter* and got a progress report for the teacher. Two of the students stayed with the task and used *PaceSetter* to help structure and manage their assignments. The third student decided it was too much trouble to continue to use the tool and felt she could do the task just by sticking with the initial outline she printed.

At the end of the assigned time, the students who used *PaceSetter,* by Mindplay, as a management tool had their class project as well as the printed reports of their progress. Both reported that using the software took more time initially; however, it was worth it because they could monitor their progress and get a better idea of how much time it took them to do the various components of the assignment. The updated reports encouraged them to continue and try to stay on the schedule they had set for themselves rather than procrastinate or turn in the assignment late. Since the reports were printed out they felt that this was an "official" note to their teacher of their taking responsibility for their own progress. One student who was working part time also used it to schedule his work duties and times so he could keep track of both.

Special Considerations   Word processing is a tremendous productivity tool for learning disabled students. It does not take the place of prewriting or editing nor can it tell students what makes a good sentence or paragraph. This must be done by a teacher. Spell checkers, grammar checkers, and thesauruses are helpful but have limitations of accuracy and still rely on the user's choice. Some word processors have built-in "clairvoyance" (*MindReader* by Kalman Toth, from Brown Bag Software, 1988, and *WriteNow* for IBM, from Airus). As the user types in the first two to three letters of a word, a window flashes on the screen with the word or alternatives the computer has determined that the user may be just about ready to type. If any one of the suggested words is correct the user may select it and it will be put into the text.

Situation 3   Several learning disabled high school students, seen by the same resource specialist, were all experiencing the same problem. They were able to do the work assigned to them with some assistance, but were receiving failing grades because of their not turning in homework and extended assignments on time. All of the students were generally disorganized with their school materials, frequently forgot to take home critical texts for an exam, or would leave necessary materials in their locker when they came for help in the resource room.

Objective(s)   After numerous discussions with the regular class teachers, a sequence of strategies was suggested for assisting these students with this problem of disorganization and poor time management. These strategies were developed: 1) to provide the students with a systematic record of their assignments, 2) to report various assignments to the resource specialist, and 3) to provide the students a structure for completing assignments.

Strategies   The team of teachers working with these students developed a plan and all were willing to cooperate to see that it was implemented and that its success was monitored. The sequence of the intervention was as follows:

1. Each morning the students reported to the resource specialist's room before their first class and received a pack of index cards with the class names written on them.
2. As they attended each class, they wrote any assignment on the appropriate index card and indicated the due date.
3. All were scheduled to receive assistance in the resource room at the end of the academic school day. Some had art, physical education, or another nonacademic classes after their resource room class, but these classes rarely had extended assignments.
4. In the resource room they were taught to use the "Calendar" feature in the software program *HomeWorker,* from Davidson and Associates, to keep track of their extended assignments. This feature allows one to create a

personalized calendar for each month and enter important dates for assignments or social events. They printed out a copy for themselves and a copy for the resource specialist. As the assignments were given or changed by the classroom teacher, the student would go in and modify the monthly calendar. An important strategy taught by the resource specialist was to break down the task into manageable units and to delineate what materials or resources would be necessary to complete each component of the task.

For example, if the extended assignment was to read a particular novel and write a book report, the first task was to secure the book and the material needed was a library card. The second task was to read the book and to make notes that could be used to finish the report. The book and a note pad were needed for this task, but the resource specialist soon found that the students were unskilled in taking notes and helped them develop a form to complete as they were reading the book. The form prompted for specific information, such as characters, setting, time, and important interactions. To ensure that each student finished the book on schedule, they broke the novel into segments and set deadlines for completion of each unit. These deadlines were entered as important dates on their personalized calendar. Once the deadline for the completion of the book was established, dates for a first draft, a conference for editing, and a final draft were entered.

5. Each time the students went to the resource room, the dates were checked against assignments to ensure that the students were on task and on time. The students developed a habit of checking their calendar each afternoon prior to leaving school to make sure they had the necessary books and materials they would need at home to complete an assignment. This constant monitoring paid off with these high school students and their grades improved significantly.

Other *Homeworker,* from Davidson and Associates, features were introduced to the students and they found the "Outliner" to be a particularly helpful program. This is an organizational tool that helps one create an outline for a paper or report.

Special Considerations When students with special needs are in the elementary and middle school grades, if they forget a book or are late with an assignment, frequently the teacher will allow them to go back to their locker for the book or will allow them to turn in the assignment late, without penalty. This teaches the student that timelines and responsibility are not critical and this attitude often generalizes to other aspects of their life. If they are to make the transition from the lower grades to high school and be successful, they must be taught strategies to overcome these difficulties. At the high school level, it is critical for students to develop organizational skills and to assume responsibility for their own learning if they are to transition from school into the work environment. The computer can be a tool to help get them started in that direction, but they must also learn to use traditional materials such as a personal calendar or notebook to compensate for these inadequate organizational skills.

Providing Access to Verbal and Written Communication

Computer Use

The sixth way in which technology currently is being used to facilitate the integration of students with special needs into the mainstream environment is through the use of assistive/adaptive devices. Although this application of technology is the least frequently used and requires the greatest amount of time and training for the educators involved, it provides by far the most dramatic opportunities for severely handicapped students to become part of regular class activities. Students who have been excluded from class discussions because of an inability to speak can participate. Students who were unable to generate written work can, with minimal assistance, produce the same quality assignments as their nonhandicapped peers.

Student Needs

Traditionally, students with severe physical limitations have been educated to a great extent in self-contained classrooms with specially trained teachers. Any interaction among them and the various other groups in a school took place only in a social context and generally, on a very limited basis. This trend is changing rapidly with the development of new microtechnology that provides verbal communication possibilities for nonoral students, writing tools for participation in language arts activities, and access to educational material through the use of the computer and educational software. Students who have benefited from this application of technology are those who:

Are nonoral or have severely limited speech skills
Have no means to produce handwritten communication
Have limited or no access to standard curriculum content and material

Intervention

An extensive assessment, experimentation, and evaluation effort on the part of a complete team of specialists usually accompanies this use of technology. Ideally, the team would be composed of teachers from both regular and special education who are responsible for the student's academic program, a speech and language specialist, an occupational therapist, a physical therapist, a computer resource person, and an educational software resource person. The example that follows is representative of the effectiveness of a team approach.

Situation Thanh is a 10-year-old Vietnamese girl who is severely physically limited. She uses a wheelchair for mobility and requires assistance for most physical activities. Thanh is unable to speak and her communication is limited to responding with head movements to yes/no questions. Her educational placement is in a self-contained special education classroom with other nonoral, physically handicapped students. Based on her performance, intellectually Thanh can function at an average or above average level.

Objective(s) The educational team responsible for Thanh's program developed an extensive plan for her integration into the mainstream at her school site. The list of goals and objectives requiring the use of technology for Thanh included: 1) educational placement for Thanh in the regular classroom for academic subjects as appropriate, 2) the selection of and training in the use of an augmentative communication aid that would allow her to participate fully in the program, and 3) provision of access to educational software and word processing through an assistive/adaptive device attached to a computer.

Strategies After intensive assessment and evaluation, the following strategies were undertaken:

1. A Touch-Talker, from Prentke Romich Company, was selected as the most appropriate communication aid for Thanh. The device was purchased and she was taught how to operate it.
2. Vocabulary for specific curriculum areas was programmed into the Touch-Talker to enable Thanh to go into the regular classroom for academics. For example, vocabulary for a given unit of study in science was programmed on the Touch-Talker for that class.
3. Thanh was taught how to program the Touch-Talker for her own needs.
4. The special education personnel worked with the regular class teacher on strategies for facilitating Thanh's integration into the class. For example, the speech and language therapist modeled some interaction situations with Thanh for the regular fourth-grade teacher. The teacher then practiced with Thanh under the therapist's direction.

5. Thanh had access to an Apple computer equipped with an Adaptive Firmware Card, from Adaptive Peripherals Incorporated, a programmable membrane keyboard (Unicorn Membrane Keyboard), from Unicorn Engineering, an Echo speech synthesizer, from Street Electronics Corporation, and a printer. Using the expanded membrane keyboard for input, Thanh was able to generate her written assignments using a word processing program and to access all the educational software programs used by the other students.

Special Considerations In order to effectively integrate severely limited, nonoral students into regular classrooms, it is critical to have the full support and cooperation of the administration and the teachers involved. Special education personnel must be available to provide information, counseling, assistance, and guidance. Careful monitoring of the student's progress is vital if the integration effort is to be successful. Constant upgrading of vocabulary is necessary until the student is capable of modifying it. Parents must be involved and encourage the expanded use of the communication aid in the home environment.

SUMMARY

Educational technology can increase education options for many students with disabilities. Five uses of computers for students with disabilities were reviewed:

1. Drill and practice—a common use that adapts previous paper-and-pencil activities to a computer format
2. Tutorial—software that acts as a "teacher" and assists students in a step-by-step sequence
3. Supplementary material—utilizes software that assists the student in the regular curriculum
4. Personal productivity—software such as word processing, database, or spreadsheets that is more process than subject oriented and serves as a vehicle for product development
5. Augmentative communication—the use of adaptive, peripheral, or stand-alone devices that assist students in overcoming problems related to physical limitations

Prior to utilizing any computer-assisted instruction the student should be assessed and a decision-making process should be employed that will ultimately match a program or equipment to a specific need. Appropriate assessment, programming, and evaluation along with strategies for the use of technology should facilitate integration and assist in educational gain.

Technology is developing so rapidly that it is impossible to write about the latest advances because the information is out of date by the time of publication. However, strategies that are based on good teaching techniques and are child oriented can be applied to new technologies as they develop, and thus benefit students with learning problems as they progress through the educational system.

STUDY QUESTIONS

1. What are some ways the computer can be used to facilitate the social integration of special learners?
2. What are some considerations in the selection of educational software to integrate special learners?
3. Develop some strategies for using the computer in a group situation to integrate a special learner.
4. For each of the following software types, describe the learner characteristics and instructional needs. When is each particular type of software appropriate?
   a. Tutorial
   b. Drill and practice

    c.   Simulation
    d.   Word processing with spell checker
5.   Describe the steps in the decision-making process for the selection and use of technology with special learners.

6.   What types of strategies could be facilitated through the use of educational software? Why is the use of strategies an important skill in problem solving, rather than simply focusing on getting the answer?

REFERENCES

Arms, V.M. (1984). A dyslexic can compose on a computer. *Educational Technology, 24* (1).

Bell, T.E. (1983). My computer, my teacher. *Personal Computing, 7* (6).

Brightman, A.J. (1988). *Apple computer resources in special education and rehabilitation.* Allen, TX: DLM Teaching Resources.

Chiang, B. (1986). Initial learning and transfer effects of microcomputer drills on LD students' multiplication skills. *Learning Disability Quarterly, 9* (2), 118–123.

Hamilton, B., & Saylor, B. (1986). *CompuTHINK: Developing thinking skills with the aid of technology.* South San Francisco, CA: South San Francisco Unified School District.

Hasselbring, T., & Crossland, C. (1981). Using microcomputers for diagnosing spelling problems in learning-handicapped children. *Educational Technology, 21* (4), 37–39.

Heck, W.P., Johnson, J., & Kansky, R.J., (1981). *Guidelines for evaluating computerized instructional materials.* Reston, VA: National Council for Teachers of Mathematics.

Kleiman, G., Humphrey, M., & Lindsay, P.H. (1983). Micro-

computers and hyperactive children. In D.O. Harper & J.H. Steward (Eds.), *Run: Computer education.* Monterey, CA: Brooks/Cole.

Mason, G. (1980, October). Computerized reading instruction: A review. *Educational Technology,* pp. 18–22.

Test, D.W. (1985). Evaluating educational software for the microcomputer. *Journal of Special Education Technology, 7* (1), 37–46.

Varnhagen, S., & Gerber, M.M. (1984). Use of microcomputers for spelling assessment: Reasons to be cautious. *Learning Disability Quarterly, 7,* 226–270.

Willis, J.W. (1987). *Education computing: A guide to practical applications.* Scottsdale, AZ: Gorsuch Scarisbrick, Publishers.

Wisenand, S., Bastanchury, M., Carlyle, A., Connors, J., Cornish, B., Halloran, K., Hamilton, S., Johnson, M., Love, L., Meyer, L., Robinson, J., & Snyder, B. (1986). *Teaching to the third power, an integrated approach to the teaching of writing and problem solving.* Goleta, CA: Goleta Union School District.

SOFTWARE PROGRAMS, EQUIPMENT, AND OTHER RESOURCES

Adaptive Firmware Card
Adaptive Peripherals Incorporated
4529 Bagley Avenue N.
Seattle, WA 98103

Apple Link: Personal Edition
Apple Computer
20525 Mariani Avenue
Cupertino, CA 95014
(800) 538-9696

Bank Street Writer III
Created by: The Bank Street College of Education, Franklin E. Smith and Intentional Educations, Inc.
Version Design: Richard R. Ruopp and Franklin E. Smith
Programmer: Gordon Riggs
Additional Programming: Charles L. Olson, Jr. and Shaun Logan
Spelling Tools: Wayne Holder
Scholastic Software

730 Broadway
New York, NY 10003
(212) 505-3000
Copyright 1986

Basic Skills in Addition
Love Publishing Company
1777 South Bellaire Street
Denver, CO 80222
Copyright 1983

Basic Skills in Division
Love Publishing Company
1777 South Bellaire Street
Denver, CO 80222
Copyright 1983

Basic Skills in Multiplication
Love Publishing Company
1777 South Bellaire Street
Denver, CO 80222
Copyright 1983

Basic Skills in Subtraction
Love Publishing Company
1777 South Bellaire Street
Denver, CO 80222
Copyright 1983

Bears, Monsters and Frogs: An Approach to Problem Solving
By: Marge Kosel and D. Stanger
Produced by: Lisa Paul
Sunburst Communications, Inc.
39 Washington Avenue
Pleasantville, NY 10570
(800) 431-1934
Copyright 1986

Decisions, Decisions
Tom Snyder Productions
90 Sherman Street
Cambridge, MA 02140
(800) 342-0236
(617) 876-4433

Echo Speech Synthesizer
Street Electronics Corporation
1470 East Valley Road
P.O. Box 50220
Santa Barbara, CA 93105

The Factory
Designers: Marge Kosel, Mike Fish
Programmers: Mike Fish, Larry Bank, Eric Grubbs,
    Jim Brayton, Adam Sherer, and Raoul Watson
Sunburst Communications, Inc.
39 Washington Avenue
Pleasantville, NY 10570
(800) 431-1934
Copyright 1983, 1984, 1985, 1986

High Wire Logic
Designed by: Donna Stanger
Programmed by: Scott Clough
Sunburst Communications, Inc.
39 Washington Avenue
Pleasantville, NY 10570
(800) 431-1934
Copyright 1985

Homeworker
By: Mike Albanese, Jan Davidson, Julie Jennett, and
    Dean Ellis
Davidson and Associates
3135 Kashiwa Street
Torrance, CA 90505
(213) 534-4070
Copyright 1986

Immigration: Maintaining the Open Door (Decisions,
    Decisions series)
Designed by: Tom Snyder, David A. Dockterman, and
    Arthur Lewbel
Programmer: Tom Snyder
Program Graphics: Peter H. Reynolds
Simulation Author: David A. Dockterman
Senior Editor: Amy R. Brodesky
Tom Snyder Productions
90 Sherman Street
Cambridge, MA 02140
(800) 342-0236
(617) 876-4433
Copyright 1986

Individualized Planning System and Curriculum
    Management System
By: Kirk Wilson
Learning Tools Inc.
686 Massachusetts Avenue
Cambridge, MA 02139
(800) 225-3003
(617) 884-8086
Copyright 1984, 1988

Math Assistant I
Program Concept: Robert Janke
Instructional Design: Robert Janke and Peter J. Pilkey
Software Design: Mike Sweet and Alice Chrystie Wyman
Programming: Peter J. Pilkey and Mike Sweet
Graphic Designer: Sandi Young
Scholastic Software
730 Broadway
New York, NY 10003
Copyright 1985

Math Assistant II
Program Concept: Robert Janke
Instructional Design: Robert Janke and Peter J. Pilkey
Software Design: Mike Sweet and Alice Chrystie Wyman
Programming: Peter J. Pilkey and Mike Sweet
Graphic Designer: Sandi Young
Scholastic Software
730 Broadway
New York, NY 10003
Copyright 1985

MicroType, The Wonderful World of PAWS
By: J. Haugo, L. Hausmann, T. Jackson
Developed by: EduSystems Inc.
Sold by: Southwestern Publishing Co.
5101 Madison Road
Cincinnati, OH 45227
Copyright 1985

MindReader, Version 1.
By: Kalman Toth
Brown Bag Software
San Diego, CA
Copyright 1985

MultiScribe
By: Kevin Harvey and Alex Perelberg
StyleWare, Inc.
5250 Gulfton, Suite 2E
Houston, TX 77081
(800) 233-4088
Copyright 1986
School version developed and distributed by:
Scholastic Software
730 Broadway
New York, NY 10003
(212) 505-3000

Pacesetter
MindPlay Division of
Methods & Solutions, Inc.
82 Montvale Avenue
Stoneham, MA 02180

(800) 221-7911
Copyright 1984

Problem Solving Workshop
By: Lois Edwards and Gail Marshall
Sunburst Communications
39 Washington Avenue
Pleasantville, NY 10570
(800) 431-1934
Copyright 1985

Rocky's Boots
Author/Designer: Warren Robinett, M.S.
The Learning Company
6493 Kaiser Drive
Fremont, CA 94555
(800) 852-2255
Copyright 1982

SpecialNet
Suite 315
2021 K Street, NW
Washington, DC 20006
(202) 296-1800

Stickybear Math
By: Richard Hefter and Susan Dubicki
Graphics by: Robert Highsmith and Dave Joly
Optimum Resource, Inc.
Station Place
Norfolk, CT 06058
(203) 542-5553
Distributed by: Weekly Reader Family Software
245 Long Hill Road
Middletown, CT 06457
Copyright 1984

Stickybear Math 2
By: Richard Hefter and Susan Dubicki
Graphics by: Robert Highsmith
Optimum Resources, Inc.
Station Place
Norfolk, CT 06058
(203) 542-5553
Distributed by: Weekly Reader Family Software
245 Long Hill Road

Middletown, CT 06457
Copyright 1986

Touch-Talker
Prentke Romich Company
1022 Heyl Road
Wooster, OH 44691
(800) 642-8255

Touch Window
Developed by: Personal Touch Corporation
Sold by: Edmark Associates
P.O. Box 3903
Bellvue, WA 98009
Copyright 1985

Unicorn Membrane Keyboard
Unicorn Engineering
6201 Harwood Avenue
Oakland, CA 94618

Using Databases in the Classroom
Videotape by: Faye Wheeler and Christie Slimak
Sunburst Communications, Inc.
39 Washington Avenue
Pleasantville, NY 10570
(800) 431-1934
Copyright 1987

WISC-R Computer Report
By: Charles L. Nicholson
Southern Micro Systems For Educators
P.O. Box 1981
Burlington, NC 27215
Copyright 1983

WriteNow for the IBM
Airus Inc.
10200 S.W. Nimbus Avenue, Suite G-5
Portland, OR 97223
(503) 620-7000

Writer's Helper
Conduit/The University of Iowa
Oakdale Campus
Iowa City, IA 52242
(319) 335-4100

THE ECOLOGY OF SERVICE DELIVERY

AN ECOLOGICAL PROCESS MODEL FOR IMPLEMENTING THE LEAST RESTRICTIVE ENVIRONMENT MANDATE IN EARLY CHILDHOOD PROGRAMS

Charles A. Peck, Sherrill A. Richarz, Karen Peterson, Laurie Hayden, Lynn Mineur, and Mary Wandschneider

Although the importance of providing services to children with disabilities in normalized settings with their nondisabled peers has been central to program design in special education and related developmental services for over a decade (Snyder, Apolloni, & Cooke, 1977; Wolfensberger, 1972), achieving widespread implementation of integrated programs remains a largely unmet goal. Too often the attempts of parents and professionals alike to implement the mandates of PL 94-142 and related legislation for the development of integrated programs in local communities are met with frustration, opposition, and inaction (Ballard-Campbell & Semmel, 1981). This state of affairs is particularly ironic given the development of a substantial number of validated strategies for educating children with a variety of characteristics in integrated or mainstreamed settings (Brady & Gunter, 1985; Gaylord-Ross, Haring, Breen, & Pitts-Conway, 1984; Peck, Apolloni, Cooke, &

Raver, 1978; Russo & Koegel, 1977; Strain, Kerr, & Ragland, 1979).

Programs may fail despite evidence of substantial investment of resources and the presence of many desirable programmatic features. Instances of discontinued programs abound, although descriptions of these are conspicuously absent from the professional literature, and therefore are likely to be overlooked in the analysis of factors necessary for the development of successful programs. For example:

In one northern California community, preschool-age children with disabilities were routinely served in regular county-run day-care centers, along with their nonhandicapped peers. Special education and related services were provided to these children within the regular classroom, and special education teachers "team taught" with regular education colleagues

The authors extend their appreciation to Edwin Helmstetter for his helpful comments on an earlier draft of this chapter.

in each classroom. Despite the fact that this service delivery system had functioned successfully for several years, had strong administrative support, and was highly consistent with the mandates of PL 94-142, the program was disbanded at the request of the *special education teachers,* and a centralized segregated preschool was created for children with disabilities.

Also, for example:

In another community, an integrated preschool was developed that relied on embedding specialized instruction into a typical preschool curriculum. A specific goal of this program was to provide a normalized preschool experience for children with disabilities, and also for the parents of those children. Thus, parents of both nondisabled and disabled children actively took part in a variety of social and educational activities associated with the preschool. Despite the overwhelming popularity of this program, it was not continued by the local school district, which chose instead to transfer the children into existing segregated special education programs.

Even when appropriate administrative decisions have been made, programs may fail to be implemented at the "hands-on" level:

In a rural community in Northern Idaho, a child with autism was "mainstreamed" full time into a regular classroom. At the request of the student's parents, who had successfully sued the district previously, the student was allocated a full-time aide to support his participation in the regular class. Despite this procedural and substantive compliance with the law, and rich allocation of resources to support implementation of the program, the student interacted little with any of the regular class teachers, and not at all with his nonhandicapped peers. Because no one was truly aware of the purpose of his presence in the regular class, his full-time aide conducted all of his instruction, and mediated all of his contacts with other students. He was ef-

fectively isolated from contact with anyone but his aide for the entire school day.

These programs did not fail so much because they were improperly designed from a pedagogical point of view (although limitations clearly existed for each of them), but because they did not adequately analyze and respond to the *social/political contexts* in which they would be implemented. A perusal of the research literature related to the development of mainstreaming programs (see Gaylord-Ross & Peck, 1985; Guralnick, 1986; Peck & Cooke, 1983; Semmel, Gottlieb, & Robinson, 1979; and Strain & Kerr, 1981, for comprehensive reviews), as well as other programs emphasizing the social integration of children with disabilities, reveals that inattention to social/political aspects of program implementation is characteristic of many of these projects. This apparently reflects the assumption that the successful implementation of programs of social integration and mainstreaming primarily represents challenges in the development of effective educational technology. Although sound educational strategies are clearly fundamental to the achievement of effective integrated programs, they represent only one aspect of the factors involved in the successful initiation and long-term survival of these programs. Indeed, as Baer (1986) has pointed out, the survival of innovative programs for children with disabilities may have little to do with the educational variables that consume the attention of most professionals in the fields of special education and developmental disabilities. Clearly a pressing need exists for both a conceptual framework and procedural strategies for identifying and shaping social/political factors related to successfully establishing integrated programs.

This chapter describes concepts and strategies for developing a base of social and political support for integrated educational programs that have been used as part of a broader federally supported model demonstration (Rural Area Model Preschool Project: RAMP) conducted at Washington

State University (Richarz, Peck, & Peterson, 1986). The purpose of the project has been to increase the availability of integrated preschool options for children with disabilities in eastern Washington State. In pursuing this project, the authors have adopted a number of "working hypotheses" that have guided their work with school districts, private agencies, and parents.

Pedagogical variables (i.e., curricula, instructional design, design of classroom environments, etc.) represent only one dimension of the "social ecology" that must be considered in the design and implementation of educational programs. Although most of the planning and negotiation of arrangements for integration carried out by parents and professionals (for example, in the context of individualized education program [IEP] meetings) focuses on pedagogical issues, there are numerous other variables that powerfully affect the implementation of any educational arrangement. These include the personal and logistical needs of parents, teachers, and administrators that may be unrelated, or even in conflict with the child's direct educational needs. The assumption here is that the program must meet the critical needs of all persons whose participation is integral to the program's operation (i.e., parents, teachers, and administrators, as well as children) if it is to succeed in the long term. Failure to explicitly consider the needs of all these individuals in the program design process only sets the occasion for nonparticipation and lack of support for the program during implementation. This point of view is often difficult for professionals and parents to accept, since it appears to violate the strongly held belief that the child must "come first." It is often quite difficult for parents, teachers, and administrators to acknowledge the factors outside of the child's direct needs that are strongly affecting their choice of programmatic arrangements (including integration).

The behavior of parents and professionals represents intelligent and active attempts to cope with problems and situations as they see them. The widespread tendency to view the behavior of teachers, parents, or administrators as deficient in dealing with certain problems often obscures the actual meaning of that behavior. For example, the behavior of a teacher who appears unwilling to have a child with disabilities added to the regular class enrollment may reflect not a lack of acceptance of that child, but a sense of not being able to serve *all* the children in the class adequately. Viewed from such a perspective, this position may represent a high level of professional integrity. An administrator who appears unresponsive to requests for aide time for the support of children with disabilities in regular class placements may in fact be responding to the needs of other children for physical therapy. A parent who appears unable to consistently implement a behavior management program in the home may be highly engaged in responding to the pressing needs of other family members or to the demands of the workplace. The point is that failing to analyze the reasons underlying behavior that conflicts with programmatic goals, including goals related to social integration, is likely to lead to attempts to implement programs that ignore or conflict with powerful social/political factors that drive the behavior of individuals who must ultimately support the program.

Social or educational policies can only be effective when the people who are in direct "hands-on" contact with children choose to implement them. The assumption here is that the day-to-day experiences of children are controlled fundamentally and incontrovertibly by parents, teachers, aides, day-care providers, and other individuals who actually spend the most time with them. Simply mandating programs at the administrative level does not assure implementation, even when relevant administrative arrangements have been instituted (Semmel, Lieber, & Peck, 1986). The situation described previously, wherein a student was "mainstreamed" into a regular classroom full time, but remained completely isolated from any actual involvement in social or educational activities in that classroom, strikingly exemplifies the extent to which actual implementation of a program is controlled by the people directly involved. In that case, the rationale and goals of integration had been neither understood nor accepted by the teachers and aides to be involved in implementing the program. The result was that the student was "mainstreamed" in an administrative sense, but was entirely isolated from social interaction with other children. Far from an unusual phenomenon, the power of the "street-level bureaucrat" to ignore or modify public policy has been amply documented (Weatherly & Lipsky, 1977).

ECOLOGICAL FRAMEWORK FOR ANALYSIS OF FACTORS AFFECTING IMPLEMENTATION OF MAINSTREAMING PROGRAMS

A major task confronting individuals wishing to implement change in existing practices is to recognize and systematically assess the influence of factors affecting the implementability of a specific program. Unfortunately, the multiplicity and complexity of sociopolitical factors that potentially affect the success of educational programs is truly intimidating, if not overwhelming to most special educators and many other would-be change agents. Responding to their own need for some conceptual framework from which to analyze the myriad of such issues, the authors have developed the model depicted in Figure 1.

This model assumes parents, administrators, teachers, and the community in general, as well as the child, have needs that will be affected by whatever programmatic policies are adopted. The term "ecological" is used to allude to the interdependence of these needs, as well as the highly local and individualized arrangements that develop in each community for meeting them. Although these needs are not often included in the process of analyzing and choosing between various programmatic and policy options, nevertheless they may strongly affect subsequent implementation. For example, many parents readily acknowledge the value of having their child in contact with non-

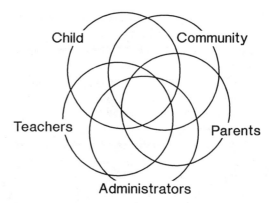

Figure 1.   Ecological model of needs that must be considered in the development of integrated programs that can be successfully implemented.

handicapped peers, but may be even more in need of a preschool program that responds to their needs for transportation, or a program that is close to their home or workplace. Teachers and other interventionists such as speech pathologists, physical therapists, and others may feel that they must have a certain amount of direct professional time with the child in order to maintain their role (and their jobs) within the system. Administrators may perceive integrated programs as representing high risks for liability or interagency problems. Community members may be very concerned about the quality of educational options available to non-handicapped children locally, and may need to be convinced that there are potential benefits for *all* children as a result of integrating children with disabilities.

The dimensions depicted above obviously do not exhaust those that might be important to consider in specific situations. Rather, the model is intended to suggest factors that are likely to have significant impact on programs in most situations. Further, the partially overlapping nature of needs and concerns that underly the behavior of parents, teachers, administrators, the community, and the children involved explicitly represented in the model underscores the fact that needs that do not directly overlap with those of the child affect the likelihood of an individual's supporting the program.

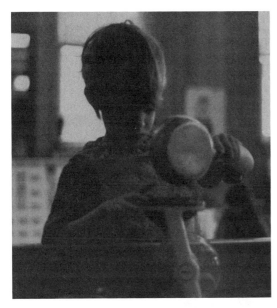

Children at varying developmental levels benefit from educational experiences such as water play.

Preliminary Data on Needs/Concerns

In order to ground their own program development activities in a general understanding of the issues related to integrated preschool programs as perceived by parents, teachers, and administrators, the authors conducted a set of interviews with 30 individuals involved with such programs in the state of Washington. The data from the interviews were analyzed using qualitative methods (Glaser & Strauss, 1967) to generate a set of categories that described the prototypical concerns of individuals in each of these constituent groups. The purpose of this process was not to define needs/concerns that would characterize all communities (which would violate some of the authors' basic assumptions regarding the highly individual nature of such communities), but rather to identify issues that should be regularly probed to assess whether they were actually concerns in the communities in which the authors were involved.

Three basic categories of concerns or needs were identified. The first category reflects concerns with adequate preparation for integration.

The second set of concerns focuses on potential loss of control over programs and children represented by shifts to more integrated program arrangements. Third, the individuals interviewed revealed considerable concern about the availability of adequate resources for operating high-quality integrated programs. Differing, but overlapping concerns regarding each of these categories were expressed by parents, teachers, and administrators.

Adequate Preparation

Parents expressed a number of concerns related to the adequacy of preparation for integration, particularly in terms of the awareness and understanding held by the children and parents to be involved. They were concerned, for example, that parents of nonhandicapped children be "informed" about the nature of the special needs of the handicapped children to be served, but that this process should be carried out in a manner that did not stigmatize children with disabilities. In addition, parents were concerned that teachers be adequately trained to recognize the similarities between children with disabilities and nondisabled children—rather than seeing children with handicaps primarily in terms of their disabilities. Many parents of children with disabilities expressed the belief that the social acceptance of their child would be strongly affected by the way in which both children and teachers were prepared for the integrated program.

Teachers were also concerned with the adequacy of preparation. They, however, identified their primary training needs to be related to curriculum and instructional strategies appropriate for integrated programs. Teachers also commented on the importance of adequate planning for effective implementation of integrated programs, including the need for working out specific role definitions and functions for the various professionals involved. The development of a cohesive program philosophy integrating the concerns of regular and special education professionals was seen as a key aspect of adequate preparation by many teachers.

Training for teachers was the predominant issue related to adequate preparation cited by administrators. In addition to skills-oriented training, administrators noted the need to change the perceptions of many teachers and parents related to expectations for outcome of integration. They indicated that if programs were to be successfully implemented, both inflated expectations for developmental change by some parents and expectations for success by some teachers were potential problems to overcome.

Loss of Control

A second category of needs and concerns expressed by parents, teachers, and administrators centered on the importance they placed on maintaining control over "their" programs. For parents (of both handicapped and nonhandicapped children), a major concern was whether their child's needs would continue to be met in an integrated program. They expressed the concern that many of the needs of the "other" group of children and parents would be substantially different from their own. One parent (of a nonhandicapped child) commented that she was initially concerned that her child's needs would be "lost in the shuffle" of an integrated program. In some cases, existing programmatic arrangements (e.g., provision of a specified amount of speech therapy) had been won through hard and conflictive negotiation, and parents were concerned that these gains might be lost as the political context of program decision making changed.

Teachers were also concerned about losing control over their programs. Both special and regular educators repeatedly expressed the fear that some of the important goals and practices of their instructional programs would be subverted in the integration process. Special educators were particularly concerned over the possible loss of individualization and direct instructional time. Regular classroom teachers expressed concern that they would not be able to implement important curric-

ula, and maintain an appropriate rate of growth for nonhandicapped children through the school year. Maintaining the integrity and cohesion of the instructional program to be offered to both special and regular education children was viewed as a major issue by most teachers.

Administrators frequently expressed needs related to control of programs. Many aspects of their need for control were focused on reducing the likelihood that conflicts of a professional or legal nature would arise. Specific areas of concern about integrated programs were: potential liability problems, conflicts in authority and resource allocation between agencies, and the potential for conflict and disruption between professionals holding differing views on programmatic issues. The need for direct and unambiguous program and teacher "accountability" was raised by a number of administrators.

Adequacy of Resources

A nearly universal concern of parents, teachers, and administrators was the availability of adequate resources to implement integrated preschool programs of high quality. However, the specific resource issues raised by each of these groups differed somewhat.

Parents of both disabled and nondisabled children saw resource issues primarily in terms of the need for adequate staffing ratios to allow teachers to respond to the divergent needs of both handicapped and nonhandicapped children. While many teachers expressed the same concern, a number of them also noted that too many staff could also cause problems. They noted, in particular, the tendency for children from "staff-rich" special education settings to rely more on adults for assistance, even in peer interaction situations.

Teachers frequently said that adequate space was a major resource issue in providing integrated programs. Typically, programs developed to serve segregated populations (either special or regular preschool programs) had acquired classroom space that was adequate for their needs, but that did not necessarily meet the needs of an expanded group of children. Teachers almost unanimously cited the need for direct support for scheduled time to ensure adequate planning, coordination, and true integration of general and special education program functions. An additional concern of many regular preschool teachers was the availability of consultative support services, as well as access to specialized curricula relevant to the needs of children with disabilities.

Administrative concerns related to integrated programs were often focused on sources of funding for such programs. A major issue for many administrators was how to reconcile the public funding structures supporting the education of children with disabilities with the predominantly private support of preschool education for nonhandicapped children. In many cases the relatively "rich" funding support available for special education programs was viewed as a potential source of conflict between regular and special educators. As long as programs remained isolated and segregated from one another, educators remained relatively unaware of many large discrepancies between private preschools and public school-supported special education programs in terms of professional salaries, availability of curriculum and instructional materials, and other resources. Putting programs and professionals into direct contact with each other made these differences clear. Finally, several administrators observed that competition for resources in their communities was keen, and that in some cases collaboration or blending of programs had come to be viewed as incompatible with maintaining sufficient "numbers" of children in individual programs to generate an adequate funding base.

Conclusion

The interview data presented above attest to the complexity of issues that potentially affect support for integrated programs. Clearly, building support for such programs requires analysis and management of a multitude of factors that reach beyond the instructional design issues that have dominated program development models to date.

Building Support Through Public Participation

The multiple and often conflictive nature of many of the perceived needs and concerns expressed by teachers, parents, and administrators the authors interviewed underscores the need for a program development process that has educational and consensus building outcomes, as well as appropriate products in terms of program design decisions. The authors assumed that such a process must be truly *transactional* in nature, that is, specifically designed to allow the viewpoints of all parties to mutually influence one another. In designing and implementing the process, the authors found that their own understanding of the issues involved in creating integrated preschools in small communities evolved considerably.

In developing such a process, the authors drew on work in the public policy planning literature that describes numerous strategies for facilitating community participation in planning decisions (Kweit & Kweit, 1981; Langton, 1978). The purpose for using public participation strategies in developing integrated preschool programs were: 1) to ensure that the needs of key constituents, not just child needs, were addressed in the design of the program; 2) to provide a context in which participants could become more aware of each other's perceptions and needs; and 3) to build a broad and diversified base of awareness, understanding, and support for the program in the local community.

It is important to note that the objective of this process is not simply to allow input, but to ensure that constituents have real influence in the design of the program. The assumption is that unless the program development process actually identifies and responds to the needs of the community, the program will not be supported over the long term.

THE RAMP PROGRAM DEVELOPMENT MODEL

The process model the authors have constructed for developing integrated preschools in small communities has been used in situations where the local base of awareness and support for such programs is either extremely narrow (e.g., limited to one teacher or administrator) or completely absent. The general outline of the model is represented in Figure 2.

In the following sections, each of the steps involved in the process model is discussed in terms of its function and specific strategies for implementation. It should be noted that the "model" has been constructed to represent the authors' general experience. It is not intended to serve as a lock-step procedure to be implemented without adjustment and modification in specific situations.

Starting the Process

A basic problem confronting individuals wishing to initiate the program development process in a

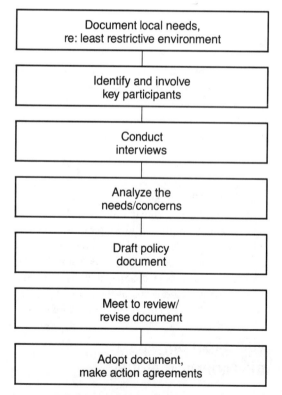

Figure 2.   Process model for program development based on local community needs.

particular community may be deciding whether they or someone else could effectively start such a process. In the authors' recent work in four communities in eastern Washington State, individuals in a variety of roles have been responsible for initiating local changes. In one community it was two parents who were concerned about the absence of contact between their children with disabilities and nonhandicapped peers. In another community the local director of special education initiated the process, while in a third community a preschool consultant from the rural special education consortium acted in this capacity.

Strategies for starting the process were the same in each case, and consisted of documenting and analyzing local needs related to preschool education and child care. While general needs and issues related to the availability of quality preschool and day care were considered, a particular focus was given to the extent to which local children with disabilities had opportunities to participate in normalized social and educational experiences in their own community. This information was obtained by contacting the local director of special education, or another local professional who was knowledgeable regarding local services.

The function of starting the process by documenting local needs and services is twofold. First, there is an obvious need to assess the extent to which local services are meeting the needs of children related to the mandates and principles of the laws related to LRE (least restrictive environments). Equally important, however, is the need to identify the basic service structure of the community in order to evaluate where possibilities and needs for integrated programs exist, and to identify key individuals for involvement in the program development process.

Identifying and Involving Key Participants

A comprehensive description of the local array of preschool and day-care services provides a wealth of suggestions for identifying key individuals for participation in the program development process.

The authors began by meeting with a director of special education in one community, with two parents in another, and with a rural superintendent of schools in a third community. Beginning with any individual who was both responsive to the integration issue and formally connected with the schools in some way, the authors' strategy was to meet with that person to discuss the needs of the local community, and to identify the need to interview other individuals whose views would be important to obtain. Key participants within a given community can be identified by asking each individual contacted to think of other people who would be concerned about preschool services, or who might have a "stake" in decisions made about integration, and whose views should be obtained through interview.

In some situations the authors found that little awareness existed regarding social integration or mainstreaming as program issues for preschool children. In those cases it was helpful to provide information about "best practices" that had been demonstrated around the state and nation. This educative process took the form of providing relevant articles from professional journals; providing a consultation/inservice; and, in one community, arranging a panel presentation by professionals and parents who had experience in preschool mainstreaming programs. Perhaps most important, however, an awareness of the goals and rationale for integrated programs was developed in the context of informal discussions with parents and teachers regarding specific children's needs and experiences, as well as their own feelings about special education.

The function of identifying and involving important individuals affecting preschool education in each community is not only to ensure that program decisions are made that reflect these individuals' concerns and needs, but also to draw them into a process that has a strong educative dimension. Participants should, thus, emerge from the process with a program that they will strongly support, as well as one for which they clearly understand the goals and rationale.

The potential makeup of a program development group or task force in a given community might include someone from virtually any personal or professional role. Particularly in small rural communities, there may be individuals who have high levels of influence in virtually any community matter—but who may have relatively little direct experience or contact with preschools in general, and special education in particular. Regardless of his or her previous background, any individual whose support of the program is likely to affect its long-term survival and level of community acceptance should be considered for inclusion. At minimum, the authors have included parents of both handicapped and nonhandicapped children, administrators of regular and special education programs, day-care and preschool teachers, special education teachers, and professional support staff.

Conducting Interviews

Once a tentative list of individuals to be involved is developed, semi-structured interviews are conducted with each person identified as a key decision maker in that community. The authors did not interview every person who later participated in program development meetings. Rather, in addition to obtaining information from each of the major constituent groups (i.e., teachers, parents, support staff), they sought interviews with individuals who were viewed as marginally involved or as potentially nonsupportive of integrated programs, or who held key decision-making roles. Often these persons were administrative personnel.

A basic assumption the authors made was that programs are most likely to survive when they reflect policies that represent "win-win" situations for key constituents. A major function of the interview process, therefore, was to gather information from which policies might be constructed for each community that achieved as many common goals and violated as few values as possible.

Interviews were conducted around three basic questions:

1. What do you see as the challenges to agencies working together to develop integrated preschool or day-care services for handicapped and nonhandicapped children in this community?
2. Ideally, what would an integrated preschool education system look like?
3. Who has to be involved in creating such a system?

The questions above were constructed specifically to avoid focusing on issues related to what was wrong with the current programs and policies. Rather, it was the authors' intention to focus the process on what people viewed as desirable in preschool programs, and how to achieve it.

In conducting the interviews, a specific effort was made to legitimize the views of the person being interviewed. This does not mean that the authors agreed with those views necessarily; they did not indicate agreement or challenge anyone's point of view. The goal was to get each person's *perceptions* of the issues, so that the focus would be on the actual issues during exchanges in subsequent meetings, or in the construction of policies and programs for that community. For example, one administrator expressed the conviction that parents of nonhandicapped children would be extremely resistant to the integration of children with disabilities into their preschool program. The authors' experience, as well as available data collected previously in that community (Peck, Killen, & Owen, 1987), suggested this was not an accurate perception. The authors later responded to this concern, however, by proposing the need for a parent education component related to the development of the integrated program in that community.

Analyzing the Data and Drafting a Policy Document

The purpose of developing a written document at this point is not to attempt to define the ultimate features of the program. Rather, the document provides a reason to bring all of the key partici-

pants together to begin dialogue about how their community should respond to the needs that have been identified. The document itself attempts to construct policies/principles on which an integrated preschool program could be based consistent with the major issues expressed by each participant during interviews.

Clearly not all concerns can be accommodated, and, indeed, some are antithetical to integration. The authors did two things in those cases. First, an active attempt was made to allude to that concern within the document in a manner that clearly showed the participant that "their" issue had been considered carefully. Second, the authors attempted to identify another issue that was important to that participant that could be "leveraged" to maintain support for the program. For example, in one community a group of speech therapists were very concerned that moving children out of a medically oriented facility into regular preschools with support services would disrupt their existing arrangements for pulling the children out to clinic rooms for therapy. Closely related to this issue, of course, were ongoing difficulties in integrating therapeutic services into programs controlled by educators. In the document written for this group, the authors attempted to "trade off" loss of the clinical setting by affirming the importance of maintaining a strong therapeutic services component for the program (see Figure 3).

The document itself may consist of a list of policy-like statements, or a set of statements about program philosophy, or a set of program design features, depending on the issues raised by participants. For example, in the community described above, which was just beginning to consider the development of integrated programs, the initial document outlined a program philosophy that reflected the values and beliefs of parents and professionals in that community. Figure 3 represents the set of program philosophy statements written for that community group.

In another community, an initial integrated program had already been established. Issues in this community were centered more on expanding the

---

Program Goals and Philosophy

The following statements represent a synthesis of the philosophical issues and goals discussed during the April 29 and May 6 meetings.

Emphasis on Providing a Normalized Preschool Environment

The basic preschool program should provide many of the learning opportunitites available in a normal preschool as well as an ongoing program of specialized educational, therapeutic, and support services as needed by individual children. This reflects an awareness that the characteristics of the normal preschool environment present important challenges and opportunities for children with handicaps that may not be available in special education programs serving handicapped children only. Several specific programmatic characteristics are viewed as important in this regard: 1) a ratio of nonhandicapped to handicapped children of at least 1:1, 2) an emphasis on teaching social interaction and social play skills in the context of normal teacher-child ratios and play group sizes, and 3) an emphasis on stable instructional groupings consisting of "family groups" (i.e., small groups of children who reflect a range of chronological and developmental ages, who consistently participate in activities together).

Emphasis on Intensive Therapeutic Services

The availability of high-quality therapeutic services (occupational therapy, physical therapy, child development, audiology, etc.) is an important part of the program. Both pull-out and in-class services have a place in the program. The ultimate test of the effects of therapy should involve child change across all environments. This implies that classroom and other "natural" settings should be the primary focus of intervention and evaluation. Pull-out services should be utilized as per demonstrated need (e.g., initial stages of auditory training, teacher/clinician training), but should not be the primary treatment delivery model.

Program Evaluation and Development

The preschool will reflect a commitment to regular internal and external evaluation. This means that program policies will be reviewed and adapted based on results of data-based evaluations of child growth and parent satisfaction with specific aspects of the program. Concomitant with this, there will be onging efforts to provide staff support and development resources to maximize the program's ability to grow and adapt to new developments in the field.

Comprehensive and Flexible Array of Services

The preschool will strive to provide an array of services within the framework of a comprehensive center for early education and family support. These services will include special education, therapeutic assessment and treatment, comprehensive day care, parent education, home visitations, teacher/clinician training, entry and exit transition services, and a resource library. Emphasis will be on maintaining sufficient programmatic and fiscal flexibility to meet the variety of community needs in the county.

Figure 3.   Example of one community's program philosophy document.

number and variety of such programs available, and on developing some guidelines for making placement decisions. Figure 4 depicts a more policy-oriented document that emerged from that community process.

In both of these documents it is worth noting that a number of statements are made that are highly redundant with existing legal mandates (e.g., the affirmation of parent involvement in placement decision making in Figure 4). The au-

1. Placement options for preschool children with special educational needs should include a wide array of choices, including delivery of special services in regular preschool and day-care programs.
2. Program placement should be based on systematic consideration of both the needs of children and their families, and should be made with input and involvement by parents, professionals from relevant disciplines, and potential service providers.
3. Any integrated program placement should be accompanied by allocation of support resources (regular consultation, aide time, tuition, etc.) sufficient to ensure that direct costs for necessary specialized program adaptations and implementation of specialized instruction are covered for that child.
4. Provisions for parent education related to rationale and potential benefits of integrated preschool programs should be made for parents of both handicapped and nonhandicapped children involved or potentially involved.
5. Specific and regular times and locations for meetings to facilitate interagency communication and coordination should accompany development of collaborative relationships with each regular preschool or day-care program.

Figure 4.   Example of one community's program policy document.

thors included such statements in local community documents even though they appeared in some sense superfluous, because the authors believed that in many cases it was important for communities to self-consciously affirm their support of specific practices. In several cases the authors observed changes in program practices in these communities that had been mandated for years, but not implemented. The most basic illustration of this phenomenon was related to the LRE principle itself, which, though legally mandated for over a decade, showed virtually no evidence of implementation in any of the rural communities the authors surveyed in eastern Washington State.

Meeting to Review and Revise Document

As just noted, the document itself is intended to initiate and guide discussion, and to provide a context for bringing all of the key decision makers into a meeting focused on the integration issue. Even if interviews have been conducted effectively to identify issues of importance to participants, and a document that represents those issues accurately has been constructed, the authors' experience has been that subsequent discussion extends and clarifies principles articulated in the written document in important ways. For exam-

ple, in one community a major issue arose regarding the legality of providing support services to children in day-care environments. While the issue was resolved easily within the document by adding the caveat that such services would only be delivered as allowed by state administrative regulations, an important outcome was that considerable "misinformation" was corrected on this issue, and a major reservation to the document (and the proposed program) was removed. In some cases issues may not be resolved so easily, and referral to "subcommittee" for further consideration and information gathering may be useful. It is important that a time and date for review of changes to be made to the document be set if such changes are deferred.

Adopting Document and Making Action Agreements

Important outcomes will have already been achieved at this point in the process in terms of educating the community to the state-of-the-art options in early childhood services, as well as to one another's values and perceptions of local issues affecting preschool-age children. For example, an issue that emerged out of one group was the unavailability of child-care services for children within that community. This itself became an important agenda item for future action with that group.

However, the most salient outcome of the process is formal adoption of the written program document, and the identification of actions to be taken by one or more members of the group toward implementation of integrated programs. A variety of outcome actions have been achieved in the communities in which the authors have worked. In one community the first step taken was to begin part-day integration of children from Head Start and special education preschool programs. In another community a major change in program philosophy took place, and three integrated programs were started, as well as a reverse mainstreaming program in the originally segregated preschool. Clearly, the "size" of the steps taken by each community toward development of a fully integrated array of preschool and day-care services has varied greatly; each of the actions taken are relevant to that community's baseline level of awareness of preschool and special education issues, as well as a myriad of other social/political factors. The authors have found, however, that the amount of change undertaken initially by a community may not predict how rapidly subsequent changes are made. For example, the community that chose to begin with only an experimental part-day integration program is now in the process of making major facility modifications to accommodate a fully integrated and comprehensive early childhood education center.

A CASE ILLUSTRATION

The program development process model identified above may be further illustrated by describing its implementation in a specific community in eastern Washington State. One purpose of such a case illustration is to underscore the individualistic nature of the actual implementation of the general model within each community. The authors' experiences in one community are reported in terms of background/context factors operating in

that community, description of the process itself, discussion of specific issues identified, and description of program outcomes to date.

Background/Context

The community of Fairview (a pseudonym) is a small rural township of about 8,000 residents in eastern Washington. The major industries in the town are logging and farming, and residents typically represent lower middle–socioeconomic status backgrounds. Although the Fairview School District is relatively small, its superintendent is quite active, and the district has attempted to develop a number of innovative programs, including several in special education. The director of special education is highly responsive to new professional trends in the field, and enjoys strong support from the superintendent. The district operates one preschool special education classroom, which is housed adjacent to both a Head Start program and a parent cooperative preschool program.

At the regional and state levels several contextual factors have also affected the authors' work in the Fairview community. First, the state had recently passed legislation mandating provision of services to all children with identified handicapping conditions age 3 to 5 years. This, coupled with strong leadership in early childhood special education from the state Office of the Superintendent of Public Instruction, had led to establishment of regional consulting and support services for preschool special education programs in eastern Washington. At the same time, the expressed willingness of university faculty in special education and child development to work with Fairview and other communities toward development of an integrated program provided a source of leadership and information for the community as it initiated the program development process.

Program Development Process in Fairview

The program development process in Fairview was initiated through a meeting between the director of special education in the Fairview school district, a university faculty person, and the regional early childhood special education consultant. The focus of this meeting was to discuss local needs related to early childhood services and the potential overlaps between these needs and integrated service delivery models for preschool programs. The need to further explore this issue was identified, and a list of key participants for future meetings was developed. This list initially included teachers and parents from each of three early childhood programs in the community, including the existing segregated special education preschool. This list was gradually expanded during the course of subsequent meetings to include regional administrators connected with each of the local programs (e.g., Head Start coordinators). The formal program planning and development process consisted of a series of five meetings interspersed over the school year. However, important informal exchanges and meetings between the teachers and parents involved took place almost constantly during this time as well. Early meetings were characterized by considerable ambiguity and tension as the group discussed the goals of integration, likely benefits, and potential problems. As the meetings continued during the year, discussion gradually shifted away from expression of concerns and toward actual planning of concrete features and arrangements for an integrated program.

Throughout this process the role of the regional consultant (and university personnel, when present) was one of facilitation and support, rather than decision making. In fact, a salient feature of this process, as well as others with which the authors were involved, was the importance of allowing the community group to define its own needs and priorities for action in the program development process. While this required enduring considerable ambiguity as the group developed its priorities and focus, avoiding a directive role in the process appeared critical in assuaging some of the concerns about loss of programmatic control held by several participants. Moreover, at several points in the process the "credibility" of the regional consultant as a facilitator and support person, rather than as an agent of an outside agency imposing change, appeared to be bolstered by her timely responsiveness to needs identified by the group. For example, at one point the group expressed a need for ideas about how a preschool environment might best be constructed to facilitate independent child learning and interaction. The regional consultant arranged for inservice training, as well as a visit from an outside consultant with specific expertise in this area.

The interviewing process that was described previously in the general model for program development was initiated after two meetings in the Fairview community. Since these meetings had been easy to arrange and had successfully involved most of the key players in the local community, the authors decided it was not imperative to conduct formal interviews with all of these individuals. However, interviews were conducted with administrators who had little direct participation in the meetings conducted in the local community (e.g., the regional Head Start director). Information from these interviews was incorporated into subsequent discussion and policy documents, to assure that the needs of these administrators (which centered on maintenance of program identity and accountability) would be represented in programmatic decisions.

Issues Identified in Fairview

A number of specific issues were raised in the Fairview process that required clarification and problem solving as the group's work progressed. Most of these resembled the types of issues and concerns expressed in the interview study described earlier in this chapter.

Adequate Preparation

Both parents and professionals expressed considerable anxiety over completing adequate preparation before initiating an integrated program. To some extent, it appeared as if many of these concerns were reduced as participants became convinced that they did, in fact, have considerable influence over the pace at which the program development process would move forward. The authors decided it was not useful to rush the group before they had time to make necessary plans and to think through the implications of planned changes. Initial action plans for cross-program visitations and partial integration of some students allowed participants to explore potential problems and plan responses to them in an incremental fashion. A specific need identified by the group related to preparation was the development of a written program philosophy that would clarify the jointly held goals for integration, as well as jointly held values for preservation of program strengths and priorities of each of the individual programs involved. A recurring issue was the difficulty of coordinating the scheduling of activities, meetings, program hours, and staffing for each of the programs to be involved.

Control

In the data from Fairview, as in the interviews the authors conducted statewide, the issue of maintaining control of individual programs was very important to most participants. Professionals and parents from both special education and regular preschool programs in Fairview were initially quite concerned about the possible loss of identity and focus for "their" program if integration occurred. For example, one of the programs, a parent cooperative preschool, emphasized much higher levels of parent influence and involvement than did the others. Understandably, parents in this program were worried that they would have little influence over a larger, integrated program.

Considerable concern was also expressed by regional administrators over maintaining control of local programs. It became routinely necessary, as word of the interagency cooperation planned at the local level spread "upward" through the administrative bureaucracy of each agency, to present the rationale and potential benefits of the integrated program, and to bring administrators into

at least indirect involvement in the process. This was accomplished in most cases by interviewing each administrator to identify his or her sources of concern, as well as goals and priorities for his or her program. In most cases, it was possible to reflect these issues in policy documents, action plans, and other observable products of the process, which reduced administrative concerns about the integrated program.

Resources

Allocation and joint use of resources in the integrated program did not develop as a conflictive issue in Fairview, perhaps because both the local school district and the regional special education consortium provided considerable resources toward creating the integrated program. Resources that were available and allocated by the local school district included classroom space, teacher release time for planning and training, and curriculum materials. The regional consortium provided consultation and inservice training related to curriculum development, design of preschool environments, and other topics requested by participants.

The social "norms" that developed among the teachers during the program development process in Fairview emphasized sharing of resources. For example, curriculum materials were exchanged, joint inservices were conducted, and complementary areas of instructional expertise were identified by the teachers involved.

Identifying Convergent and Divergent Interests

A strategic goal held for the program development process was the identification of convergent interests of participating agencies and individuals that could be met through an integrated program. Many of these involved augmentation of resources available to all of the programs when they operated jointly. For example, the integrated program model allowed pooling of resources for inservice training and consultation. Integrating the programs also allowed increased flexibility in staffing arrangements. For example, staff members from the parent co-op were able to conduct intake staffings occasionally by having staff from the "other" programs supervise all of the children during specific times.

In some cases jointly held values became the basis for emphasizing specific program features. For example, both the parent co-op and the special education program placed a high priority on parent involvement. This became a salient aspect of the program philosophy for the integrated program.

Conversely, some interests were not jointly held across the participating agencies and programs. The authors' goals in such situations were to identify other interests that could be used to motivate commitment to the integrated program. For example, the interest in facilitating high levels of parent participation described above was not shared by the Head Start staff, who were concerned that such a policy might reduce their control over curriculum and instructional decisions. The Head Start staff had, however, a strong interest in augmenting consultative services for their program, particularly in the area of speech pathology. The commitment of the special education program to utilize their communication disorders specialist within a classroom-based service model emphasizing work with integrated groups of children and consultation to teachers rather than a clinical "pull-out" model, was thus a major benefit to the Head Start program that could be used as leverage against their concerns about high levels of parent influence over the program.

Outcomes

The process described in Fairview has been ongoing for 1 year, and is still underway. Outcomes to date have been modest, but there appears to be a broad base of support from the diverse group of individuals and agencies involved. Children from each of the three programs are integrated for free-play activities on a daily basis. In addition, integrated language and other instructional groups are operated on a regular schedule throughout the week. Perhaps most significantly, the decision has been made to remodel the early education facility for the specific purpose of permitting more complete integration of the programs. Although it is planned that each program will remain under its own administrative aegis, a substantial investment has been made toward replacing the original separate and segregated service models with a coordinated array of services emphasizing integration of children, staff, and resources.

CONCLUSION

The activities described in this chapter are focused on analysis and intervention strategies related to essentially nonpedagogical aspects of implementing integrated programs at the preschool level. The authors believe that these issues have been seriously underplayed in the professional literature on the development of integrated programs—resulting in programs that do not have the social/political support base necessary for long-term survival. It should not be inferred, however, that the authors believe that the actual educational experiences designed for children within integrated programs are not important. The effective development of strong community support for integrated programs is clearly necessary, but is hardly a sufficient condition for providing quality programs. The development of pedagogically sound, integrated programs is in itself a highly complex task, one that requires careful consideration of a host of programmatic variables (see Guralnick, 1981, 1986, for particularly comprehensive analyses of these issues).

Segregated special education programs were not invented, nor have they ever been justified, as a pedagogically superior arrangement for meeting the needs of children. Rather, they have historically represented a socially and politically acceptable response to pressures from parents and other advocates seeking access to services for a traditionally disenfranchised group of children. The LRE concept, however, goes far beyond issues of simple access to public school services. Efforts to achieve true social integration open a much wider front of social and ethical issues that challenge closely held cultural assumptions about the worth and appropriate treatment of human beings who have disabilities. The problems of implementing the LRE principle are thus seriously misconstrued when framed in purely pedagogical terms, and barriers to implementation will not be resolved by narrowly pedagogical means. Including children with disabilities in the mainstream of American life will require alteration of the basic social/political values on which communities have based educational policy decisions. It is in this context that the authors hope the issues they have raised and the processes they have described here have value.

STUDY QUESTIONS

1. Given the conceptual model for implementing an LRE shown in this chapter, list and discuss aspects affecting teachers and administrators, and generate ideas about how to cope with perceived difficulties.

2. Write a sample letter to parents of nonhandicapped children explaining any special needs or information concerning a child who has a particular impairment (your choice).

3. Compare and contrast the ecological process described in the chapter to a strictly pedagogical approach to designing an integrated preschool program.

4. Select one of the three "working hypotheses" described in the early section of this chapter and describe why you would consider it the most important to use in drafting a model for implementing an LRE program.

5. Briefly explain why an LRE program is best supported through public participation. Why is this necessary?

6. In regard to your own experiences in working with human service agencies/programs, consider the process model outlined in the chapter and generate a list of individuals who might be key players for the situation you have experienced.

REFERENCES

Baer, D. (1986). Exemplary service to what outcome? [Review of *Education of learners with severe handicaps: Exemplary service strategies*]. *Journal of The Association for Persons with Severe Handicaps, 11*, 145–147.

Ballard-Campbell, M., & Semmel, M.I. (1981). Policy research and special education: Research issues affecting policy formation and implementation. *Exceptional Education Quarterly, 2*, 59–67.

Brady, M., & Gunter, P. (Eds.). (1985). *Integrating moderately and severely handicapped learners: Strategies that work*. Springfield, IL: Charles C Thomas.

Gaylord-Ross, R., Haring, T.G., Breen, C., & Pitts-Conway, V. (1984). The training and generalization of social interaction skills with autistic youth. *Journal of Applied Behavior Analysis, 17*, 229–249.

Gaylord-Ross, R., & Peck, C.A. (1985). Social integration of students with severe mental retardation. In D. Bricker & J. Filler (Eds.), *Serving students with severe retardation: From research to practice*. Reston, VA: Council for Exceptional Children.

Glaser, B.G., & Strauss, A.L. (1967). *The discovery of grounded theory: Strategies for qualitative research*. Chicago: Aldine Press.

Guralnick, M.J. (1981). Programmatic factors affecting child-child social interactions in mainstreamed preschool programs. *Exceptional Education Quarterly, 1*(4), 71–91.

Guralnick, M.J. (1986). The application of child development principles and research to preschool mainstreaming. In C.J. Meisel (Ed.), *Mainstreaming handicapped children: Outcomes, controversies, and new directions* (pp. 21–41). Hillsdale, NJ: Lawrence Erlbaum Associates.

Kweit, M.G., & Kweit, R.W. (1981). *Implementing citizen participation in a bureaucratic society: A contingency approach*. New York: Praeger.

Langton, S. (Ed.). (1978). *Citizen participation in America: Essays on the state of the art*. Lexington, MA: Lexington Books.

Peck, C.A., Apolloni, T., Cooke, T.P., & Raver, S. (1978). Teaching retarded preschool children to imitate nonhandicapped peers: Training and generalized effects. *Journal of Special Education, 12*, 195–207.

Peck, C.A., & Cooke, T.P. (1983). Benefits of mainstreaming

at the early childhood level: How much can we expect? *Analysis & Intervention in Developmental Disabilities, 3,* 1–22.

Peck, C.A., Killen, C., & Owen, S. (1987). *Evaluating preschool mainstreaming programs: A conceptual model and case study.* Unpublished manuscript, Washington State University, Pullman.

Richarz, S.A., Peck, C.A., & Peterson, K. (1986). *Developing integrated preschools in rural communities.* Proposal funded by the U.S. Department of Education, Handicapped Children's Early Education Program, to Washington State University, Department of Child and Family Studies.

Russo, D.C., & Koegel, R.L. (1977). A method for integrating an autistic child into a normal public school classroom. *Journal of Applied Behavior Analysis, 10,* 579–590.

Semmel, M.I., Gottlieb, J., & Robinson, N.M. (1979). Mainstreaming: Perspectives on educating handicapped children in the public schools. In D. Berliner (Ed.), *Review of research in education* (Vol. 7). (pp. 223–276). American Educational Research Association, Peacock Publishers.

Semmel, M.I., Lieber, J., & Peck, C.A. (1986). Effects of special education environments: Beyond mainstreaming. In C.J. Meisel (Ed.), *Mainstreaming handicapped children: Outcomes, controversies, and new directions* (pp. 165–192). Hillsdale, NJ: Lawrence Erlbaum Associates.

Snyder, L., Apolloni, T., & Cooke, T.P. (1977). Integrated settings at the early childhood level: The role of nonretarded peers. *Exceptional Children, 43,* 262–266.

Strain, P.S., & Kerr, M.M. (1981). *Mainstreaming of children in schools: Research programmatic issues.* New York: Academic Press.

Strain, P.S., Kerr, M.M., & Ragland, E.V. (1979). Effects of peer-mediated social initiations and prompting/reinforcement procedures on the social behavior of autistic children. *Journal of Autism and Developmental Disorders, 9,* 41–54.

Weatherley, R., & Lipsky, M. (1977). Street-level bureaucrats and institutional instruction: Implementing special education reform. *Harvard Educational Review, 47,* 171–197.

Wolfensberger, W. (1972). *The principle of normalization in human services.* Toronto, Canada: National Institute on Mental Retardation.

CHAPTER 14

ADMINISTRATIVE STRATEGIES FOR INTEGRATION

William C. Wilson

A school district's or state education agency's (SEA) understanding of "mainstreaming" or "integration" often serves as the basis for employing administrative strategies to develop an integrated service system. Although not identified or defined within the Education for All Handicapped Children Act (Public Law 94-142, 1975), the terms have evolved around the concept of the least restrictive environment (LRE) and have specific meaning to administrators within the context of service delivery. Mainstreaming usually refers to placing children with mild disabilities in the regular education program. The term is misleading in that identified children who are placed in regular education classrooms are also often taken from the classroom for special intervention in a resource room, in a "pull-out" program. Therefore, depending on the time of day one observes, these students can be viewed as receiving their education in the mainstream through regular education, or they can be viewed as receiving their education in a special education situation. Resource room instruction may be intricately tied to regular class activities. However, more often than not, the activities relate only tangentially, if at all, to the regular education curriculum. Thus, in many cases the resource room has become a part-time self-contained program for many students with mild disabilities (Meyen, 1982). The term integration has had a broader interpretation and has referred to a program design that brings a proportionate number of students (e.g., students with severe disabilities) from a previously segregated environment to the regular school campus and then extends the program beyond the campus to the community and workplace.

With regard to school integration, the term has evolved to mean: the location of students with disabilities on a regular campus, in an age-appropriate setting, with integrated transportation; where special classes are in immediate proximity of regular classes; where frequent interactions occur between students with disabilities and their nondisabled peers; where there is a natural proportion of students with disabilities to their nondisabled peers; and where there is inclusion of students with disabilities in all school activities (Sailor, 1989). The least restrictive environment concept as described within the statute (Public Law 94-142, 1975) provides the undergirding for both mainstreaming and integration. Administrators desiring to promote integration should not get lost in terminology but should move ahead with programs that are true to the spirit of these words. It is easy to find loopholes in laws and to interpret meanings in order to avoid program changes. It is difficult to take critical steps that, although they may not be embraced by fellow educators, ensure that students are truly being provided their education in the least restrictive educational setting.

Prior to discussing administrative strategies, a brief review of the service implications of federal law is provided. State laws, while important, follow federal provisions once the state participates in a federal educational program such as the Education of the Handicapped Act. Thus the reader should refer to specific state laws for information pertaining to state procedures. Following this discussion, the remainder of the chapter is devoted to strategies that can be utilized by local administrators desiring to provide an integrated and complete range of services for students with disabilities. The intention of the chapter is to provide practical strategies related to the central theme of all special education programs; that is, to ensure that high-quality services are provided to individuals within the historical concept of "normalcy" (Nirje, 1969).

The reader should keep in mind that the delivery of integrated services is a complex issue and cannot be reduced to five or six strategies that will guarantee success. However, the suggested strategies should provide a prototype that can be expanded or dealt with as part of a systems approach in order to allow students with disabilities to receive the best services possible within the same educational environment as their nondisabled peers.

LEGAL AND ADMINISTRATIVE IMPLICATIONS FOR INTEGRATION

Prior to the passage of PL 94-142 in November, 1975, there were no real incentives for serving students with mild or severe disabilities into the regular education service system. Although California had developed a *Master Plan for Special Education* (1974), Massachusetts had passed the Bartley-Daly Act, Chapter 766 (1974), and the plaintiffs had prevailed in the *PARC* (1971) and *Mills* (1972) cases, on the whole, parents of students receiving special education services were mostly concerned about whether services were available through the public schools and not whether they were being provided within the educational mainstream.

Regulations for the landmark legislation were published in 1977 (*Federal Register,* 1977, August

23). Those regulations clarified and interpreted the provisions pertaining to the least restrictive environment. The regulations implied that a disabled child should be able to enroll at his or her neighborhood school and receive the necessary assessment and services as delineated on the individualized education program (IEP). Success was met in many locations, but all too often program decisions resulted in segregated, isolated, pull-out placements. Placing students in situations with nondisabled peers became a minor concern rather than a foundation of the service program. This situation occurred for a variety of reasons, not the least of which was the determination of "appropriateness." Many IEP committees interpreted the phrase "to the maximum extent appropriate" (*Federal Register,* 1977, August 23) to mean appropriate as deemed by the committee that developed the IEP. The result was a conservative interpretation that ultimately was based on the child's handicapping condition (e.g., if learning disabled, it meant resource room; if mentally retarded, it meant self-contained). Although the majority of children identified as handicapped under the current definitions are in fact now receiving most of their education within the regular educational environment, no data collection procedures of the government document the number of children who are actually receiving *special education* within the regular education classroom (*Reports to Congress,* 1982–1987).

The LRE provisions became the most controversial aspect of the new law and were often the subject of debate among scholars, discussion among program administrators, and frustration for parents and advocates for services to be provided in the most normal educational environment (i.e., the regular education program). In many instances even the most logical service pattern for a compliant service delivery program was met with a great deal of resistance.

While program administrators grappled with the concept of LRE and integrated educational service delivery, advocates pressed the administration to publish regulations for Section 504 of the Rehabilitation Act of 1973 (*Federal Register,* 1977, May 4), a provision that ultimately had more of a consequence on LRE than the Education of the Handicapped Act (1977). Simply stated this section said:

> no otherwise qualified handicapped individual . . . shall, solely by reason of his handicap, be excluded from the participation in, be denied the benefits of, or be subjected to discrimination under any program or activity receiving federal financial assistance. (Public Law 93-112, 1973)

Section 504 became a standard not only in educational programs but in all programs receiving federal financial assistance, such as recreation, work, and welfare programs. Buildings were remodeled, plans for buildings were modified, toilet spaces were reconfigured, ramps were built, drinking fountains were lowered, and a host of other physical measures were undertaken that resulted in allowing for more independence for disabled individuals. The dream of participating in normal activity with nondisabled peers came closer to reality. It appeared as though Section 504, when applied with the LRE provisions of PL 94-142, would assure more mainstreaming and integration.

Yet resistance continued from many communities and school systems. Arguments supporting specialized yet segregated facilities were presented utilizing the rationale that a central location would be more cost-effective and could house complete services such as speech therapy, occupational therapy, physical therapy, and psychological services at one location. Although this argument was used by many public agencies, others offered an even more drastic alternative in that the school system stated that they could only provide special education services that were currently available within the district. If a child's assessment indicated that it was necessary for him or her to have a self-contained room with a teacher who was qualified to instruct students with disabilities that manifested themselves in autistic behaviors and the district did not currently employ such a person, the services were often arranged through a

contract with an outside vendor or private school. Many localities felt that children could be placed in special schools outside the district if the IEP committee agreed to such a placement. The tragic result of this interpretation was that many children classified as learning disabled were placed in private schools specifically designed for children with learning disabilities. When this action was taken, the referring local school district or the state usually paid the bill and thus avoided having to build an integrated service delivery model. The mildly handicapped student was thus totally removed from the regular education environment and placed in a segregated and isolated setting. This placement seldom resulted in movement back to a school district special education program, and even more rarely resulted in integration into the educational mainstream.

Once the Department of Education began conducting program reviews in states that had submitted approved program plans for PL 94-142, LRE was often cited as an area of noncompliance (*Letters of Findings,* 1980–1981). Indeed, when state education agencies monitored local districts, they found many segregated programs, particularly for students with severe disabilities. Students who received special education services through contracts developed with private or outside agencies were found to be in isolated rather than integrated educational environments. The U.S. Office for Civil Rights (OCR) began acting on complaints filed with the federal agency by parents or advocacy groups. The OCR, which acted independently from SEAs, also found a proliferation of segregated programs.

If programs were reviewed or complaints were investigated and noncompliance with LRE was discovered, formal letters from the U.S. Department of Education were sent to state officials indicating the violation with specifications for necessary corrective actions and a timeline for meeting compliance standards. This procedure was effective in that, often, states would modify service programs merely after receiving notice that their state would be visited, before the visit actually took place. In addition, when state agencies were cited through the program review process, actions were usually taken that corrected PL 94-142 violations.

During the late 1970s and early 1980s, service delivery patterns throughout the United States slowly changed. Segregated services for the students with severe disabilities became a less-frequent occurrence and programs were integrated onto regular school campuses. Even with such activities, in 1988, only 30% of students with severe disabilities were being served on integrated sites (Gaylord-Ross, 1988). Students with learning disabilities who were also emotionally disturbed, although initially allowed "contract" status, began to be reassessed and placed within the local school system. Some of these students were placed with regular education students for at least a portion of the day but students with behavior disorders were more commonly placed within segregated programs or self-contained classrooms.

An interesting phenomenon occurred in service delivery during the late 1980s. As programs providing services to severely disabled students changed the pattern and method for service delivery from segregated to integrated settings, the goal for these students became ultimately associated with the community-at-large as well as the school system. Students with severe disabilities began to be integrated into the community, thus extending beyond the educational system into the adult service system, the working world, and recreational activities.

During this time of change for students with severe disabilities, services for learning disabled and mildly handicapped children remained essentially the same (i.e., resource rooms [pull-out programs] and self-contained classes). Service in the least restrictive environment for learning disabled children was seldom challenged, as resource rooms were almost always located on a regular school campus and even self-contained rooms for mildly handicapped students were usually located in regular elementary or secondary schools. Reports revealed that when a child was labeled learning disabled, the service was usually delivered via the resource room; and most students labeled as emotionally disturbed were served in a self-contained situation (*Eighth Annual Report to Congress,* 1986).

The original intention of resource programs was to provide short-term services that would allow the child to function more effectively within the regular educational environment (Adamson & Van Etten, 1972; Lilly, 1971). The early models emphasized regular classroom placement and periodic criterion-referenced monitoring. Many teachers implementing these models kept behavioral records and frequency counts in order to note each child's educational gains. Although the method was time-consuming, the rate of the child's educational progress was measured and subsequently, children were allowed to move toward more service in the regular classroom. The goal was regular classroom placement. This goal became somewhat distorted once the resource model became widespread in that the referral to special education was often based on a discipline problem rather than a learning problem, and placement was long term rather than short term. Thus, a student labeled as learning disabled became a responsibility of the special education system. A quick tour of many school buildings in the early 1980s would lead one to believe that very little mainstreaming existed. It was not unusual to find a sign such as the following above a door in the hallway of an elementary school building: *Miss Franks, Special Education.* Special education was both labeled and segregated.

PL 94-142 not only did little to alleviate the stigma of the label, it created a financial incentive for increasing the number of handicapped students labeled as receiving special education services. States and districts were allocated dollars based on the count of handicapped children receiving special education services. Therefore, instead of striving for service within the regular education continuum, school districts increased the count by qualifying large numbers of children with learning disabilities for special education. The legislation placed a cap on the number of children that could be counted as learning disabled by a state at 2% of the number of all children age 5–17 in the state (Federal Register, 1977, August 23). However, in December, 1977, the federal government published criteria for labeling a child as learning disabled (*Federal Register,* 1977, December 29). The regulation also lifted the cap on the count. Once the regulation was published, a guaranteed method for increasing the child count existed. Although the federal mandate provided the incentive for program integration through the LRE provisions, the funding mechanism within PL 94-142 provided no incentive for special education in the regular classroom. In fact a disincentive was in place in that once a child received 100% service from regular education with no supplemental services, he or she was no longer considered handicapped. If the student was re-evaluated and determined to be ineligible for special education services he or she was dropped from the count. This resulted in less state and federal funding for the program and guaranteed that the student would no longer receive services of any kind from special education personnel. Thus the learning disabilities child count was increased (*Reports to Congress,* 1982–1987) and students who were so labeled and placed became valuable to the district because they increased the state and federal allotment for the program.

The Regular Education Initiative

Recently, service delivery to students with learning problems has been an issue of national discussion. The regular education initiative (REI) (Will, 1986) caused program administrators, direct service personnel, and even higher education training programs to question, debate, or become entrenched in positions regarding service to this large group of students. While some felt this to be a financial tactic and others felt it to be the beginning of the end of special education for children with learning problems, Madeleine Will, the U.S. Assistant Secretary for Education for the Office of

Special Education and Rehabilitative Services, indicated that many mildly handicapped children being served within the special education system could be better served in alternative ways through regular education. Will challenged that children with learning problems were the responsibility of the general education system and that education options for these children were often never fully explored, especially with regard to receiving services in regular classrooms. The work of Wang and Birch (1984), Reynolds, Wang, and Walberg (1986), Reschly (1987), and others supported this position. Wang, Reynolds, and Walberg edited the *Handbook of Special Education: Research and Practice* (1987), which became controversial in that it was seen as supporting the notion that education for students with learning problems should be provided by regular education.

Professionals working in the field of special education began to interpret and misinterpret the information. Enthusiastic supporters of the REI saw a new role for special education in either a consulting or peer support capacity, while others felt that the federal government was advocating elimination of special education for children with learning disabilities. For example, the *Journal of Learning Disabilities* published a special issue that presented articles by well-known authors that essentially supported the continuation of the status quo (Hallahan, Keller, McKinney, Lloyd, & Bryan, 1988; Kauffman, Gerber, & Semmel, 1988; McKinney & Hocutt, 1988).

The debate, which will continue at least for a few years, will have a definite impact on service delivery. Although it can be said that one group believes that service delivery to children with learning problems should be provided within the regular education system while the other group believes that pull-out programs are the best approach, this oversimplifies the issue and ignores a complex problem that addresses financial considerations, human rights, parental concerns, and educational effectiveness. Further, while findings can be presented validating or invalidating each side of the argument, sadly enough, the courts may determine the service pattern, based on single-case and group litigation. Indeed, the law itself is sufficiently vague as to allow for a number of placement decisions to be made on the part of judges. On the positive side, the REI has caused the field to look internally to the services currently being provided to students with mild disabilities and has caused questions to arise, research to be conducted, and intellectual as well as practical discussion to take place.

The New Integration

As one develops or attends to administrative strategies for integration, one should notice that, once again, a new event in special education has taken place with only minimal involvement of regular education. At the national level, the emphasis in regular education has been on education reform measures and very little has been said about special education in, for example, *A Nation Prepared* (1986), Goodlad's work (1984), the Holmes group (1986), or other U.S. Department of Education publications pertaining to reform. In fact, the REI has only received the attention devoted to it thus far as a result of the Office of Special Education Programs within the U.S. Department of Education.

If the education of handicapped students in the least restrictive environment is viewed within the same context as the civil rights of minorities, then it is logical that the field of special education should be approaching a *true* integration of services (i.e., service in the regular classroom). This cannot be accomplished without an integration of administrative plans and strategies as students begin to receive special education services in the regular classroom. The difficulty lies in the lack of a mandate or a history of litigation efforts. The integration of students with learning problems into the educational mainstream is a progressive step, yet school systems do not have a history of taking high risks and progressive steps. The entire movement in special education services has been the result of pressure on the system to do what school systems traditionally do not like to do, that is,

serve students who do not fall into the normal education pattern.

Figure 1 shows the history of integrating the child with learning problems into the educational mainstream. This diagram clearly shows that the field is now approaching a service pattern similar to that that was available before special education was mandated—students with learning problems are being served with their nondisabled peers. The service pattern is different in the sense that services, as well as children, are now beginning to be integrated.

The new integration (integration of the special education service system) will only be supported by special education administrators when they see themselves as an important part of the total educational service system, rather than an independent entity. If students with learning problems are to be

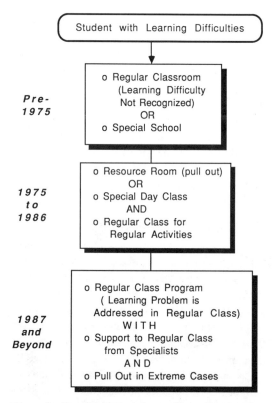

Figure 1. Service pattern for students with learning difficulties.

served through regular education, a program that includes both special educators and regular educators as one basic component should be more effective in serving the special needs of students than the current configuration in most school districts.

Prior to embarking on a new mission or developing strategies for integration, special educators should agree on the premise that children with disabilities are entitled to the same rights and educational privileges as their nondisabled peers. Therefore, special educators should support the regular system so that it can work for students with learning problems and prevent their removal from the system and the subsequent labeling, if at all possible. This is not to say that all mildly disabled children will be served 100% of the time in the regular classroom; it is a commitment to changing the configuration of most special education service systems. First, however, administrators must ask some practical questions about the consequences of providing services to mildly disabled students through a more integrated service system.

1. How can information be presented that shows the benefits of an integrated service system?
2. What will be the impact on the referral and assessment process?
3. Can assurances for due process be maintained?
4. How can individualized education programs be established for the entire school population? Should IEPs be eliminated for children with learning problems who are being served in the educational mainstream?
5. What are the projected personnel needs?
6. Are teacher preparation programs ready to provide the district with elementary, secondary, and special education personnel with the skills that will be necessary to successfully implement alternative services?
7. Have enrollment projections provided a fairly accurate count of the numbers of students with learning problems that can be expected?
8. How can parents and others responsible for the students be assured that at least the same if not improved educational progress will be made through a change in the service system?
9. When can one expect the system to become totally integrated?
10. Will labeling (if only for internal purposes) be necessary? If so will fewer categories exist?
11. How will all special education services function within an integrated system and how will student progress and social integration be measured?
12. Will a totally integrated system be in compliance with federal and state laws as they currently exist, or will the district be requesting waivers at the state level?
13. Have arrangements been made with the state department of education that will assure ongoing funding and not less funding if students are served in the regular classroom?

Answers to these questions are complex, and simply to incorporate a new administrative design will only add to the complexity. The questions have been presented in order to illustrate the difficulty in progressing to a new level of service, even when such a move receives widespread support. However, when administrators, teachers, and parents address these issues systematically, better programs with a greater capacity to serve children with disabilities can result.

STRATEGIES FOR INTEGRATION

Although emphasis at the federal level during the mid-1980s was on severely disabled individuals, the late eighties and early nineties will see evidence of the new integration for students with mild disabilities—to put it simply; there will be more mainstreaming, prevention of labeling, and less pull out. The remainder of this chapter is devoted to the key administrative strategies for facilitating a service system that provides all disabled individuals, from those with severe multiple disabilities to students with learning problems, a high-quality educational program. (However, in order to limit the length of this chapter, the example given focuses only on students with mild disabilities.) The strategies discussed provide a *practical application,* not a panacea. Furthermore, the list of strategies is not exhaustive, nor does it specifically apply to planning for special education programs. Some of these same strategies have been utilized in business (Lewis, 1985, 1986a) and special education management (Burrello & Sage, 1975; Sage & Burrello, 1986). The focus, however, is on using the strategies in the context of the integration and mainstreaming of individuals with disabilities into the regular education and community milieu.

In order for the reader to operationalize the various strategies, and in order to provide a context for the administrative strategies, an example of a particular school system undergoing change is utilized from time to time. A description of the community and the school system is provided below:

Pacific Bay is a scenic community of 75,000 in the northwestern United States, located along the Pacific Ocean. The main industries in the community are agriculture and fishing. The population comprises commuters to a large city, residents engaged in the occupations of fishing or agriculture, and a number of migrant workers. Tourism is not a major industry as the cool climate and the rough water are not conducive to water sports or swimming.

The school system provides special education and related services to students identified as handicapped, as per state criteria, but there are also a number of students with learning problems who may eventually be identified as in need of special education services. The su-

perintendent of schools is aware that the state legislature is concerned about two important considerations concerning special education: 1) the growing number of children labeled as learning disabled, and 2) the amount of state dollars contributed to special education and related services programs. The state Department of Education is in the process of endorsing special education services through the regular education modality. The superintendent knows some changes will be made in the near future but he desires to anticipate rather than be surprised by those changes so as not to disrupt the overall program.

Strategy 1: Become Knowledgeable of the Issues

Knowledge is a key factor for anyone desiring to effect a change in a system (McCormack, 1984). Special education as a field has a history of debate and literature pertaining to where and by whom the child with mild disabilities should be served (Affleck, Madge, Adams, & Lowenbraun, 1988; Dunn, 1963; Reynolds et al., 1986; Stainback & Stainback, 1984). As one examines the various pieces of literature it becomes clear that researchers, practitioners, administrators, and parents have mixed emotions about the best service options (Gerber, 1988; Reschly, 1987; Wang & Birch, 1984; Will, 1986). The administrator desiring to offer total integrated services within the district should lead the staff to be open to the different options and not to be "stuck" in the current service pattern. It is critical to all who may be affected not to be closed to the issues and to realize that in any situation, data may be presented in strong rational ways, both for and against. The following suggested steps should help to implement this particular strategy:

1. Have an assistant or lead teacher develop an annotated bibliography, and distribute it to district staff along with information indicating that the district will soon be engaging in

discussions about improving the service system for students with learning problems. This list should include articles that will be informative. Assuming that a number of personnel will not seek out the information, the administration may choose to distribute key articles, chapters, reports, or monographs.

2. Make sure that any information provided on initiatives that may affect the service configuration is distributed through the regular education program rather than the special education program. This demonstrates responsibility on the part of the administration and allows special education to function in a supportive rather than a dominant role.

3. Follow up by asking teachers and administrators what they think and let them know that the administration is interested in their views on the issues from a curricular as well as a sociopolitical standpoint.

4. Contact persons who have had experience or conducted research and see if they would be willing to address the staff, PTA, school board, or other groups within the constituency in order to carry out an inservice information-gathering effort.

The intent of this strategy is to provide information about the issues to individuals who will be making decisions about program service patterns. At this point, officials within Pacific Bay want to move forward in the planning process. The juncture presents some excellent opportunities for failure before the project is off the ground, or it can lift spirits and generate enthusiasm—depending on how it is handled.

Strategy 2: Involve Teachers and Parents in the Input

When job descriptions change, when service systems change, when rooms change, and when transportation arrangements change, administrators can be certain that resistance (to put it mildly) will come from individuals as well as groups. Because services to students with mild disabilities are such highly emotional issues, just investigating the possibility of change can damage the credibility of the administration. It is rather obvious that all steps cannot be completed through consensus, and many times each day administrators have to make decisions based on what they think is the most logical approach. However, involvement of those who will live with the decision is critical. There are a number of different ways to do this. Some approaches are:

1. Move from building to building and talk to teachers. Be informal but sincere in asking questions. Ask "What do you think would happen if . . . ?" questions. This style of interacting has been utilized in successful companies and undoubtedly school systems could benefit from it as well (Peters & Waterman, 1984).

2. Meet with parents in groups and individually. On the one hand, if the administrator provides a notice to parents that the special education services will be modified and children with learning problems will now be served through regular education, several lawsuits may be filed. On the other hand, if the administrator approaches parents for their participation in developing a plan to provide a full range of services at the building level to serve all children with learning problems, another reaction can be expected. Parents in general do not like their child to be labeled in order for the child to receive special services. However, if a choice has to be made, parents will probably choose the label rather than lose the service. This type of alternative is damaging to the program and the student. Parents should be involved in decision making about programs, not manipulated or tricked into believing that something will work when it is unproven. Administrators should seek input initially during planning, and later during implementation and evaluation.

Pacific Bay school officials recognize that each strategy may have an effect on another strategy.

Therefore, regardless of which strategy is being utilized, change should be viewed as a system rather than as a single event or an independent entity. Many mistakes will be encountered if one decides to develop and implement Strategy 1 until it has reached completion, and then move to Strategy 2, and so on. During implementation of PL 94-142, many SEA officials chose to hire a "child find specialist" in order to meet the location and identification provisions of the law. Subsequently, the majority of the task fell to one person who had to develop a system. Once the system was in place and children were located, job titles had to be changed, descriptions of duties had to be modified, and personnel had to change their areas of emphasis. Thus, implementation had been viewed as an event under one person's control that had a beginning and an end, rather than many persons sharing in the responsibility of different parts of a system. Some strategies should be initiated at different times, while others should be started simultaneously. Although there is no formula to determine timing, it can be critical and can contribute to the success or failure of the project. Pacific Bay officials recognize this danger and have chosen to simultaneously conduct Strategy 2 with Strategy 3.

Strategy 3: Gain the Support of Principals

Effective schools are managed by effective principals. Successful expansion of the service system will depend on principals. Meet the principals and define the task so that they have a clear understanding of the rationale and are offered the opportunity to provide their thoughts on the issues involved. One only has to move from building to building and review IEPs to discover that the "good ones" are written when the principal believes in the provisions of PL 94-142 and does his or her best to implement the law in the spirit intended.

Principals may face angry parents in the morning and meet with upset community leaders in the afternoon. In between, they try to motivate faculty by being the instructional leader of the school. With the multiple responsibilities and duties to which they must attend, one must realize that it will be difficult to expect principals to be enthusiastic about modifying a special education service system that took several years to implement. However, most principals want to improve their services and there is a sense of pride involved in implementing a program that will serve students with disabilities in a more complete manner. If the task is defined as expanding the service continuum and reconfiguring the pattern of services so as to prevent the need for labeling and a lifelong attachment to special education for children with learning problems, most will be willing to learn and to participate in "brainstorming" sessions. The following tips are helpful to remember about principals:

1. They can be the instructional leader of the school—or they can lead the resistance against new ideas.
2. They can motivate teachers—or they can be controlling and insensitive.
3. They can make decisions based on input or consensus of faculty—or they can be authoritarian.
4. They can involve parents in decision-making activities—or they can exclude them from any real role in the educational process.
5. They can be respected by the students—or they can be ridiculed.
6. They can participate in community activities—or they can ignore them.
7. They can arrange high-quality inservice training—or they can do only what the system requires.
8. They can be aware of situations at the classroom level—or they can remain aloof.
9. They can be knowledgeable of current education literature and its implications—or they can be completely unaware of research.
10. They can resolve conflict in a sensitive, problem-solving manner—or they can ignore problems and let them grow larger.

These are only 10 items; the reader may wish to add to the list. Educational systems have evolved into what they are today without any true design or intent (Skrtic, 1988). Children are placed in grades, teachers teach a group of children, and the principal is the administrator or "boss" of the school. Unions have not changed this scenario, nor have a host of innovative organizational system ideas. The result has been that principals affect the instructional attitude in their building, provide the leadership or lack of it, and, to an extent, may even control teacher behavior during nonschool school hours. Their authority is often unquestioned within the building and if one expects to successfully expand the service continuum, the principals must cooperate.

Officials in the Pacific Bay system have long recognized the real as well as the perceived authority of principals. Thus, careful hiring and promotion practices have resulted in a group of sensitive leaders. The system has chosen to seek their ideas, to find the right time to provide the stimulus, and to follow through with the necessary support.

Strategy 4: Form a Representative Group to Develop the Plan

As most administrators know, it is difficult to write in committee. However, it is imperative to plan in committee. Choosing the individuals who will represent a working group is a strategically difficult task and the administrator must recognize that no matter how fairly the group is chosen and no matter who is in the group, the administration will be criticized for not having a representative sample. One does not want to disenfranchise various groups or individuals who have contributed to the success of the special education program. Yet, if the goal is to develop a plan for integrated services in order to expand the continuum, the following should be helpful:

1. Select individuals who can analyze and discuss a problem without getting highly emotional.

2. Base representation according to groups such as regular teachers, special teachers, related services personnel, parents, principals, aides, and so forth. Avoid selection by disability labels. (Why? You are seeking to develop an integrated program, and labels will provide a rationale for separate programs. However, this does not mean that any disability area should lack the appropriate resources necessary to provide high-quality services.)

3. Keep the group as small as you can but large enough to be representative. In some cases groups may need to have as many as 25 individuals. If this is the case it is important to break the group into several working subgroups once tasks are defined.

4. If at all possible, recruit an outside facilitator who has done a substantial amount of preparation and has had group experience. This person can remain detached from political issues and assist the group in avoiding the "we've tried that before and it didn't work" mentality.

Pacific Bay Schools, desiring to move forward in the planning process, selected the following group to assist in the development of a plan to integrate special education services and expand the continuum available to all students: three principals, five parents, one director of special education, five regular education teachers, five special education teachers, one assistant superintendent of curriculum, one school attorney, one school psychologist, and one related services personnel (speech pathologist, occupational therapist, etc.). Although this may seem too large a group to accomplish the task, the most important aspect is that the group is representative; that is, it is composed of those who will be affected most by the outcome.

Strategy 5: Analyze the Current Special Education Service System

When meeting with the group that has been selected it is important to indicate that the task that the group will undertake is to develop a service system for special education that provides a range of services within an integrated environment. Another way to state the mission of the group is to challenge them to integrate the current special education service system into regular education. At this point it is very tempting for administrators to explain the new system as they see it and try to obtain group agreement. To take such action would be a serious mistake and cause a credibility gap to develop between the administration and the service providers.

The group may decide the procedure. However, a plan of operation that follows the child sequentially through the system allows participants to notice how the regular system handles each phase and to compare this set of activities with the procedures of the special education system.

Pacific Bay Schools chose to follow the path of service provision as presented below. Key questions or comments follow each step.

Identification   How is the student identified? Has the initial concern come from parents, regular education teachers, school nurse, or other sources? Is the child identified as having a learning problem, socialization problem, or behavior problem; or is the student just initially identified as someone who doesn't "fit"?

Referral   Once the child has been referred for an assessment, this usually means that the student is on his or her way to being labeled as a special education student. Has a prereferral process taken place? Has a professional worked with the child's current teacher to see if the problem can be resolved before a formal evaluation? Usually the answer is "no." It is important for any group examining the current service system to ask probing questions rather than to indicate that an identification and referral system is in place. The key question is "Why is this student being referred?"

Assessment   If the system is receiving any funds from the SEA or the federal government for the education of handicapped students, there should be evidence that assessment procedures are in compliance with the various statutes. Assessment should be unbiased, should evaluate the student's strengths as well as his or her deficiencies,

should include more than one instrument, should be explained to and approved by parents, should be administered in the child's native language, and so forth. When evaluating the assessment system the administrator should be sure to indicate to the group the importance of knowing if there is a good observational and behavioral assessment of the child in a variety of settings. In addition, it would be interesting to know whether assessment procedures have done nothing more than to confirm an original reason for referral, or whether assessment procedures have positively contributed to program decisions. Pertinent questions are: What is the average amount of time that elapses between the time the child is initially referred and the time that the child begins to get instructional assistance with the problem? (The concern is not with the legal limit in number of days but actual instructional time; that is, time spent working on the problem that the regular education teacher identified in the first place!) What actions, other than formal referral for assessment, could have been taken that would have addressed the learning problem? Did any professional examine commercially available computer programs or other technology that might have been available to assist with the learning problem prior to assessment? It should be noted, however, that the federal mandate is concerned with the protection of the student's rights during assessment and evaluation procedures, not the quality of the assessment. A system can be in compliance with federal law without knowing if the referring teacher could have addressed a learning problem through alternative instructional strategies.

Programming (Instruction and Placement)   How did the committee that developed the IEP decide which services were necessary and where the services should be provided? The group examining the existing system should be aware that all program decisions should be made within the context of the least restrictive environment. The school nearest to the child's home and the regular class should be the first placement option. All too often the IEP committee assumes that a mild handicapping condition means that the student should receive special education via a "pull-out" or segregated model, thus ignoring the school nearest to the home and the regular classroom option. If the student needs help with a learning problem, and even if the student has a true learning disability (however the term is defined within the school district), committees should remember that the student is not to be removed from the regular classroom unless he or she cannot function, even with the use of supplementary aides and services (Public Law 94-142, 1975).

Evaluation How is the student re-evaluated? How often is the IEP monitored? Does the special education teacher ever suggest that the child should go back to the regular classroom? Is the child making adequate progress vocationally? Does the student truly have access to the regular education curriculum? Is the student making subject matter progress? How many times does the resource teacher consult with the regular teacher? How does the student feel about him or herself? What is the percentage of students who were initially referred to special education who receive all of their education in the regular classroom before graduation? This series of questions suggests that special education should consistently evaluate the student's progress and should strive to return the student to regular education whenever possible. Unfortunately, most special education referrals stay in special education. Models presented in the early 1970s (e.g., Fail-Save system [Adamson & Van Etten, 1972, 1973], and the Zero Reject Model [Lilly, 1971]) were based on the premise that referred students should return to the regular classroom. Both models emphasized training and sought to serve the student with special needs prior to labeling. Ultimately, these models were the forerunner of the resource room. However, although students in resource rooms are reviewed annually, few are returned to 100% service through the regular education system.

Strategy 6: Develop the Ideal Service System

After the working group has examined the current service system in light of the points and questions listed above, the same group should develop the ideal service system in which all students would be able to meet their educational needs through an integrated continuum of services. Special education and regular education would be service providers to children identified through the assessment process as needing special education as well as students who are experiencing other learning problems that are keeping them from succeeding in school. By expanding the provisions of PL 94-142, both federal and state special education laws would be met. The result should be a stronger service system that can provide more instructional time for working with the child and his or her learning problem.

Items to Consider

In addition to alternatives that could be developed within the sequence of events discussed in Strategy 5, consideration should also be given to the following:

Infant and Preschool Program Any system to be developed should insure that infant and preschool services for handicapped children are made available. Services should be integrated, especially at a young age. This is especially important in assisting parents in the normalization process. Services should include a variety of professionals who may be involved with both the infant and preschool continuum.

Organization of the Regular and Special Education System The standard should be a working system where children with learning problems are educated by the professionals most capable to meet their needs. Political and philosophical points of view should not be a guide. The system should offer all services required by federal law and the ideal system would expand the service continuum. The new continuum should meet the needs of slow learners not identified as needing special education services but needing some additional instructional assistance. All service providers should be seen as having educational and social responsibilities for children with learning problems, whether these students are identified as disabled or with some other problem.

Integration of Related Services Related services are often extremely difficult to negotiate. Questions about the service to be provided, where it will be provided, and who will provide it frequently cloud the issue of what the student really needs. If proper referral and assessment procedures have been completed, the appropriateness of related services should not be an issue. Of importance in the development of integrated services is the environment or mode in which these services will be provided. Clearly, service provision in an integrated model should be more practical than clinical in nature.

Transdisciplinary Team The heart of the ideal service system should be a transdisciplinary approach that includes special education, related services, health services, and regular education without differentiating between the systems. A transdisciplinary team is one whose individual disciplinary roles overlap, thus allowing for service provision through a number of professionals rather than a specific individual or area (Bigge, 1988). An example of a transdisciplinary approach would be a teacher who has been trained by an occupational therapist (OT) to carry out certain prescribed therapeutic activities with a child who previously might have been the exclusive responsibility of the occupational therapist in a multidisciplinary approach.

Students' Choice of Services An ideal system should include the students in the decision-making process. Often students are seen as receivers of services, and they do not participate in decisions about their education. While the educational curriculum choices for regular education students are limited, these same choices are practically nonexistent for special education students. Note the following testimonial of a high school student-athlete who was placed in a "pull-out" situation to remediate his learning difficulty. The comment was made to a university graduate class in "Mainstreaming for Secondary Education":

I feel like a second class citizen. It's bad enough feeling stupid and knowing that others know it, but it is worse when I have to leave the class that I'm in, to go with the special education teacher. I do 'mickey mouse' things that don't relate to my other class; and when I return I am further behind than I would have been if I had never had special education. (anonymous personal communication)

Curriculum Adaptation An ideal system should be current in educational methods and curriculum adaptations should be made for students with learning problems. If this approach becomes reality, the first step would be prereferral or prevention, rather than referral to the special education system.

Rate of Educational Gain An ideal system should be accountable. Students, parents, and teachers should know the child's rate of learning. All should be aware of the student's success.

Socialization The student as well as his nondisabled peers should feel comfortable with the environment. Normal socialization processes should develop. Positive peer interactions should be more evident than ridicule or labeling.

Preparation for Employment or Postsecondary Education An ideal system should provide different curricular emphasis areas from which students and parents may choose. This will assist in an appropriate transition from school to the postsecondary situation or work. This requires a continuum of vocational education opportunities for all students.

Parent Satisfaction with the Program An ideal service system should include parents as participants in the educational process, not just receivers of information. Their ideas should be sought, their opinions valued, and their participation welcomed.

Granting of a Diploma The diploma should not be a meaningless document. Many special education students who experience learning problems may be labled as learning disabled and subsequently, may not receive training in the basic skills that would entitle them to receive a high school diploma. There are other special education students who may be awarded a special diploma. However, many special education students can learn basic skills and meet high school competency requirements as well, if they are provided with the appropriate educational opportunities (Gloeckler, 1988).

Athletics and Extracurricular Activities Athletics, while not a part of students' academic education, may enhance the students' perceptions of self-direction or locus of control. Perhaps the only comment pertaining to athletics worth considering is "inclusion." If a system is to be in compliance with Section 504 of the Rehabilitation Act of 1973, then all services offered to nondisabled students must be offered to students with disabilities. Obviously, adaptations of the athletic curriculum will have to be made. A specialist may be needed to consult with the athletic staff in order for appropriate activities to be offered.

Access to Technology Section 603 of PL 99-506, an amendment to the Rehabilitation Act of 1973, was passed by the U.S. Congress in 1985. This amendment created Section 508 of the Rehabilitation Act, which is basically a restatement of Section 504 as pertaining to electronic equipment. It is directed specifically to technology and directs the Secretary of Education to develop guidelines to ensure that handicapped individuals have access to electronic equipment and the supporting peripherals. Technology can render great assistance in helping school systems develop more integrated programs in that the whole idea behind the application of technology is to assist persons with disabilities to function in the mainstreamed or normal environment. Much has been accomplished utilizing technology. A new professional discipline within the field of disability, the rehabilitation engineer, has emerged, providing knowledge and skills to technological applications for individuals with disabilities. Technology services for students have been disjointed in that roles and responsibilities of various public agencies sharing the financial costs have yet to be determined and implemented. The Office of Special Education Programs within the U.S. Department of Education issued a proposal to be implemented in 1988 to develop plans for expanding technological services. The primary interest of the government was to ensure that these services are available and integrated within the continuum of services available.

Instructional Time and Strategies Provided to Students with Learning Problems Deschler and Schumaker (1984) have developed an entire system of strategies that can be incorporated in school systems by teachers. The key to success in applying the strategies is a thorough understanding of the concept and its application. The strategies are practical and ultimately teach self-responsibility. Although these strategies have yet to be applied in a general education situation on a broad scale, an ideal service system could include a suggestion that regular education personnel attend to the development of learning strategies for all children when appropriate.

Severely and Multiply Involved Students The focus of this chapter is on mildly disabled students, yet in developing the ideal service plan, the successful research within the severe disabilities area should be acknowledged and incorporated if possible. Great strides have been made toward deinstitutionalization, integration of age-appropriate programs, assisting local education agencies in providing less restrictive environments for disabled students (Sailor, 1989; Sailor & Guess, 1983), and implementing supported work and transition programs (Gaylord-Ross, 1988; Wehman, 1981).

Pitfalls

The above list covers items that need to be considered when developing the ideal service plan. If left without sensitive leadership, groups can often become negative about an ideal plan. Once this occurs it is difficult for a facilitator to assist the group toward the accomplishment of this goal. As previously stated, the group needs to feel that they are engaged in a genuine planning activity that will be seriously considered. Examples of comments that can detract from the task at hand are:

Administrator: "This plan is going to cost this school district more money than we are currently budgeting."

Regular Education Teacher: "I already have 4 troublemakers in a group of 30 and I don't believe that I will get the needed resources.

Why should I want a special education kid back when I referred him so I could have more order in my classroom?"

Special Education Teacher: "It took me three years to obtain the resources I need and to understand the referral process. Now you are asking me to change the thing I really want to do—work directly with handicapped children."

All of the above comments express how individual professionals feel. However, comments such as these can set a negative attitude for the entire group. When similar comments begin to be heard, participants need to be reminded that they are part of a planning effort for the entire district and they should continue on task in order to develop the "ideal system."

The ideal service system may have other components and may operate somewhat differently from what was presented here. The direction and form is not as important as having a participatory group address the crucial areas in a way that will

actually promote change. As emphasized previously, this is a high-risk activity that requires a skillful facilitator and a dedicated group of individuals. The process could prove to be a useful strategy when, as in the case of a Pacific Bay schools, a commitment exists to move toward a compliant and integrated special education system.

Overcoming Barriers

Once the group has addressed all components of the ideal plan, they should note the discrepancies that exist between the current service system and the ideal service system. This should take a relatively short amount of time since the differences will be obvious. The strategic move that the group needs to make if they expect the district to implement the plan is to rewrite the discrepancy statements into barrier statements, and lay out steps to overcome the barrier. Figure 2 presents an abbreviated component of the Pacific Bay plan pertain-

---

PACIFIC BAY FULL SERVICES PLAN

Assessment

Current

The system provides all of the appropriate notices and receives the appropriate signatures as required by law. However, the number of days required to provide notice and to obtain the appropriate signatures is maximal. In the meantime little or nothing is done for the child and his learning problem.

Ideal

A prereferral system will be implemented whereby a specialist will work with the regular education teacher to see if the child's educational deficit can be addressed in the regular classroom prior to referral.

Discrepancy

The system does not have a prereferral system.

Barrier

Regular education teachers do not want a prereferral system.

Strategy

Principals will meet with staff in order to describe a prereferral system. Additionally, the principals will obtain suggestions as to how such a system could be implemented at a building level. Specialist staff will be assigned to work with regular education teachers in order to see if the children's learning problems can be solved before referral and assessment are required.

Figure 2. Abbreviated version of the Pacific Bay plan dealing with assessment and service.

ing to assessment and service. Keep in mind that it is for illustrative purposes only.

Strategy 7: Develop a Concomitant Training Plan

Although the majority of higher education programs in this country are in existence for training individuals for various professions, there are few that are truly working with local school systems in a cooperative fashion to develop the necessary inservice training program. Training can be of importance when implementing a plan for integrated services. Many regular education teachers lack some but certainly not all of the technical skills required. Many specialists are unaware of the changes in regular education as a result of educational reform publications such as *A Nation At Risk* (1983), *What Works—Research about Teaching and Learning*, (1986), *Who will Teach Our Children?* (Commons et al., 1985), *Cooperative Learning* (Slavin, 1980) or other techniques that have been recently been incorporated in regular education training programs. New university training models are currently being developed that address the regular education/special education interface (Hudson, Correa, Morsink, & Dykes, 1987; Stainback & Stainback, 1987).

A statewide training plan should be developed as a part of the comprehensive system for personnel development required under PL 94-142. In developing a comprehensive plan, credentialing authorities and legislators may be requested to modify current credential requirements in order for the credential to reflect the service system rather than specific categories. Because these are state-level activities, local administrators may be influential in determining the skills teachers must have that will contribute to program integration. In order for the local system to meet their needs with teachers already employed within the system, a local plan for training must be developed. A training plan is critical if a new integrated service model evolves. Successful business and industry organizations have always considered training to be important (Lewis, 1986b). Yet,

school systems often neglect training or organize it in a piecemeal fashion. The Pacific Bay school system followed a standard plan and incorporated the following basic components of a training plan:

Conduct a Needs Assessment Most administrators know how to conduct this activity. However, care should be taken to include questions that will provide true, rather than perceived needs. Construction of the instruments and asking the right questions will save dollars for direct service, shorten the time of analysis, and possibly reduce the need. As the opinions of staff are not necessarily going to provide a true picture, plans that include a comprehensive look at the backgrounds and experiences of the professional staff could prove very beneficial.

Rank the Needs Little comment is necessary other than to consider the groups that have been surveyed in order to ascertain overall training needs.

Determine How Needs will be Addressed and Implement Training Remember that most discipline and learning problems are already handled in regular education and that expansion of the service continuum should provide alternative instructional strategies for both the regular education teacher and the special education teacher. Strategy sessions with key individuals may be more helpful than the traditional consultant oriented 1-day workshop. Specialists, regular educators, and administrators could develop their own individualized professional inservice training program that will meet their needs. A variety of alternatives exists. The local university might be of assistance. However, universities are often constrained by procedures and budget limitations and thus cannot provide the necessary inservice training. Finally, request the State Department of Education to assist in providing the necessary inservice training in order to ensure success.

Evaluate Training Traditional questionnaires that are distributed following inservice training programs are of little value in determining the long-range impact that training may have on the participants. One must monitor the entire training process in order to ensure that appropriate needs have been assessed, that correct training has taken place, and that training has been cost-effective. The most important question to ask is: "Did participants acquire usable skills as a result of the training?"

Strategy 8: Develop an Appropriate Financing Plan

Costs seem to relate directly to the kind and quality of education provided in a system. Education programs for children and youth with disabilities have been accused of encroachment upon the regular education program, unnecessary expenditures, excessive costs, and unjustifiable program growth. The federal program for education of handicapped students has been the fastest growing appropriation in education at the national level for the past 10 years, yet it has not kept up with authorized levels of funding (Public Law 94-142, 1975). Many districts and states provide the primary source of funding for special education programs and the federal share may amount to less than 10%.

Given these constraints and accusations, one cannot expect special education administrators to immediately embrace the idea of program integration without a specific, accountable auditing trail. The federal law has been specific with regard to eligibility, service, and protection of rights. Indeed, these are important provisions that should only be modified if the resultant services will reach more, rather than fewer students with learning problems. Merging budgets of various programs has been difficult at the federal level, so many may believe it will prove to be tremendously complex at the state and local level with respect to service position. Suspicion and paranoia on the part of special educators may bring forth comments such as: "The State Superintendent's agenda is to reduce the finances for special education, therefore the regular education initiative plays right into his hands." This may be a valid comment in that the academic merits of mainstreaming, while commendable, could result in fewer available services received from less than competent professionals if schools do not plan effectively.

The financing plan for Pacific Bay Schools as well as other districts across the United States can only be workable if:

1. Federal counting procedures are amended to include identified children receiving 100% service in the regular classroom (without pull out).
2. Assessment procedures prove to be less costly than they are now.
3. Assurances are received that affirm that regular education programs will be accountable for the appropriate use of special education dollars allocated to the regular education system.
4. Children receive appropriate services from qualified personnel.
5. Overall compliance with the original intent and integrity of special education statutes is maintained.

Conclusion

All of the cautions listed in Strategy 8 can be viewed as opportunities if the basic premise that all disabled children have a right to an education with their nondisabled peers is not lost. Validated models are necessary. However, many states are moving toward a consultant approach, which is only one alternative. Regardless of the direction in which a district chooses to proceed, the following principles should be kept in mind:

1. Engage in a continuous self-questioning process.
2. Communicate issues with administrators, practitioners, and parents.
3. Demonstrate educational leadership within the community.
4. Have a flexible administration.
5. Be ready to modify service patterns if the need arises.
6. Incorporate sound ideas in any model developed.

7. Provide a child-centered service system with transdisciplinary involvement.

SUMMARY

Public laws that have had an impact on the integration of children with disabilities are, primarily, PL 94-142, the Education for All Handicapped Act of 1975, and PL 93-112, the Rehabilitation Act of 1973 (Section 504). These laws had a profound effect on the configuration of services as well as teacher training programs and the due process rights of persons with disabilities and their families. Prior to implementation of these mandates, students were served mostly in segregated environments and parents had very little choice about the program in which their child was placed. Beginning in 1977, students placed in special education programs had to have an appropriate assessment battery, an individualized education program, placement in the least restrictive environment, and periodic evaluation of their educational progress. In addition, students and parents were able to question procedures through due process and were ensured that the student's rights were protected throughout the entire educational process.

Although PL 94-142 required school districts to provide a full continuum of services, most children diagnosed as learning disabled were placed in resource programs that pulled them out and away from the educational mainstream, for at least a portion of the day, for special services. A new trend has emerged as a result of action taken by the U.S. Department of Education's Office of Special Education and Rehabilitative Services. The regular education initiative is based on the premise that there are large numbers of children who are experiencing learning problems that could be more adequately and appropriately served in the regular classroom. Convincing research on both sides of the issue has been presented, as well as a possible cost-savings prediction. New models for service are being tested in several states and some states have changed their teacher credential requirements in order for the training to fit the service pattern.

Many administrators are concerned about providing a totally integrated program not only because of the REI, but because when more children are served within the regular education program, a more normal environment is established. The task is complex and appropriate strategies must be utilized in order to ensure the participation of those affected by possible program changes. School systems must plan for adequate dissemination of information about integration; employ group decision-making processes; include a cross-section of parents, teachers, ancillary personnel, and administrators; and systematically develop a plan. If these activities are conducted, the chances for success are greatly enhanced. The future may or may not see totally integrated service programs for students with disabilities. However, logical and sincere problem-solving strategies should be recognized and used by any school system desiring to move in a progressive direction.

STUDY QUESTIONS

1. Discuss the concept of integration of services and how it has evolved from the integration of the student.
2. Assume that you are a school administrator and you have been assigned the task of integrating special services. What strategies and procedures would you employ in order to make a smooth transition?
3. Why, and in what form, would you retain special services if your school system is moving toward a noncategorical, integrated model?
4. How would you conduct a 1-day workshop for principals on administrative strategies on the topic of integration? Keep the following in mind: pertinent articles and texts, large and small group sessions, administrative plans, and opportunities for professional discussion of the issues.

REFERENCES

Adamson, G., & Van Etten, G. (1972). Zero reject model revisited: A workable alternative. Exceptional Children, 38, 735–740.

Adamson, G., & Van Etten, G. (1973). *The fail-save program: A special education continuum*. In E. Deno (Ed.), *Instructional alternatives for exceptional children*. Arlington, VA: Council for Exceptional Children.

Affleck, J., Madge, S., Adams, A., & Lowenbraun, S. (1988). Integrated classroom versus resource model: Academic viability and effectiveness. *Exceptional Children, 54*(4), 339–348.

Bartley-Daly Act, Chapter 766. (1974). Massachusetts Regulations, Section 322, Massachusetts Department of Education.

Bigge, J. (1988). *Curriculum based instruction for special education students*. Mountain View, CA: Mayfield.

Bryan, T., Bay, M., & Donahue, M. (1988, January). Implications of the learning disabilities definition for the regular education initiative. *Journal of Learning Disabilities, 21*(1), 23–28.

Burello, L.C., & Sage, D. (1975). *Leadership and change in special education*. Englewood Cliffs, NJ: Prentice-Hall.

Commons, D.L., et al. (1985, November). *Who will teach our children?* Sacramento: The Report of the California Commission on the Teaching Profession.

Deschler, D., & Schumaker, J. (1984). Learning strategies: An instructional alternative for low achieving adolescents. *Exceptional Children, 52*(6), 583–590.

Dunn, L.D. (1963). *Exceptional children in the schools*. New York: Holt, Rinehart and Winston.

Federal Register. (1977, May 4). Regulations for P.L. 93-112, Rehabilitation Act of 1973. Washington, DC: Department of Health, Education, and Welfare, Office of Education.

Federal Register. (1977, August 23). Education of Handicapped Children: Implementation of Part B of EHA, P.L. 94-142, Education for All Handicapped Children Act of 1975. Washington, DC: U.S. Department of Education.

Federal Register. (1977, December 29). Assistance to States for Education of Handicapped Children, Procedures for Evaluating Specific Learning Disabilities. Washington, DC: Department of Health, Education, and Welfare.

Gaylord-Ross, R. (Ed.). (1988). *Vocational education for persons with handicaps*. Mountain View, CA: Mayfield.

Gerber, M.M. (1988). Weighing the 'regular education initiative: Recent calls for change lead to 'slippery slope'. *Education Week*, 32 VII.

Gloeckler, L.C. (1988, January 14). *Implementation of state-wide policy change: Goals, strategies and considerations*. Presentation to the California State Task Force on Regular Education/Special Education Initiatives, Monterey.

Goodlad, J. (1984). *A place called school*. New York: McGraw-Hill.

Hallahan, D.P., Keller, C.E., McKinney, J.D., Lloyd, J.W., & Bryan, T. (1988, January). Examining the research base of the regular education initiative: Efficacy studies and the adaptive learning environments model. *Journal of Learning Disabilities, 21*(1), 29–35.

Hewett, F.M. (1967). Educational engineering with emotionally disturbed children. *Exceptional Children, 33*, 459–471.

Holmes Group, Inc. (1986). *Tomorrow's teachers: A report of the Holmes Group*. East Lansing, MI: Author.

Hudson, P.J., Correa, V.I., Morsink, C.V., & Dykes, M.K. (1987). A new model for preservice training-teacher as collaborator. *Teacher Education and Special Education, 10*(4), 191–193.

Kauffman, J., Gerber, M., & Semmel, M. (1988). Arguable assumptions underlying the regular education initiative. *Journal of Learning Disabilities, 21*(1), 3–11.

Letters of findings to state education agencies, pertaining to compliance with P.L. 94–142 Regulations. (1980–1981). Washington, DC: U.S. Department of Education.

Lewis, J.L., Jr. (1985). *Excellent organizations*. Westbury, NY: J.L. Wilkerson.

Lewis, J.L., Jr. (1986a). *Achieving excellence in our schools*. Westbury, NY: Wilkerson.

Lewis, J.L., Jr., (1986b). *Creating excellence in our schools*. Westbury, NY: J.L. Wilkerson.

Lilly, S. (1971). A training based model for special education. *Exceptional Children, 37*, 745–749.

Master plan for special education [AB 404, Chapter 1532]. (1974). Sacramento: California State Legislature.

McCormack, M. (1984). *What they don't teach you at the Harvard Business School*. New York: Bantam.

McKinney, J.D., & Hocutt, A.M. (1988, January). The need for policy analysis in evaluating the regular education initiative. *Journal of Learning Disabilities, 21*(1), 6–12.

Meyen, E.L. (Ed.). (1982). *Exceptional children in today's schools: An alternative resource book*. Denver: Love Publishing.

Mills v. Board of Education of The District of Columbia, 348 F. Supp. 866 (D.D.C. 1972).

A nation prepared: Teachers for the 21st century. (1986). New York: Carnegie Task Force on Teaching as a Profession, New Carnegie Forum on Education and Economy.

A nation at risk: The imperative for educational reform. (1983). Washington, DC: The National Commission on Excellence in Education.

Nirje, B. (1969). The normalization principle and its human management implications. In W. Wolfensberger (Ed.), *Changing patterns in residential services for the mentally retarded*. Washington, DC: President's Committee on Mental Retardation.

Pennsylvania Association for Retarded Children (PARC) v. Commonwealth of Pennsylvania, Civil Action No. 71-42 (1971).

Peters, T.J., & Waterman, R.H., Jr. (1984). *In search of excellence*. New York: Warner Books.

Public Law 93-112, Rehabilitation Act of 1973, Section 504. (1973). Washington, DC: U.S. Department of Rehabilitation Services.

Public Law 94-142, The Education for All Handicapped Children Act of 1975. (1975, November). Washington, DC: U.S. Department of Education.

Public Law 99-506, Rehabilitation Act Amendments of 1986, Section 603. (1986, October). Washington, DC: U.S. Department of Rehabilitation Services.

Reports to Congress on the implementation of P.L. 94-142. (1982–1987). Washington, DC: U.S. Department of Education.

Reschly, D. (1987). *Learning characteristics of mildly handicapped students: Implications for classification, placement, and programming.* In M. Wang, M. Reynolds, & H. Walberg (Eds.), *Handbook of special education: Research and practice.* (Vol. 1, pp. 35–58). New York: Pergamon Press.

Reynolds, M.C., Wang, M.C., & Walberg, H.J. (1986). The necessary restructuring of special and regular education. *Exceptional Children, 53*(5), 391–398.

Sage, D., & Burrello, L.C. (1986). *Policy and management in special education.* Englewood Cliffs, NJ: Prentice-Hall.

Sailor, W. (in press). The educational, social, and vocational integration of students with the most severe disabilities. In D.K. Lipsky & A. Gartner (Eds.), *Beyond separate education: Quality education for all.* Baltimore: Paul H. Brookes Publishing Co.

Sailor, W., & Guess, D. (1983). *Severely handicapped students: An instructional design.* Boston: Houghton Mifflin.

Skrtic, T. (1988). An organizational analysis of special education reform. In *Conference proceedings: Policy Analysis on Special Education Reform, General Education/Special Education Interface Task Force for the California State Department of Education.* Sacramento: California Department of Education.

Slavin, R. (1980). Cooperative learning. *Review of Educational Research, 50,* 315–342.

Stainback, W., & Stainback, S. (1984). A rationale for the merger of special and regular education. *Exceptional Children, 51,* 102–111.

Stainback, W., & Stainback, S. (1987). Facilitating merger through personnel preparation. *Teacher Education and Special Education, 10*(4), 185–190.

U.S. Department of Education (1985). Eighth Annual Report to Congress on the Implementation of Public Law 94-142, *The Education for All Handicapped Children Act.* Washington, DC: Author.

Wang, M.C., & Birch, J.W. (1984). Effective special education in regular classes. *Exceptional Children, 50,* 391–398.

Wang, M., Reynolds, M., & Walberg, H. (Eds.). (1987). *Handbook of special education: Research and practice* (Vol. 1). New York: Pergamon Press.

Wehman, P. (1981). *Competitive employment: New horizons for severely disabled individuals.* Baltimore: Paul H. Brookes Publishing Co.

What works—Research about teaching and learning. (1986). Washington, DC: U.S. Department of Education.

Will, M.C. (1986). *Educating students with learning problems: A shared responsibility.* Washington, DC: U.S. Department of Education, Office of Special Education and Rehabilitative Services.

CHAPTER 15

COMMUNITY LIVING AND THE EDUCATION OF STUDENTS WITH SEVERE DISABILITIES

Steven J. Taylor and James A. Knoll

Harvey and Sam (all names have been changed) live on the first floor of a typical apartment building in Madison, Wisconsin. The one distinctive characteristic of their house is the ramp that Harvey needs to get in and out of the building in his electric wheelchair. When the authors visited Harvey he was adjusting to his new home after having spent most of his 50-plus years in a state institution. Using his communication board and one-word symbols, he made it quite clear that he was enjoying his new life and looking forward to his new job as a 15-hour-a-week clerical volunteer in the local library. His talkative, gregarious roommate Sam (about 60 years old) has been living in the community since he was, as he puts it, "paroled" from the institution years ago. These two men lease a three-bedroom apartment—their home. They share it with Bob, their "paid roommate," who pays one third of the household expenses. Options in Community Living, a local agency that provides residential supports to people with disabilities, helped to set up this living arrangement and offers some of the other in-home services (e.g., relief for Bob; physical therapist, occupational therapist, and visiting nurse for Harvey) that enable these two men to live in their own home and not in an agency-run facility.

Throughout the United States people like Harvey and Sam, who were deprived of the benefits of a "free, appropriate, public education" and often have spent years in sterile, deprived environments, where they never had the opportunity to develop the necessary "prerequisite skills" for community living, are defining the state of the art in residential services. They are helping to form a vision of the future for all people with disabilities that should act as a guide for everyone involved in their lives.

TRANSITION TO WHAT?

"Transition" has become a buzz word used to characterize the need that many special education

Preparation of this chapter was supported by the Research and Training Center on Community Integration, Center on Human Policy, Division of Special Education and Rehabilitation, School of Education, Syracuse University. The Research and Training Center (Cooperative Agreement No. G0085C03503) is funded by the U.S. Department of Education, Office of Special Education and Rehabilitative Services, National Institute on Disability and Rehabilitation Research. The opinions expressed herein do not necessarily reflect the position of the U.S. Department of Education and no official endorsement should be inferred.

The authors would like to thank Robert Bogdan, Douglas Biklen, Henry Bersani, Jr., Bonnie Shoultz, Julie Racino, Pamela Walker, Zana Lutfiyya, Dianne Ferguson, Rebecca Salon, Stan Searl, and Parnel Wickham-Searl for their participation in the site visits and interviews cited in this chapter.

graduates have for supportive services as they move from a school system to adulthood. There is now a generation of students, graduating from special education, who challenge the existing adult service system. They have had an education that prepared them to be active participants in their communities. Many of these students, including those with very severe disabilities, have been educated in integrated settings, alongside nondisabled peers. Many of them have received a functional, community-based education that has prepared them to continue, as adults, to work with nondisabled people. And, it is just this type of employment that their teachers and parents expect the vocational service sector to aid them in finding.

The importance of transition reflects the fact that as the educational system was changing, the vocational sector was not keeping pace—so the necessary system of supports was not there. Now, after students have begun to graduate, it becomes necessary to set up the structure needed to meet the needs of this new generation of special education graduates; that is, to create task forces, formulate interagency agreements, and develop regulations governing "supported work." In the meantime some of these same students, whose education reflects the hard-won victories of the last decade, spend their young adult years either sitting at home doing nothing, performing some type of vocational task in a segregated sheltered workshop, or doing "prevocational" activities in an adult day center. The importance of transition is that it is not about students becoming adults, it is about changing the system of adult services to meet the heightened expectations of students, parents, teachers, and advocates.

Most of the discussion on transition has centered on vocational issues. This does not mean that the other systems of support for adults with disabilities are any less in need of renovation. This situation probably reflects the direct connection that has developed between school and the workplace. Numerous students, not in special education, have used vocational education as their transition into the world of work. Furthermore, the

approach of the functional community-based curriculum is uniquely oriented toward developing job skills in people whom adult vocational services had traditionally defined as "unemployable." In residential services the school-home connection was and is much less clear. Certainly educators teach their students skills related to household management and self-care, but it is not readily apparent that the educational system can make a substantive contribution to a fundamental transformation—a transitioning—of residential supports for adults. Indeed, most special education teachers probably are not even aware of the need to transform residential services; instead, they think of residential services in terms of helping parents to get their children on the waiting list for a group home.

The authors of this chapter do not intend to outline the elements of a curriculum in community living for people with disabilities (for this, see, for example: Brown et al., 1983; Ford et al., 1986; Hamre-Nietupski, Nietupski, Bates, & Maurer, 1982; Horner, Meyer, & Fredericks, 1986; Wehman, Renzaglia, & Bates, 1985). The functional community-based approach to education, which uses ecological inventories, individual adaptations, and partial participation strategies, provides a solid framework within which to design individualized education programs (IEPs) for students with a wide range of handicapping conditions. Such an approach provides a model for developing the specific skills that each student will need to meet the demands of the actual community environments within which he or she will have to function. What this chapter addresses is the discontinuity that exists in most locales between this approach to education and the realities of the system of adult residential supports. The bad news is that, if anything, residential services are even less well prepared than the vocational service system to meet the individualized needs of this generation of special education graduates. The good news is that people like Sam and Harvey are leading lives that illustrate the kind of transition residential support services need to undergo. The remainder of this chapter briefly outlines the present state of the residential service system; discusses the major characteristics of individualized, integrated residential supports; and cites some of the implications of community integration for educators.

DEINSTITUTIONALIZATION, COMMUNITY LIVING, AND COMMUNITY INTEGRATION

Throughout the 1970s and early 1980s, the major issue dominating the field of developmental disabilities was that of institutions versus community. With over 100,000 people with developmental disabilities living in public institutions (Braddock, Hemp, & Howes, 1986), the debate has obviously not yet been resolved.

Yet the state of the art in services for people with developmental disabilities has moved beyond this issue. That people with severe disabilities can live in the community is not just an idea—It is a reality in a growing number of places across the country. The critical issue today has to do with how people with disabilities, including individuals with severe or multiple disabilities, challenging behaviors, and complex medical needs, should be served in the community and what arrangements foster the greatest degree of community participation.

Deinstitutionalization has proceeded at a steady pace. While several studies have documented that there has been a gradual movement of people from public institutions to the community, the overall number of people living in the U.S. system of residential services has remained relatively constant at about 250,000 (Braddock, Hemp, & Howes, 1984; Hauber et al., 1984; Lakin, Hill, & Bruininks, 1985). As useful as these studies are for revealing national trends, they do not say much about what community living really means for the people within the residential service system.

The meaning of community living varies widely from place to place and from person to person. Indeed, some practices associated with de-institutionalization do not seem to represent community integration at all. In New York, for example, newly constructed "small residential units" on the grounds of several state institutions are being converted to the status of "community facilities." In many states, the term "community" is used to refer to anything other than a public institution. Thus, deinstitutionalization has often meant "transinstitutionalization"; that is, the movement of people from large public institutions to smaller, but equally restrictive private ones, including nursing homes (Warren, 1981). According to Lakin, Bruininks, Doth, Hill, and Hauber (1982), as of 1980, over 69,000 people with mental retardation were living in nursing homes. In many regions community living for people with developmental disabilities is translated by the general public, and by special educators, to mean group homes. Yet even in some of these relatively small facilities, life may be just as segregated as in public institutions (Bercovici, 1983).

Today most states describe their residential services in terms of a "continuum of options" (see Figure 1) ranging from the most restrictive setting (i.e., traditional institutions) to the least restrictive (i.e., independent living where the person is no longer a client of the residential service system). As initially formulated, this model is intended to provide for an orderly process of de-institutionalization. People leaving institutions were supposed to move gradually through the continuum as they developed the necessary skills to enable them to live more and more independently. While a continuum of services has a certain conceptual appeal, in practice this ideal system quickly breaks down.

In his analysis Taylor (1987b) highlights six conceptual and practical "pitfalls" in the continuum of residential services.

1. As an organizing principle the continuum legitimizes the most restrictive settings. It provides a basis for justifying institutions and other segregated settings as the least restrictive setting for some people.

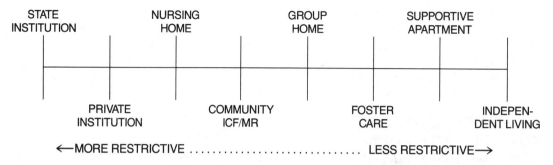

Figure 1.   A simplified continuum of residential services.

2. The continuum confuses intensity of services with restrictiveness of a setting. In fact, any support service that is offered in an institution can be and is provided for people in their homes.

3. The continuum implies that people must be made ready to live in the community. Because the demands of the environment are so different, more restrictive settings do not help people develop the skills required to live in a less restrictive setting.

4. The continuum suggests that as people develop new skills they must move to a new setting. This constant state of flux undercuts a sense of stability and the development of enduring relationships.

5. The continuum and its adjunct, the legal principle of the least restrictive environment, deflect attention from a fundamental underlying question of human rights: Why is there any need to infringe on the right of people with disabilities to freedom and community participation? The principle of the least restrictive alternative misleadingly diverts attention from this issue and focuses on ascertaining the least obnoxious level of infringement.

6. The continuum places an emphasis on facilities (buildings) rather than on services to people. Under this model people are placed in the type of facility that meets their needs rather than having supports provided to them where they need them.

In summary the continuum of residential services transfers the bureaucratic management practices of the institutional system of service into the community. The emphasis on the management of a range of options and the need to keep the beds in each facility occupied takes priority over creating the unique array of services to support an individual in the community.

The concept of community integration offers an alternative to the continuum of services. On the one hand, community services based on the continuum model are often described as offering residents a range of "residential settings" that are "homelike" and "normalized," primarily because they are smaller and geographically less isolated than the large institutions of the past. On the other hand, integrated services support people with disabilities in their homes and communities where they are full and active members.

Unfortunately, the ideal of community integration does not tell us what difference it makes in the day-to-day functioning of service providers and in the lives of people with disabilities. One way to begin to answer this question is to look in depth at state, regional, county, and private agencies nominated as "model" community programs. By examining these programs, observing settings, reviewing documents and policies, and interviewing administrators, staff, and parent and advocacy organizations, one can identify that that is state of the art and begin to answer the question of what community integration means.

As part of a larger study of promising practices for integrating people with severe disabilities into the community, the authors conducted detailed phone interviews with 40 programs across the country nominated by researchers, service providers, advocates, state administrators, and parents as examples of community integration (Community Integration Project, 1986). In addition, they visited the following locations around the country to gain a detailed understanding of how community integration is actually being achieved.

1. The state of Michigan, which stands out among states for its rapid depopulation of institutions
2. The Macomb-Oakland Regional Center in Michigan, widely heralded for serving a large number of people with severe disabilities in the community
3. Seven Counties Services in Louisville, Kentucky, a regional agency that has a reputation for integrating people with severe medical and behavioral involvements in the community
4. Region V Mental Retardation Services, based in Lincoln, Nebraska
5. The Working Organization for Retarded Children, a small agency in New York City that serves people with severe multiple disabilities, including former Willowbrook residents
6. Several counties, state programs, and private agencies in Wisconsin
7. Boise Group Home in Idaho
8. A number of small residential programs in the state of Washington
9. Westport Associates, an agency running three residential programs in Massachusetts
10. The Vecchione home in Vermont
11. The residential support services in Weld County, Colorado
12. The foster home and supported apartment program in Washington County, Vermont
13. The family support program administered by the Calvert County, Maryland, Association for Retarded Citizens

These interviews and site visits were based on an open-ended, descriptive, qualitative approach that attempts to understand how the people involved in these programs think about what they are doing (Taylor & Bogdan, 1984).

PRINCIPLES FOR COMMUNITY INTEGRATION

Those states, regional agencies, and private agencies that are serving people with severe disabilities in the community are committed to a clear set of principles. To be sure, no program stacks up perfectly against its principles. No state, no region, and no agency has developed ideal or perfect services. Yet some are moving in a clear direction. For these programs, principles are not merely lip service. Rather, they provide guidelines for day-to-day decision making and a way to gauge progress toward an optimal situation. These principles reveal what community integration means in practice.

Principles

All people with developmental disabilities belong in the community.

People in the Macomb-Oakland region in Michigan; Region V around Lincoln, Nebraska; and other places across the country do not believe simply in the "least restrictive environment." They believe that all people, regardless of the severity of disability, belong in the community. As Lyn Rucker (1987), the Executive Director of Region V Community Mental Retardation Services in Nebraska, has written, "If decision makers believe that *everyone* will be served and integrated in the community, half the struggle is over. In systems where that attitude is not embraced, I have seen every conceivable artificial barrier thrown up as a block to providing appropriate, integrated services for everyone" (p. 121).

Translated into practice, the belief that all people can and should live in the community means several things. First of all, Macomb-Oakland, Region V, and many other systems and agencies do not reject people as being "too severely disabled." In fact, one can find people with extremely severe disabilities, including children with complex medical needs (tube-feeding, suctioning, etc.) and people with a history of self-abuse and violence, living in the community there. Macomb-Oakland no longer admits children to institutions of any kind. Second, when placements do not work out for whatever reason (parental misgivings, resource limitations, etc.), which is rare, this is viewed as a failure of the service system, rather than an inability of the person to adjust to the community. Finally, the philosophy of these programs is not that people with the most severe disabilities should wait until everyone else is placed out of institutions before they have the opportunity to live in the community, but rather that they should be among the first. As Rucker (1987) explains, this helps a service system develop the capacity to serve people with more challenging needs early in its development.

People with severe disabilities should be integrated into typical neighborhoods, work environments, and community settings.

This principle gets at the heart of community integration. Community integration does not just mean physical placement in the community, but social integration as well. Some people living in group homes, community intermediate care facilities for the mentally retarded (ICFs/MR), and other facilities are as segregated as people in institutions. They live in a facility with 8 or 10 or 12 other people, board a van in the morning, go to a sheltered workshop or day activity center, return to the facility in mid-afternoon, and perhaps go on field trips as a group in the evening or on weekends. In short, these people are just as cut off from the life of the community as they would be in a setting for 500 people with a barbed wire fence around it.

To varying degrees, many agencies are attempting to integrate people with developmental disabilities, including those with severe disabilities, into typical community settings. At many small group homes and apartments in Wisconsin, for example, staff members take clients individually or in small groups to grocery stores, shopping centers, local churches, restaurants, community recreational centers, and other places.

Community living arrangements should be family scale.

As Rothman and Rothman (1984) point out, the field of developmental disabilities has been obsessed with trying to determine the optimal size of a community residence. Depending on how they designed their studies, researchers have reached different conclusions on the effects of size (Baroff, 1980; Landesman-Dwyer, 1981). Although small size alone, considered in isolation from other factors, will not guarantee a high quality of life or a high degree of integration, large groupings do seem to invite an institutional atmosphere and discourage community participation.

The state of the art for people with severe disabilities is defined as settings with six or less residents. Most Michigan group homes and community ICFs/MR (referred to as "Alternative Intermediate Services for the Mentally Retarded") have six people. Region V in Nebraska is moving to settings of no more than three or four people.

Many service systems currently are exploring alternatives to group homes for people with moderate and severe disabilities. Seven Counties Services in Kentucky, Nebraska's Region V, and agencies throughout Michigan and Wisconsin are developing supportive living arrangements for one to three people, with live-in or occasional staff support. Options in Community Living, a private agency in Dane County, Wisconsin, which was mentioned in the opening paragraph of this chapter, supports approximately 100 people with a wide range of disabilities in their own homes.

The development of relationships between people with severe disabilities and other people should be encouraged.

A community is not only a place, it also implies a feeling of belonging. Historically, there has been a lack of opportunities for people with severe disabilities to have close, mutual, and ongoing relationships with other people. Many agencies are attempting to foster such relationships. This takes many forms: citizen advocacy; permanency planning (to ensure that children have stable homes and families); placement policies that encourage proximity to family and friends; supportive living arrangements that enable people to live in their own homes with friends, as opposed to being transitioned through a continuum of residential placements; and the encouragement of relationships with typical people in schools, neighborhoods, and community settings.

The development of community living skills should be fostered.

The field of special education has witnessed a revolution in instructional approaches for students

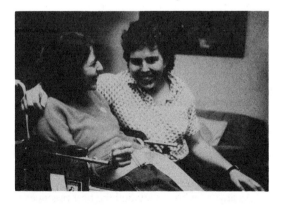

A visit from a friend.

with severe disabilities (Biklen, 1985; Brown et al., 1977). In Madison, Wisconsin, Dekalb, Illinois, and dozens of other school districts across the country, students with severe disabilities are learning practical, "functional" life skills in school and community settings (Taylor, 1982). Curricula have been developed to teach students with severe disabilities to use public transportation, order in restaurants, select and pay for groceries, cook, clean houses, and perform hundreds of other tasks once deemed impossible for them to learn. Similarly, vocational agencies have begun to explore ways to support people with severe disabilities in typical jobs in the community.

The field of residential services has lagged behind special education and vocational services in directing serious attention to teaching people with severe disabilities practical community living skills. Many community residences are defined as places to live, rather than places to learn. Others, especially ICF/MR-certified facilities, focus exclusively on teaching people personal care skills. However, some community service systems and agencies are beginning to focus on teaching people a range of skills necessary to function as independently as possible in the community. Options in Community Living is an example of an agency that attempts to strike a balance between respecting people's autonomy and right to relax in their own homes, and helping them to develop domestic and community living skills. The agency employs life skills trainers, independent of attendants and direct care staff, who work with people on learning practical skills such as budgeting, cooking, and grocery shopping.

Planning should be person-centered.

The traditional approach to human services provides a limited number of options. Within this model, individuals in need of support services are expected to fit into the available spaces and accept the services that are connected with a particular setting. When individual life situations change and people are deemed to be in need of either more or less intense supports, they will be required to move to another option—if a space happens to be available. An awareness of the basic fallacy in this facility-centered approach to residential services, with its predisposition for disrupting people's lives, has led the most innovative service systems to explore new ways of planning and organizing their systems of supports.

While traditional services play lip service to the specific needs of the individual by requiring Individualized Program Plans (IPPs), the best services actually structure their services around the person. As a way of underscoring this different focus, some of these services consciously avoid referring to themselves as residential providers and speak in terms of being an agency that supports individuals in their own homes. Services are determined based on a person-centered approach to planning that looks at the individual within the context of the community. Consideration is given to the person's network of relationships, functional limitations, strengths, weaknesses, and personal preferences—all with a focus on providing the individual with a future that will ensure a good quality of life as a member of the community (see O'Brien, 1987b for a detailed description of one approach to this type of planning). Two of the hallmarks of services that have adopted this approach are a flexibility to meet the ever-changing needs of people and an enduring commitment to always be there to provide support.

Parents and consumers should be involved in the design, operation, and monitoring of services.

Many service systems and agencies are starting to regard parents and consumers not merely as passive clients, but as partners in developing and operating services. Since 1980, Macomb-Oakland has actively supported a parent monitoring committee that reviews all community residential settings in the region. Macomb-Oakland provides parent photo identification cards; pays parents'

mileage for trips to group homes; and donates office space, a telephone, postage, stationery, and photocopying to the parent monitoring committee. Region V in Nebraska maintains a consumer advisory committee, which comprises recipients of its services, and surveys both parents and consumers as part of an annual quality assurance review. Options in Community Living has done as much, if not more, as any other agency in the country to ensure direct consumer involvement in and control over services. Its approach to serving people with disabilities lends itself to this: In contrast to the traditional group home approach, in which people are expected to fit the program, Options in Community Living supports people in individualized living arrangements that enable them to have a say in where and with whom they will live. It also encourages people to hire their own staff, called attendants.

Parent and consumer involvement is not merely a nice thing to encourage. In looking at innovative programs, it becomes clear that parents and consumers have played a major role in ensuring the quality of services.

Summary

In a service system that has almost from its inception concentrated on creating environments and services to meet the special needs of people with disabilities, it is clear that the success of community integration hinges on refocusing on basic human needs. The authors asked people about innovative services and they told stories about individuals. The authors went looking for the state of the art in residential services and they found out about homes. They tried to define the essential support services and they kept hearing about the importance of enduring relationships. The service providers with whom the authors talked did not discount the special needs of the people with disabilities for whom they worked, but they refused to allow those needs to obscure basic human equality.

As anyone who has studied the best practices in education knows, basic philosophical principles and the underlying themes of commitment, flexibility, individualization, accountability, and the importance of personal relationships have much to do with the success of any program. How can any human service based on such fundamental principles help but achieve its goal? The problem is that like so many "best practices," community integration is not accomplished by a new instructional technology, a better monitoring instrument, an innovative approach to staff training, or a creative model of management. The success of community integration depends on the ever-elusive human factor. It happens when people believe in it and work very hard for it. It is achieved when people without disabilities value people with disabilities as their peers. In the end it depends more on what those who are not disabled learn from people with disabilities than on what they teach to people with disabilities.

Kathy Bartholomew, the former director of Options for Individuals, a Louisville, Kentucky, agency committed to community integration for all of the people it serves, describes how an approach to services that strives to build the community connection has worked out in the lives of two people:

John [all names have been changed] is a man in his mid-twenties. His one great love is music, especially gospel music. John is very shy and although he stutters when he talks, we have found that he can sing along with gospel tunes. We contacted a local gospel radio station and now John goes to the station several times a week to do odd jobs, hang out, and listen to music. He is accompanied by one of our staff who is supporting a growing relationship between John and the employees of WSSS. We envision John associating with a gospel choir; traveling and maybe singing. The people at the radio station care about John and we plan to reduce our presence there soon.

Betsy, a woman thirty-three years old, began volunteering her time dishwashing at a local diner. Betsy is accompanied by one of our staff because of her fear of new situations and her tendency to have tantrums when she is unhappy. Although Betsy works at Bonnie's diner clearing tables and washing dishes, we have focused primarily on Betsy's feeling comfortable, and on nurturing an understanding relationship between Betsy and Bonnie. Bonnie's diner is a small "down home" place. It's a place where women come in each afternoon to drink coffee, smoke cigarettes and talk about their life. Betsy spends most of her time as a part of this informal association of women. Over the past nine months, they have become very comfortable with Betsy and Betsy with them. Betsy doesn't talk but Mary (our staff member) has helped Bonnie and the other women develop a better understanding of Betsy and her ways.

We haven't changed Betsy. She still has tantrums and in fact, has had a couple at Bonnie's. But Bonnie hasn't asked her to leave. Instead, she has tried to understand her more. Last week, our staff member mentioned that we were starting to wonder if staff presence was necessary and Bonnie suggested that Betsy start coming by herself. She said that she thought that Betsy trusted her now. In time we know she will go every afternoon by herself. But this will not be because we have made her "independent." Betsy is not independent. She stays at Bonnie's without a paid service worker *because she can depend on the other people there.* (1985, pp. 2–3)

EDUCATING FOR COMMUNITY INTEGRATION

While all of the above provides an informative overview of some of the major issues in residential services, what are the implications for special educators? After all, what can an individual teacher really do to affect the system of residential services for adults?

The discussion of transition in the introduction to this chapter points to the potential power of educators to reform adult services. Once a shared vision of real work for students with severe disabilities became the guiding principle for educators, and they began to resolve the practical problems involved in the attainment of that goal, the traditional system of segregated "make-work" vocational services was doomed. The vast expansion of job opportunities for people with disabilities that is now developing can be traced to a guiding vision shared by teachers—and others—and not to some new technology of instruction or sudden awakening of adult services. This new system stands as eloquent testimony to the ability of educators to change the way services are designed.

Nurturing a Vision

Knoll and Ford (1987) point out that the guiding vision in most residential agencies is the need to maintain a smoothly running facility. Few providers have a clearly articulated goal that looks beyond the walls of the residential setting. Most of them see themselves either as behavioral technicians in treatment settings or as personal care attendants in enhanced boarding houses. They are so caught up in the day-to-day problems of making group homes work that they do not have the opportunity for a fundamental re-examination of their priorities. The exceptions are the scattered agencies or small systems that have taken the time to reflectively evaluate their mission (see O'Brien, 1987a for a description of this process; see also Bogdan, 1986; Taylor, 1985, 1987a). It is these reflective agencies that emerged in the interviews and site visits discussed in the previous section.

When agencies and service systems have come to redefine their role as supporting people with disabilities in becoming part of the community, they have taken a major step toward balancing an individual's special learning needs with the basic human needs for a home and human relationships. Once this goal is clearly articulated, the providers gain a basis for establishing priorities for the people they serve and a more precise definition of the agency role as a facilitator of integration. In this new role, the provider will gradually become a less pervasive presence in a person's life, rather like a job coach in vocational services who fades into the background as skills and natural supports develop.

Just as they have helped to shape the future of vocational services, educators can influence what residential support services will become. By educating themselves about adult residential services and developing a vision of the best possible future for their students, teachers can lay the groundwork for the growth of a system that supports people in their own homes rather than a system of group-home beds. What follows is an outline of some of the elements in a "curriculum" that you as a teacher can use to learn about and foster community integration in adult services for your students.

Strive for fully integrated schools.

A basic premise underlying the discussion here is that in school all students with disabilities are integrated with nondisabled students. In the long run this will have the most profound effect on the system of residential supports. Certainly anyone who has had regular involvement during their school career with people with disabilities will, as a parent or a service provider, have a perspective on what constitutes an adequate system of residential support that is very different from the point of view of someone who has been raised in a segregated environment. So, make attainment of the goal of school integration the initial item on your agenda for assuring community integration for your students.

Know the community.

The traditional approach to special education placed great store on the professional clinical model. Operating from this perspective, the teacher was the skilled professional with the specialized knowledge needed to identify and remediate a student's educational deficits. This model essentially emulates, in the classroom, the clinical approach of psychologists who provided the theoretical and practical underpinnings for much of special education. Recent years have seen this narrow clinical focus challenged as greater emphasis has been placed on understanding the learning needs of students as determined by the demands of their environment. This changing perspective has had a particularly profound effect on the education of students with severe disabilities. A growing awareness of the importance of integration makes an education that is solely confined to the classroom increasingly untenable. As a teacher who is concerned for the lifelong integration of your students in the community, you cannot afford to be a detached professional. Get to know the community environments within which your students need to function now and in the future.

Learn the service system.

As a force for change in the community, educators need to know what type of residential supports presently exist and to have a sense of where the potential allies and major barriers to change are located.

A good first step in learning about your local system of services is to contact your local (state/county/regional) developmental disabilities office and find out what agencies provide residential and other support services. Be sure to ask about the range of supports that are available (e.g., Are family support services limited to respite care as opposed to the individual supports families need?). As a follow-up, interview agency officials to gain an understanding of their perspective. For example, you might ask about their vision of the future, what new services they feel are needed, what services take priority in their mind, and how large the local waiting lists are. This process will give you a sense of the people who will be potential allies as resources for parents and sources of information on constraints on developing innovative programs.

Try to visit the full range of "residential options" available in your community. Be sure to include nursing homes and traditional institutions in your rounds. It is important to have a personal sense of what segregation is like and why it is wrong. In visiting and evaluating residential settings, remember the following question: Would I like to live here, and if not, why not?

Interview parents and other members of your students' families to gain an understanding of their perception of the service system, their hopes for the future, and their fears regarding the family member with a disability. Ask them: What supports are they currently receiving? What else do they need? Who has been their greatest help/hindrance in regard to their family member with a disability? How have the schools helped or hindered them? Where do they think their child will be living in 5, 10, 15, and 20 years? How much do they know about the adult service system?

As a final and most crucial step in understanding your local service system, interview adults with disabilities about their experiences living in institutions, group homes, or on their own. Some questions might include: What do you like most/least about your current situation? Who have been the most important people in your life? How did schools help/hinder your ability to live in the community?

Although this process is rather involved, it will reward you by providing a perspective on the service system from every possible angle. As a result, you will be able to tell the difference between the reality of services and the official description. This gives you a firm basis for critiquing existing services and offering innovative alternatives for your students.

Foster relationships—Maintain the community connnection.

Increasingly, the most forward-looking residential support providers are becoming aware of the fallacy underlying any attempt to quantify the degree to which people are integrated into the community. They point out that integration is not measured by a frequency count of how often a person leaves the place of residence. The keystone of real integration is enduring relationships with other members of the community. The realities of attempting to reintegrate people into a community when they have had their bonds severed by the service system are an ever-increasing source of frustration. The recurring question is: How do you become a member of the community when you are always the new person on the block?

The truth is that there is no quick fix. Residential neighborhoods do not always assimilate newcomers. In fact, many of the characteristics of households that aid in assimilation—the presence of young children, for example—are absent in the case of people with moderate to severe disabilities. In addition, the structures of the residential service system often erect subtle barriers that even further hamper the possibility of acceptance. For example, some agencies, because of the regulatory demands for documented active treatment, schedule group recreation activities in which everyone in the house is expected to participate. This practice cuts down on the opportunities for less formal individual use of community resources and hence limits the possibility for interacting with other members of the community. When confronted by such systemic barriers to integration the first line of defense is the development of a consciousness attuned to seeing them. The service provider can then act to minimize the effect of these barriers and provide opportunities for people with disabilities to be seen as good neighbors. Nevertheless, the process of becoming integrated into a community will still take time.

A primary aim of the education of students with disabilities should be a conscious effort to nurture the students' connections to their neighborhoods and communities. Just as school integration affirms the need for the local school to take responsibility for all the students in its area, community integration is based on the premise that the best protection of disabled people lies in the responsibility that a community feels for it members. Therefore, your educational program should consistently demonstrate to the community, by using neighborhood merchants and other resources, that your students with disabilities are integral to its life. Your students will then have a constituency that can be called on to question any effort to cut them off from their community, their home, and their neighbors. Remember—Relationships are far easier to maintain than they are to build from scratch.

Create a cooperative environment.

A great deal of the academic research literature still addresses the question of determining the optimal living environment for people with severe disabilities. Most of this material is written from a perspective that buys into the continuum of services and sees a residential setting as a training environment for the next less restrictive option. Each resident of such a system has an individualized program plan with a set of specific goals to be mastered. These goals are often derived from a set of pre-established exit criteria. Like so much in this system, goals are determined by the facility and not by the individual's specific needs.

In a system that attempts to support people in their homes, the learning needs and formal goals are determined by the real demands of daily life, not by a predetermined list of skills. For example, an individual may not need to master a skill if a roommate has that skill, or two roommates may split a task that would be an overwhelming effort for each of them to master in isolation. In this type of system, people and their skills are not considered in isolation. Like all homes, these residential supports place an emphasis on a model of mutual interdependence rather than narrowly focusing on an abstract goal of individual independence.

The lesson in this for you as a teacher is the need to help students with disabilities to develop cooperative behavior by structuring cooperative learning situations in your classroom. The research on school integration (e.g., Johnson & Johnson, 1983) has shown that this type of classroom organization is a way of nurturing integration and developing positive relationships between students with and without disabilities. Moreover, the experience of service providers, who have recognized the contribution an interdependent life-style makes to a high quality of life, suggests that learning how to interact cooperatively is a crucial skill for students who will need to receive support services in their homes.

Recognize individual preferences and support real choices.

"Home" may have many different definitions but control of the environment, individual preferences, and the ability to make substantive choices all seem to be necessary aspects. Although the need for students to learn how to make decisions responsibly has long been identified as an important component of the educational process, the realities of the special education system indicate a high degree of classroom management and a low

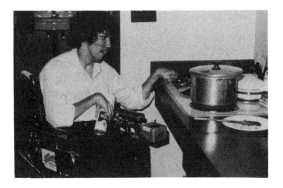

Making choices and doing things for yourself.

level of student control (cf. Houghton, Bronicki, & Guess, 1987). This creates just the type of educational situation needed to prepare people for life in a highly managed residential facility.

If you as a teacher intend to prepare your students for life in their own homes, their educational programs must be geared toward fostering basic skills in expressing preferences and making choices that have real meaning to them. This is essential for students with mild and moderate disabilities, who may be able to decide whether to live alone or with someone else, as well as for students with severe disabilities, who may simply be choosing what to eat or what TV show to watch. Both decisions have major implications for the control that the individual can exercise over his or her environment.

Develop management skills.

One important support provided by some of the most forward-looking supportive living agencies involves helping people with disabilities develop organizational and managerial skills. These skills are usually associated with independent living centers and educating people with physical disabilities to manage their own attendant care. However, there is an increasing awareness that these same skills are relevant to the lives of people with severe and multiple disabilities who are receiving support from mental retardation and mental health agencies. The skills needed to interview, manage,

and schedule an aide are applicable, in at least an adapted form, to the long-term needs of any students who are likely to be involved with service providers for most their lives. In fact, an increasing number of relatively traditional group homes for people with moderate and severe disabilities are structuring their hiring process so the residents have direct involvement in deciding who works in their home. Needless to say, providers who have adopted this approach can recount stories of job interviews filled with irrelevant questions and instances where the wrong person got hired. They also affirm that people, who for most of their lives have been powerless when it comes to such fundamental decisions as who should assist them, can and do learn how to become more effective employers.

Support self-advocacy.

Self-advocacy, that is, people with disabilities supporting one another and speaking up for their rights, is a major force in adult services that is only beginning to have a real impact on service providers and bureaucrats. At this point self-advocacy within the service system has largely been limited to the role of a grievance committee, as in the case of a group of sheltered workshop employees who informed the agency director that they were adults and did not appreciate working in a place that proclaimed to the world that it helped children.

In a community-based service system, the potential effects of this movement are far reaching, provided some of the current barriers are overcome. In some areas self-advocacy has been co-opted; for example, it is used as a label for a recreation program within a system of segregated services. In other locales self-advocacy is not happening at all because of a lack of information and an absence of even minimal initial support from nondisabled people who are not connected with the system of services. If this movement is to grow, the schools need to provide an initial forum for students to learn about it, begin to organize, and in the last years of school make a connection with active self-advocates in their own community. In addition, interested special education teachers, who are not involved in adult services, should be providing a ready pool of advisors for adult self-advocacy groups.

Be an advocate.

To the maximum extent possible, be an active presence in your community. Let parents and providers understand your vision of the future, and make it clear to them that it is guiding the education of your students with disabilities. However, do not assume that providers, bureaucrats, and planners have a clear sense of the ramifications of a curriculum focused on community integration. You must show them that their system of services does not meet the needs of the students who will be graduating from your program. Find out about different and innovative models of residential support and offer one as an alternative, being sure to point out how you are preparing students to live with that type of support. If necessary, provide a forum for parents to organize a challenge to the existing system.

Shaping the Future for Individual Students

While all of what was just discussed is important and is intimately involved with your role as a teacher, it could be regarded merely as preparation for working with your students. After all, your primary responsibilities as a teacher revolve around developing an individualized education program for each of your students that prepares them to live in their own home and be actively involved with the service providers who support them there.

The principles of community integration lead directly to some basic questions that can be used by teachers, parents, advocates, service providers, and others who have a relationship with a student with disabilities to organize an education plan that will prepare the student to live in his or her own home. The following questions should

become part of the planning process for each student who will need support from a service provider as an adult:

Should this person live alone or with others?
Who are the person's closest friends?
How will contact with friends and family members be maintained?
Is there someone who wants to live with the person?
Is there someone with whom the person wants to live?
What staff supports would be necessary for this person to live in his or her own place?
What level of support does the person need in interpersonal relationships? Will assistance be needed here?
What skills will the person need to live in his or her own home?
To what extent can this person manage his or her own staff?
What aspects of the person's day provide opportunities for making choices?
What furnishings, household goods, and appliances will the person need?
What adaptations will have to be made to accommodate the person?
What are the person's preferences regarding housing and furnishings?
What will a typical week be like in this person's life in the future?
Where and when will the person go shopping?
When will the person see family and friends?
Where will the person spend leisure time?
To what community associations will the person belong?
Where will the person work?

This list is not exhaustive but it does reflect the fact that some people will need a rather detailed level of long-term planning to begin relatively early in their educational career. As an alternative to this the teacher, who is educated about the residential service system, should compare the ideal vision of the person's life with what will happen if he or she lives in an institution, group home, or some other facility.

Consider the following example.

Michelle, Gloria, and Mary (all names have been changed) are three young women in their early 20s who are moving into an apartment together. They became good friends during the 4 years they spent together in high school. Since they now all have, respectively, entry-level jobs in a restaurant, a motel, and an office in their hometown, they have pooled their resources so they can move out of their family homes and get set up on their own. Not an unusual scenario, except that these three young women are labeled as moderately or severely mentally retarded. And the person most responsible for this fairly typical progression into an adult life-style is their high school homeroom teacher, Sarah Lord.

Almost 4 years ago, a full year and a half before Michelle and Gloria were scheduled to graduate from high school, Sarah, along with the women, their parents, and a supportive school district administrator, developed a vision of what their life should look like after graduation. All three of the women, along with all of their classmates, had been involved in community job-training sites for several years and two of the employers had indicated that they were favorably disposed to employing Michelle and Gloria when they were no longer being supported by school personnel. The one unknown quantity in the vision was exactly where the women would live and who would supply the supports that they would need.

The ideal called for an apartment to be rented at some time during the last year in school. Michelle and Gloria could live there during the week, with agency support, and work on their household management skills *in their own home* as part of their school program. Mary would also spend part of her day with them and

then move in about a year later during her last year of school. For several years their school program had focused on developing household skills in one of the staff's homes and using the community resources in the surrounding neighborhood. So, it was important to find an apartment in the same area.

Unfortunately, the ideal, well-ordered vision that Sarah had fostered quickly ran into the slow-moving, inflexible residential service system in her state. Up to this point Sarah's knowledge of the residential service system was limited to her dealings with the group home where two of her students lived. She now began a 4-year course in the intricacies of how the system functions. In the process of seemingly endless meetings with a residential planner from a local advocacy group, university consultants, and public and private providers, Sarah heard about all of the barriers to a typical young adult life-style for Michelle, Gloria, and Mary.

Now over a year after Mary graduated from Sarah's class, a living situation that roughly resembles the original plan is being realized. There have been some major compromises—a fourth person will live in the apartment, and it is being defined as a group home by the agency "managing" it—and numerous missed opportunities. Nonetheless, this transition in the life of these three women has been much more orderly and their life-style is far more typical than that experienced by most other people in their area with moderate or severe disabilities. And all of this is because of Sarah's vision as an educator and tenacity as an advocate.

CONCLUSION

Integration is a word that has been used in a multitude of contexts by educators, social planners, scientists, jurists, and politicians. Integrated housing, integrated schools, integrated theory, integrated planning, integrated therapy, integrated personality—the list could go on and on. The central meaning of the word "integration" that lies behind all these diverse concepts is the process of forming a coherent whole.

This chapter has attempted to underscore the need for all the pieces of an individual's life to fit together. When participation in the community is only a goal in one segment of people's lives they are not really integrated. Educators working with students with severe disabilities have, for quite some time, been aware of the need to take a holistic perspective on the lives of their students and begin longitudinal planning early in a child's educational career so precious school time is not lost in teaching nonfunctional skills. Recently, the holistic functional perspective has begun to change the opportunities for work available to many special education graduates. Students who have been prepared to do real work now are getting that chance. Those pieces of people's lives have started to come together. The last piece of the educational, vocational, and residential triad now must be addressed, so all graduates from special education can have the chance for a truly integrated life.

Once this vision is realized and everyone goes to school together, works side by side, and lives in neighboring homes, then integration will no longer be a topic for discussion—it will be a reality.

STUDY QUESTIONS

1. What are the problems with a continuum model of services for people with disabilities?
2. What principles should guide the design of community services for people with disabilites?
3. What steps can teachers take to influence the future community living options for their students with disabilities?
4. What questions should teachers ask themselves about their students with disabilities to help plan for their futures in the community?
5. Why is it important for teachers to know about adult community living options?
6. What is the difference between deinstitutionalization and community integration?

REFERENCES

Baroff, G.S. (1980) On "size" and the quality of residential care: A second look. *Mental Retardation, 18,* 113–117.

Bartholomew, K. (1985, November). Options for individuals. *Institutions, Etc.*, pp. 2–3.

Bercovici, S. (1983). *Barriers to normalization: The restrictive management of retarded persons.* Baltimore: University Park Press.

Biklen, D. (Ed.). (1985). *Achieving the complete school: Strategies for effective mainstreaming.* New York: Teacher's College Press.

Bogdan, R. (1986). *The no name program.* Syracuse, NY: Center on Human Policy, Research and Training Center on Community Integration.

Braddock, D., Hemp, R., & Howes, R. (1984). *Public expenditures for mental retardation and developmental disabilities in the United States: State profiles.* Chicago: University of Illinois at Chicago, Institute for the Study of Developmental Disabilities, Evaluation and Public Policy Analysis Program.

Braddock, D., Hemp, R., & Howes, R. (1986). Direct costs of institutional care in the United States. *Mental Retardation, 24* (1), 9–17.

Brown, L., Nisbet, J., Ford, A., Sweet, M., Shiraga, B.,

York, J., & Loomis, R. (1983). The critical need for non-school instruction in educational programs for severely handicapped students. *Journal of the Association for the Severely Handicapped, 8* (3), 71–77.

Brown, L., Wilcox, B., Sontag, E., Vincent, B., Dodd, N., & Grunewald, L. (1977). Towards the realization of the least restrictive educational environment for severely handicapped students. *Journal of the Association for the Severely Handicapped, 2* (4), 195–201.

Community Integration Project. (1986). *Programs demonstrating model practices for integrating people with severe disabilities into the community.* Syracuse, NY: Center on Human Policy.

Ford, A., Dempsey, P., Black, J., Davern, L., Schnorr, R., & Meyer, L. (1986). *The Syracuse community-referenced curriculum guide for students with moderate and severe handicaps.* Syracuse, NY: Syracuse City School District.

Hamre-Nietupski, S., Nietupski, J., Bates, P., & Maurer, S. (1982). Implementing a community-based educational model for moderately/severely handicapped students: Common problems and suggested solutions. *Journal of the Association for the Severely Handicapped, 7* (4), 38–43.

Hauber, F.A., Bruininks, R.H., Hill, B.K., Lakin, C., Scheerenberger, R., & White, C.C. (1984). National census of residential facilities: A 1982 profile of facilities and residents. *American Journal of Mental Deficiency, 89,* 236–245.

Horner, R.H., Meyer, L.H., & Fredericks, H.D.B. (Eds.). (1986). *Education of learners with severe handicaps: Exemplary service strategies.* Baltimore: Paul H. Brookes Publishing Co.

Houghton, J., Bronicki, G.J.B., & Guess, D. (1987). Opportunities to express preferences and make choices among students with severe disabilities in classroom settings. *Journal of the Association for Persons with Severe Handicaps, 12,* 18–27.

Johnson, R.T., & Johnson, D.W. (1983). Effects of cooperative, competitive, and individualistic learning experiences on social development. *Exceptional Children, 49,* 323–330.

Knoll, J., & Ford, A. (1987). Beyond caregiving: A reconceptualization of the role of the residential service provider. In S.J. Taylor, D. Biklen, & J. Knoll (Eds.), *Community integration for people with severe disabilities* (pp. 129–146). New York: Teacher's College Press.

Lakin, K.C., Bruininks, R.H., Doth, D., Hill, B., & Hauber, F. (1982). *Sourcebook on long-term care for developmentally disabled people.* Minneapolis: University of Minnesota, Center for Residential and Community Services.

Lakin, K.C., Hill, B., & Bruininks, R. (1985). *An analysis of Medicaid's intermediate care facility for the mentally retarded (ICF/MR) program.* Minneapolis: University of Minnesota, Center for Residential and Community Services.

Landesman-Dwyer, S. (1981). Living in the community. *American Journal of Mental Deficiency, 86,* 223–234.

O'Brien, J. (1987a). Embracing ignorance, error, and fallibility: Competencies for leadership of effective services. In S.J. Taylor, D. Biklen, & J. Knoll (Eds.), *Community integration for people with severe disabilities* (pp. 85–108). New York: Teacher's College Press.

O'Brien, J. (1987b). A guide to life-style planning: Using *The Activities Catalog* to integrate services and natural suport systems. In B. Wilcox & G.T. Bellamy, *A comprehensive guide to The Activities Catalog: An alternative curriculum for youth and adults with severe disabilities* (pp. 175–189). Baltimore: Paul H. Brookes Publishing Co.

Rothman, D.J., & Rothman, S.M. (1984). *The Willowbrook wars: A decade long struggle for social justice.* New York: Harper & Row.

Rucker, L. (1987). A difference you can see: One example of services to persons with severe mental retardation in the community. In S.J. Taylor, D. Biklen, & J. Knoll (Eds.), *Community integration for people with severe disabilities* (pp. 109–125). New York: Teacher's College Press.

Sailor & Guess (1983).

Taylor, S.J. (1982). From segregation to integration: Strategies for integrating severely handicapped students in normal schools and community settings. *The Journal of the Association for the Severely Handicapped, 7* (3), 42–49.

Taylor, S.J. (1985). *Site visit report: Region V mental retardation services, Nebraska.* Syracuse, NY: Center on Human Policy, Community Integration Project.

Taylor, S.J. (1987a). *Community living in three Wisconsin counties.* Syracuse, NY: Center on Human Policy, Community Integration Project.

Taylor, S.J. (1987b). Continuum traps. In S.J. Taylor, D. Biklen, & J. Knoll (Eds.), *Community integration for people with severe disabilities* (pp. 25–35). New York: Teacher's College Press.

Taylor, S.J., & Bogdan, R. (1984). *An introduction of qualitative research methods* (2nd ed.). New York: John Wiley & Sons.

Warren, C.A.B. (1981). New forms of social control. *American Behavioral Scientist, 24* (6), 724–740.

Wehman, P., Renzaglia, A., & Bates, P. (1985). *Functional living skills for moderately and severely handicapped individuals.* Austin, TX: PRO-ED.

CHAPTER 16

INTEGRATION STRATEGIES FOR PARENTS OF STUDENTS WITH HANDICAPS

Addie Comegys

That summer our refrigerator chilled a variety of tonic cans. And the kitchen counter housed a generous stash of pretzels, potato chips, and other snacks. Doors banged. Voices rose and fell with activity. It was a teenage scene for sure.

The summer before had been quite different. Our refrigerator was filled with fruit juices, not soda pop. Any voices and banging doors would have been the result of much planning on our part with the mothers (usually) of other teens who were also handicapped.

What caused the change? The hearing officer of our state Bureau of Special Education Appeals had just presided over an agreement reached between our public school system and ourselves: Our 17-year-old daughter Kate, who experiences severe multiple challenges, was to start attending *our* high school in the fall!

What a contrast! The thrill of going to school was back for this family. Although cerebral palsy, severe mental retardation, severe dual hearing loss, and absence of speech have each made their mark on Kate, her ability to partially participate in regular school life has blossomed. Kate's integration into our local high school has changed the lives and attitudes in our house, in our neighborhood, in our school system, and in our suburban community of Wenham, Massachusetts. For example, one Saturday Kate and 11 of her new high school friends had a pool party and cookout at our house. Kate's teachers were also invited. If it rained, they planned to retrench in the garage to eat and then into the den to watch tapes on the VCR (video cassette recorder). My husband Brock and I were *not* invited—we enjoyed those hours together.

Parents, generally, have hopes and visions for their children: health, happiness, a good job, friends, acceptance, stature in the community, and the educational experiences that prepare for these goals. This is true for parents of regular education students and this is true for parents of special education students. We all want our children to succeed. We want to be proud of their achievements.

But all too often, when an individual is diagnosed as having a handicap, whether mild or severe, single or multiple, he or she is immediately labeled and enveloped in a bubble of isolation by society. Because the child is special, parents are told, the bubble is special. As a result, their child's special education will be separated from instead of integrated into regular education. From that point in time, parents are subtly told not to expect their youngster to have feelings or preferences, skills or spirit. He or she must receive special therapies to compensate for his or her deficiencies. He or she will need special equipment at very special prices. He or she will need special education at a special school for persons with handicaps—

due to his or her retardation and perhaps due to his or her conduct.

But sometimes, whether by pure luck or dogged work on the parents' part, children with all types of handicaps are leading integrated lives in their homes, their public schools, and their communities. When this happens, those parents want to share their joys and practical experiences that have helped achieve that precious integration with those parents whose children are still in segregated schools, segregated classrooms, segregated workshops, segregated living arrangements, and segregated leisure activities.

The moment that parents first experience that shattering realization that their offspring is handicapped is *exactly* when they will need the positive support of family, friends, and community. And the critical first step toward positive support is raising the option of integration. These parents need to have hope for the future through the example and experience of other integrated families. Parents without that positive knowledge soon learn to suppress their original dreams for their child of health, happiness, self-worth, friends, and stature in the community.

Integrated parents know that their family unit is a happier, more productive one than a segregated family. They experience the joys of watching their youngster progress functionally, and be accepted by his or her peers and the community. Parents can work *with* the school system to think creatively in planning for the education of their child.

If knowing the option of integration is the first step, then knowing the methods and strategies that have proved integration successful is the next. The ideas for achieving and maintaining integration that follow in this chapter are suitable for all types of handicaps. Appropriate modifications to fit particular needs can be made by parents, professionals, and the community.

EDUCATIONAL PHILOSOPHY

This parent believes firmly in the integration of *all* persons with severe challenges into *all* aspects of

life, from birth to death. Society needs to learn how to see the many similarities, not just the differences, between regular peers and those with handicaps—similarities such as the deep desire to love and be loved, the deep desire to be needed and yet to be as independent as possible. Yet the joy of demonstrating the option of integration is not limited to parents who have experienced that option. Regular and special educators today have the unparalleled opportunity to show new parents of a child with a handicap as well as society at large that integration works.

At the end of Kate's first year in our school system, her teacher demonstrated her professional support for integration in an article printed in our regional high school's newsletter.

> When I accepted the job of integrating a high school student (who had been in out-of-district placements for years) into her local high school, I had mixed feelings. Could I ever put into words how strongly committed I am to the goal of having all students educated together? Could those words influence anyone else to even *think* about the issue? What could I help Kate to learn?
>
> Although I had spent a year studying about integration, the closest I'd come to working in such a setting was a self-contained classroom in a local high school. In education, as in so many fields, it is rare to find a direct correlation between what's studied in graduate school and the reality of the working world. Often one is way ahead or way behind the other in theory and/or practice. Armed mainly with my convictions and, until now, merely textbook lingo about how things could or should proceed, I decided to give this job a shot!
>
> What I had suspected to be true became reality during this school year. I have witnessed both the progress Kate has made and the growth in acceptance by staff and students. I am thrilled to realize that integration *really does work*—not just in an "ivory tower" textbook, but in a *real* high school with *real* people.
>
> Kate learned, and friendships formed that were previously impossible in the segregated schools she had attended. Through the year, students and teachers alike asked tons of questions so that they could learn more. People wanted to know what they could do to help out and to make Kate more a part of the school.
>
> If you look back in time, you can see a pattern of growing acceptance of differences. Historically, so-

ciety has always had its scapegoats, its devalued persons. Each new wave of immigrants has experienced rejection, segregation, ridicule and prejudice, often based on the "fear of the unknown," before finally being accepted into integrated American life.

Changes *have* occurred for those in groups that have held their ground and pushed for equality. With each group's successes, small victories are won for *every* American, for what is our country based upon but many diverse and heterogeneous groups of individuals?

Changes for the better have obviously been made because people were active, hopeful and unaccepting of the status quo. Luckily, there were some people that did not sit idly by and allow segregation to occur; thus we now have legal racial equality. Likewise, acceptance of people with handicaps is traveling the same route towards complete integration into our society. We at the Regional have taken the important first step.

We have a long way to go, but we are definitely on our way. We should welcome criticism from opponents as an opportunity to react and educate. Ideas and ideals will die without dissent, for it is this tension that strengthens convictions. We may not be able to teach society everything about integration, but we *can* add our little piece to complete the entire puzzle that much sooner. (Considine, 1987, pp. 4–5)

Parents, the medical profession, and educators all have the responsibility to guide and support families early on so that they may be aware of their present and future options for integration. It is important that this be discussed immediately upon diagnosis, even though it is a stressful time. For that is when the option of integration for their handicapped member is a reality, not a dream.

During my years as a parent of a young person with multiple handicaps, I have come to understand the value of thinking through and writing down how we want to raise our daughter. It is helpful to back away from the day-to-day decisions and look at the broader picture. I have found the following questions to be helpful:

1. Will this child experience as much of life as his or her siblings have?
2. If he or she needs medical attention, will he or she receive as much of it as possible from the local medical profession, and go into city medical complexes only when necessary?
3. Will I be prepared to be patient with others

when they appear not to be skilled enough to interact with my child—will I teach by my example?
4. Will I educate myself about the kind of resources and people I will probably call on from time to time?
5. Will I make every attempt to draw as many friends, extended family members, and others in our community into our circle, so that they can appreciate our philosophy and follow it without hesitation—particularly including "hands on" interactions?
6. Will I post a note on my refrigerator that says: "The glass is half *full*"?

This is a starting point.

INTEGRATION ACTIVITIES

The following are seven successful activities to help in the integration process of people with all types and levels of disability, which can be performed by families, extended families, and educators.

Integrated Day Care

Integrated day care is a logical starting option for working parents of younger children. However, because it is not yet readily available in all areas, the creative parent must make suggestions to the day-care staff as to how integration can work. This sends a clear message to other caregivers and professionals down the line as to the philosophy of the family.

Marcie Brost of Madison, Wisconsin, is the foster parent of 7-year-old Andre, who is nonverbal. Andre has been integrated for 3 years through Winnebago Child Care and the prekindergarten and kindergarten classes of Red Caboose. Marcie states emphatically (M. Brost, personal communication, January 20, 1988) that she will never accept anything less than integration in the future!

Marcie describes how, at group sharing time, one of Andre's classmates often reads aloud a story, written by Marcie in what would be Andre's language style, that describes what Andre might have done during a school vacation (M. Brost, personal communication, January 20, 1988). And whenever Marcie and Andre go on a trip, they collect postcards for Andre to show at school (Andre often brings a friend along on these trips).

Functional sign language used with Andre has always been taught informally and simultaneously to his classmates. Andre now sleeps over at his friends' houses, swims, and "ice skates" on a sled guided by his peers—he is an integrated and happy youngster because he is surrounded by friends.

Dale B. Fink, of the Wellesley College Center for Research on Women, has conducted a study on child-care options for children with disabilities. His articles appeared in the March, April, and May, 1987 issues of *The Exceptional Parent*.

Educationally, the main topics of concern are the training of staff and their resources. It would appear that some integrated day-care centers are attached to clinics or medical facilities for this reason. It is important to progress beyond these medical models—integrated day care must be developed locally, within the community, through a cooperative effort by knowledgeable parents and professionals. Youngsters can receive the therapies they need in day care and they can partially participate in integrated play sessions with friends in the community.

Listing of Realms

A listing of Realms is a tool that is based on both philosophy and performance. It should clearly state how the family hopes to see their child functioning in his or her community in 3–5-year increments in each of the following integrated *realms* or areas:

1. Family life
2. School
3. Recreation/leisure
4. Real job
5. Living arrangements
6. Real friendships

These goals and activities should be shared and discussed with regular and special educators, and with parents of children in regular and special education. This should be done as early as possible in order to prevent the seeds of isolation and segregation from taking root. (Figure 1 shows how our family filled out Realms for Kate in 1984.) Realms will also give the thoughtful special education director a sense of the family's high standards and involvement, as well as their expectations of the program.

No learner as severely involved as our child had ever been admitted to any class in our school system. It is generally thought that integration at the high school level is more difficult than lower classes. But our Realms gave the director time and a platform from which to inform and persuade other school administrators about Kate's right to go to school in her own hometown in an integrated setting. In our case, the Realms persuaded the school system to take the "risk" of integration.

"My Story" Booklet

A "My Story" booklet is another useful tool, which Dr. Alison Ford of Syracuse University helped me compile. This is a booklet of basic information with photographs, composed by the family but written as though the student is telling his or her own story. There should be a copy by the student's school desk for teachers and peers; a copy at home for companions, friends, and therapists; and an extra copy for travel, medical appointments, and community gatherings.

Because the booklet describes the learner's *abilities,* the reader comes to see the *similarities* between him or herself and the student. The booklet also serves as a tool for parents who are constantly asked for the same information by the numerous therapists and professionals who move in and out of their lives.

A looseleaf binder or photo album that has plastic-covered pages is quite useful in creating a booklet for your child. It allows typed pages to be removed for updating (and to be protected from fingers) and it also allows photographs to be inserted. Figure 2 shows the main headings used in

---

Realms

School Integrated public high school in our town. Buddy system and peer tutoring. Prepare for competitive community employment. Partial participation. No sheltered workshops. 12-month educational IEP, containing quality hearing-impaired instruction, Phonic Ear Auditory Trainer, expanded use of rebus communication board. Reduce drooling, tongue thrust, grinding. Current music therapist effective in all areas. ADL skills to continue. PT essential. Parents integral part of team. Computer skills to begin immediately.

Home Home-school carryover. Continue ADL emphasis with parents consciously increasing Kate's independence. Future adoption by large family preferred over group home.

Community School and parents must achieve age-appropriate, partial participation, community involvement with/by Kate: friends, movies, shopping, public transportation, crossing streets—all on daily basis with supervision.

Leisure Planning to eradicate current dead time. Allow (and encourage) Kate to make daily rebus choices for: bike, swing, walk; or, indoors—tape recorder, TV switch, Kodak Ectagraphic slides with sound and on/off switch, books. Summer swimming and horseback riding. Local ARC's segregated recreational programs not scaled to Kate. Overnight camp annually for a week. Yearly vacation with and without family (respite vital).

Vocation We envision Kate at age 21 in a local, structured, supported, partial participatory, competitive work situation (e.g., library with computer). Results of AT, to be initiated in 2 weeks, could be an overall positive factor. The AT must be really tried by all for a year and closely monitored.

Figure 1. Sample of Realms, completed for Kate Comegys in 1984. (IEP = individualized education program; PT = physical therapy; ADL = activities of daily living; ARC = Association for Retarded Citizens; AT = Auditory Trainer)

creating a "My Story" booklet for Kate. Figure 3 contains excerpts from the sections "My Goals," and "My Interests," and "I May Not Speak—But I Do Communicate." Not including photographs, Kate's 1986–1987 booklet contained over 30 typewritten pages. Yours may be shorter or it may be longer—the important thing to remember is that the booklet should be written in concrete, descriptive terms and should be as thorough as possible. It will provide the first impression others have of your child—and you want your child to make the best first impression he or she can!

Also, the "My Story" booklet may be used in ways you do not anticipate. In our case, when the new special education director was hiring new staff, it was suggested that Kate's booklet be shown to prospective applicants. Kate's current teacher commented later that it gave her a good picture of Kate and because of that she wanted to be her teacher.

The "My Story" booklet has also been used to introduce Kate to her school peers. They have invariably expressed pleasure and a kind of reassurance in finding the *similarities* between themselves and Kate. Consequently, Kate's friendships have increased and are continuing to increase. This is one of the direct benefits of integration. (For further information see the writings of Marsha Forest.)

Solving Dressing and Grooming Difficulties

Dressing and grooming are important for all of us. Age-appropriate clothes, shoes, and hairstyles help the handicapped individual to blend into his or her social environment. Clothes need not be designed by Christian Dior or Ralph Lauren! In fact, stylish hand-me-downs can make good sense both visually and economically.

Particular grooming problems *can* be solved

"My Name is Kate Comegys"

Contents

My name is Kate Comegys

How I spend my time
　School
　Work
　After Work
　Evenings
　Weekends

My Goals

My Interests

Getting to Know Me Better
　Please Do!

I May Not Speak—But I Do Communicate
　Line Drawings
　Signs
　Body Language and Sounds

Hearing Aids and The Auditory Trainer

How I Get Around

Functional Daily Physical Exercise

Frustrations

Mealtimes
　How I Eat
　How I Drink
　Likes
　Foods to Avoid

Adapted Materials

Additional Notes

Photographs

Figure 2.   Table of contents page from the "My Story" booklet for Kate Comegys for 1986–1987.

creatively and attractively. For example, our daughter drools, which is a "turn off" for others. Any bibbing is stigmatizing, and so should be avoided or concealed—but the thought of a damp shirt in New England winters is maternally bothersome. The high school teacher helped us problem solve and we all agreed to the following: a clear plastic bib (Fred Sammons Crumb Catcher Bib, #BK 1382) with its pocket and ties removed and a V-neck cut into the rounded neckline. With double-sided adhesive tape the bib is stuck to the blouse at the shoulders. Then comes the zippered sweat jacket. When that visible jacket becomes damp, it can be changed easily so as, for example, not to interfere with Kate's Auditory Trainer or otherwise draw attention. Another advantage is that dampness is not making continued contact with the student's skin or his or her peers, and peo-

My Goals

1. I want to be as independent as I can possibly be.
2. I want to make friends with my nonhandicapped peers, at the high school, and participate in all school activities which interest me, including afterschool activities.
3. I want to be included in community functions such as recreational and park activities; church and social functions.
4. I plan on living and working in my home town after I graduate from high school.
5. I plan to work in the community (with support)—*not* in a sheltered workshop.
6. I want to learn to communicate with people better (eye contact, smile, and actions).
7. I want to learn to do things *for* people.
8. I want to learn to do more things for myself such as feed myself and participate more fully in dressing.
9. I want to develop my own sense of worth.
10. I want to be able to ride my bike by myself.
11. I am eager to operate the computer for my recreation now (*Fire Organ, Sticky Bears,* and *Musicomp* are some of the software used at home). Later I hope to apply these skills to a real job. I enjoy working a Xerox machine now.
12. I want to make choices for: partners in activities; when to stop or start an activity, etc.; my clothes, leisure, food.
13. I want to be asked to go out by a friend spontaneously—not always preplanned.

My Interests

I enjoy lights, windows, the computer, photographs and slides of familiar activities and people, and TV (nature, sports, comedy), and watching a fire in the fireplace.

I enjoy books, magazines, newspapers and catalogues, and maps. Geometric designs, too.

I like to swim, ride horseback, ride my bike around town.

I like to go places in a car. I like the school bus.

I like warmth much better than cold—it helps my muscles—spring and summer, sunbathing, warm baths, warm feet and hands are important to me.

I like to be at the piano with people who can play it.

I like to be read to.

I like to be hugged—if you know me well enough. I also like to be tickled.

I like birds and fish, very much! I have a parakeet: Pete!

I have long enjoyed many family slides on the Ectagraphic which I can fully operate alone with a special switch.

I am very interested in cookies and good things to drink (frappes, tonics, etc.)!

I like lots of daily physical exercise—walking two city blocks is prescribed—it helps me sleep and helps my digestion.

I May Not Speak—But I Do Communicate

I use total communication (visual, audiological, physical cues). I communicate in many ways: here are three—

Line Drawings

I use both single and multiple line drawings (called "Commenting Boards") which are black and white or lightly colored. They enable me to both give and receive cues. If you show me a line drawing for *car,* I

continued

will know we are going out for a drive and I will start to move toward the door. I tap some line drawings to let *you* know what I want. I use many line drawings. A few of them appear in this booklet. [not shown here]

Signs

I understand some of your signs. I am learning to make some signs. Some are my own gestures and others are formal signs. Here is a list: [not shown here]

Body Language and Sounds

Please *watch* me closely and you will see that I:

    1—point with my knuckles, or a finger, or a sweep of my arm.
    2—nod my head "yes".
    3—pull you when I want you to do something.
    4—push an object away (I may or may not want it).
    5—pull or push the bathroom door shut for privacy.
    6—tilt my head up and back which can mean I want to get up.
    7—rotate my head which can mean that it's time to get moving.

Please *listen* to my tone of voice. It changes constantly, and indicates pleasure, frustration, humming, questioning, loneliness, hunger. It helps when you pair these directions with a gesture, sign, or line drawing. For example, when it is time for me to get up from the chair and go somewhere, you might sign *stand* and show me the line drawing of *car*.

Please do not talk "around or through" me as though I am not in the room. It hurts my feelings. Include me by asking my opinion, questioning me, and showing me the appropriate line drawings and signs. It will make both of us much happier.

Figure 3.   Excerpts from Kate Comegy's "My Story" booklet for 1986–1987.

ple do not see the bibbing. The low-cost bib dries overnight and is reusable for extended periods of time. It is an economical, sensible solution for a student such as Kate.

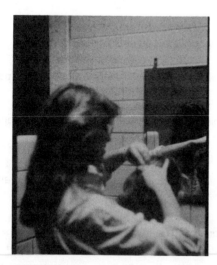

High school pal styles Kate's hair.

Involving Others

Enlightening the attitudes of the various repair/workmen who may come to your house over the years should also be considered. In our case, we carefully, graphically, and calmly explained to the carpenter that 5-year-old Kate was having difficulty rolling her walker over the thresholds in our home. He suggested and then installed roofing shingles on either side of each threshold—He was proud to have developed this solution by himself. And I am sure that his newfound awareness was shared with his associates, his family, and his community. Over time, the plumber, the house painters, the meter readers, and even the snow plow man came to understand the needs of our learner. As the ancient Chinese proverb says, "Tell me, I forget; Show me, I remember; Involve me, I understand."

Involving Parents

Because Kate had always been educated out-of-district until she was 16, we were not familiar with the inner workings of our school system. So when she started in our high school, I naturally wanted to observe her peers as well as her generic life in school. But that is not appropriate for the parent of a high-schooler, except for the couple of times each year that are designated "parents nights." I was, in reality, a "segregated" parent! So when our local newspaper ran an item calling for school library volunteers, I jumped at the chance. Cheerfully and quietly I accepted the job of volunteer library aide. I could observe peer behaviors, clothing styles, school codes, fads, spirit, and so forth. My fellow workers came to understand that I had preferences, concerns, and abilities, as did they; I was included as a member with something to contribute. It had nothing directly to do with my learner, but rather occurred as a result of my helping the improvement of the school library. (This lesson is easily transferable to other community endeavors.)

Supported Work

Supportive employment is a vocational option for individuals with severe disabilities who need ongoing support to become competitively employed. It's real work for real wages . . . integrated side-by-side with nondisabled individuals . . . with a variety of continuing support services. It's an alternative for persons in sheltered work shops—day activity programs—and persons who may have been turned down by vocational rehabilitation. It's a community effort that depends upon individuals with disabilities, parents, advocates, vocational rehabilitation services, developmental disabilities councils, mental health/mental retardation services, school systems, employers, and volunteers.

We began to push for supported employment and training in the community through the school system. It was obviously a new concept to administrators. Resistance was strong. After all, there were several sheltered workshops in the area run by either the State Department of Mental Health and Mental Retardation or the local ARC (Association for Retarded Citizens) and other organiza-

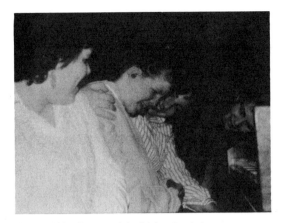

Circle of friends around the high school piano.

tions. But we knew that Kate needed to expand her participation in her hometown. Because many of our school personnel commute to work and are not familiar with the community's business world, we conducted an ecological job survey by simply listing existing businesses, by category and phone number, and presented it amicably to the special education director. She had wanted Kate assessed by a sheltered workshop employee and we would not permit it. Once again, we had presented our philosophy. By looking through the Yellow Pages and making a few contacts with business leaders, we showed her that supported work was a possibility for Kate. We learned that parents must do their homework prior to improving a social system! Table 1 lists the basic headings for our original ecological job survey for Kate in her own community.

Table 1. Types of local businesses contacted for supported work possibilities for Kate Comegys

Government	Landscapers
Drug Stores	Retail shops
Markets	Veterinarians
Gas Stations	Hairdressers
Restaurants	Real estate offices
Banks	Stables
Churches	

SUMMARY AND CONCLUSION

Seven activities for promoting family and social integration have been described. They provide some examples of activities that have been proven to help integrate a multiply challenged teen into her community, and at high school, where we saw *real* friendships develop with her classmates. These activities can be tailored to your own needs by simply filling in the blanks in your Realms (refer to Figure 1) and letting your imagination go.

Most parents want for their children the same life-style that they themselves enjoy. But when an individual is diagnosed with handicaps, the tendency has been to become entangled in a segregated approach.

But the good word is spreading! The notion that people with handicaps have abilities and are able to partially participate and contribute productively in integrated functional and ordinary realms is becoming accepted. Parents are realizing that the documentation based on research is there and that there is a national network of information and support available to help in making changes for integration (e.g., TASH: The Association for Persons with Severe Handicaps, 7010 Roosevelt Way, NE, Seattle, WA 98115, 206-523-8446; NICHCY: National Information Center for Handicapped Children and Youth, P.O. Box 1492, Washington, DC 20013; and TAPP: Technical Assistance for Parent Programs, 312 Stuart Street, 2nd Floor, Boston, MA 02116, 617-482-2915). It is no longer acceptable to allow segregated environments to exist. Both regular and special educators appreciate the opportunities they now have to educate all students in the local schools and neighborhoods.

Although this chapter has been based on experiences with Kate, a teenager with severe multiple handicaps, its philosophies can be applied to people with a wide range of challenges, and its activities and strategies can be adjusted to their skills and needs—and fine-tuned and readjusted as time goes along. The point is to set out, for all to see, a direction and a stride toward individual fulfillment in the realms of family, school, leisure, job, living situation, and friendship—the fabric of human society. This approach is possible. It should be done. It can be done.

When the foundation is *integration,* the joy of parenting returns.

Future Directions

Continued efforts must be made to raise public awareness about the following:

1. Early intervention for children 0–3 years old
2. Integrated day care
3. Public observations of integrated public schools
4. Competitive and supported work
5. Restructuring of recreation programs to include handicapped individuals of all ages
6. Use of local cable TV for educational purposes (such as the video *Regular Lives* [1987] produced and directed by Tom Goodwin and Geraldine Wurzburg, State of the Art Production Company, Washington, DC)
7. Integrated PTAs (Parent Teacher Associations) and integrated parent support groups
8. Devising creative ways to tap into the resources and individual talents of the community to interact with the handicapped population in all regular environments, including natural and lasting friendships
9. Encouraging the community to take the time to perceive and respond to the constant attempts of nonverbal individuals to communicate without misinterpretation

Final Remarks

Having the refrigerator chilling cans of tonic while bags of chips cover the kitchen counter and voices of school friends ring in the background, are the truly joyous and rightful outcomes of normalization and integration. Kate now rides the regular school bus (except when the walk to the bus stop is too snowy and icy) and attends the high school art club with her friend Corina. Several of her girl friends go swimming with her occasionally, at her invitation. Soon, I'm sure, a friend will call and ask Kate to go to the mall or the movies or whatever!

The willing collaboration of parents and professionals to educate the public to see the *similarities* between themselves and individuals with severe to mild challenges is the main strategy we need to embrace in the future. The rewards of such a collaboration are boundless and enduring!

STUDY QUESTIONS

Imagine that you have a child with handicaps:

1. Ordinary day care *is* available in your community. What strategies will you use to develop a quality integrated program there for your youngster with severe challenges?

2. It is January. Your 13-year-old has been tuitioned out-of-district for several years and your family wants him to attend his own school system in the fall. After a meeting with your special education director at which your request has been rejected, you start planning how you are going to change all that. What steps will you take?

3. List the local trades and repair men with whom you come in contact regularly. Specifically plan how you will help each of them become conversant and comfortable with your child with handicaps.

4. List the categories of businesses located in your town or neighborhood. Include cottage industries. Which ones do you feel are going to be a match for your child's future on-site job training and eventual supported employment? Will you be flexible and broaden your opinions as your child matures and his or her skills develop?

5. What are the hopes and visions you and your spouse have for your child with handicaps? for your "normal" children?

6. Make a list of successful techniques that could be used by parents and professionals to change the attitudes of society about people with challenges.

REFERENCES AND SUGGESTED READINGS

Brinker, R.P. (1983). *Why integration for severely handicapped students?*, Princeton, NJ: Educational Testing Service, Division of Education Policy Research and Services.

Brown, L., Shiraga, B., York, J., Zanella, K., & Rogan, P. (1984). Ecological inventory strategies for students with severe intellectual disabilities. In N.L. Brown, M. Sweet, B. Shiraga, J. York, K. Zanella, P. Rogan, & R. Loomis (Eds.), *Educational programs for students with severe handicaps.* (Vol. XIV, pp. 33–41). Madison, WI: Madison Metropolitan School District.

Considine, M. (1987, June 18). The first step . . . *Syllabus* [A newsletter for the Hamilton-Wenham school community], pp. 4–5.

Fink, D.B. (1987a, March). Child care dilemma: Family day care is one option for parents seeking child care. *The Exceptional Parent*, pp. 18–21.

Fink, D.B. (1987b, April). Child care dilemma: Schools are beginning to respond to demands for child care. *The Exceptional Parent*, pp. 54–59.

Fink, D.B. (1987c, May). Child care dilemma: Austin, Texas has been particularly responsive to the needs of disabled children. *The Exceptional Parent*, pp. 42–46.

Forest, M. (1987). *Integration means being together* [audio tape]. Langmont, CO: Expectations Unlimited.

Goodwin, T., & Wurzburg, G. (Producer and Director). (1987). *Regular lives* [videotape]. Washington, DC: State of the Art. (Available from WETA Educational Activities, Box 2626, Washington, DC 20013, 800-445-1964)

Perske, R. (1987). *What good is integration if you don't have any friends?* (Available from Robert Perske, 159 Hollow Tree Ridge Road, Darien, CT 06820).

Schleien, S.J., & Ray, M.T. (1988). *Community recreation and persons with disabilities: Strategies for integration.* Baltimore: Paul H. Brookes Publishing Co.

Simons, R. (1987). *After the tears.* New York: Harcourt Brace Javanovich.

Smith, P. (1984, March). You are not alone: For parents when they learn that their child has a handicap. *NICHCY Newsletter.*

Snow, J., & Forest, M. (1987). Circles. In M. Forest (Ed.), *More education/integration* (pp. 169–176). Downsview, Ontario, Canada: The G. Allan Roeher Institute.

Stainsback, W., & Stainback, S. (1987, April). Educating all students in regular education. *Newsletter of The Association for Persons with Severe Handicaps,* pp. 1, 7.

Strully, J., & Strully, C. (1985, Winter). Friendship and our children. *Journal of The Association for Persons with Severe Handicaps,* pp. 224–227.

Tracy, E. (1987). Friends, neighbors, and extended family members: Powerful resources for families of children with special needs. *Sibling Information Network Newsletter, 5*(3), 4–5. (Available from University of Connecticut, School of Education, Box U-64, Storrs, CT 06268).

With a little help from my friends. [videotape]. (1988). (Available from Marsha Forest, Ed.D., Frontier College, 35 Jackes Avenue, Toronto, Canada, M4T 1E2, 416-923-3591).

Wilcox, B. (1987, March). What should parents expect?, *Newsletter of The Association for Persons with Severe Handicaps,* pp. 1, 3.

INDEX